Macular Surgery

Fabio Patelli · Stanislao Rizzo · Carl Awh
Editors

Macular Surgery

A Clinical Guide

Springer

Editors
Fabio Patelli
ASST Santi Paolo e Carlo Hospital,
University of Milan
Milan, Italy

Carl Awh
Tennessee Retina
Nashville, TN, USA

Stanislao Rizzo
Fondazione Policlinico Universitario
A.Gemelli IRCCS, Catholic University
of Rome
Rome, Italy

ISBN 978-3-031-63507-6 ISBN 978-3-031-63508-3 (eBook)
https://doi.org/10.1007/978-3-031-63508-3

This Springer imprint is published by the registered company Springer Nature Switzerland AG
The registered company address is: Gewerbestrasse 11, 6330 Cham, Switzerland

Preface

Robert Machemer performed the first pars plana vitrectomy in 1970, and within a few years, he and others described peeling membranes from the retina and macula. Since those early days, vitreoretinal surgery has experienced dramatic growth in technology and techniques, with tremendous benefit for patients with sight-threatening retinal conditions.

Since the earliest days of vitreoretinal surgery, preservation of macular function has been paramount. However, modern vitreoretinal surgeons seek not only to preserve but to improve macular function in patients with a continually expanding list of indications.

We have assembled a group of expert and innovative surgeons who provide insights into current state-of-the-art macular surgery. These chapters are an excellent resource for both novice and veteran vitreoretinal surgeons.

Textbooks are necessarily a snapshot in time, so some of what is written in this book may one day be considered quaint, obsolete, or even distressing. If not, our vibrant field will have stagnated!

In describing his first human pars plana vitrectomy, Robert Machemer stated, "This meant the principle worked. *Now* it comes to refinement." We are grateful to the contributors to this book, who are among the many retinal specialists who continue to refine and elevate our field.

Rome, Italy — Stanislao Rizzo
Milan, Italy — Fabio Patelli
Nashville, USA — Carl Awh

Contents

A Brief History of Macular Surgery 1
Donald J. D'Amico

History of Dye 9
Kazuaki Kadonosono

Efficacy and Safety Profile of Vital Dyes 23
Mario R. Romano, Daniele Criscuolo, and Mariantonia Ferrara

Use of Intraoperative Optical Coherence Tomography in Retinal Surgery 51
S. Tammy Hsu, Vahid Ownagh, and Lejla Vajzovic

Macular Pucker Staging System and Surgery 65
Andrea Govetto and Paolo Radice

Macular Proliferative Vitreoretinopathy 79
Jose García Arumí, A. Luis Miguel Salazar, and Claudia Garcia Arumi Fusté

Macular Hole Classifications 93
Flavio A. Rezende and Bruna Gil Ferreira

Use of the Inverted ILM Flap Technique for Macular Hole Closure 111
Zofia Anna Nawrocka and Jerzy Nawrocki

Use of Amniotic Membrane for MH Closure 129
Stanislao Rizzo, Tomaso Caporossi, and Alfonso Savastano

Autologous Retinal Transplant for Macular Holes 141
Zujaja Tauqeer and Tamer H. Mahmoud

Traumatic Macular Hole 157
Fabio Patelli, Mahmoud Leila, and Ehab N. El Rayes

Myopic Traction Maculopathy 169
Giacomo Panozzo and Giovanni Bellisario

Macular Surgery in Highly Myopic Eyes 205
Mª Cristina Bohórquez, Anniken Burés-Jelstrup, Luis Miguel Salazar, and Carlos Mateo

Macular Surgery for Diabetic Macular Edema 239
Ricarda Gisela Schumann, Armin Wolf, and Denise Vogt

Index 251

A Brief History of Macular Surgery

Donald J. D'Amico

Abstract The history of macular surgery is a testament to continuous innovation in ophthalmology, marked by key milestones such as the introduction of pars plana vitrectomy and subsequent advancements in surgical techniques. Innovations like macular hole surgery, internal limiting membrane (ILM) peeling, and the development of membrane dyes have transformed the treatment landscape for various macular pathologies. Despite challenges in addressing conditions like myopic foveoschisis and lamellar macular hole, recent techniques such as the inverted ILM flap have expanded surgical options. Additionally, breakthroughs in electronic retinal prostheses and retinal gene therapy have revolutionized the management of inherited retinal conditions. Looking forward, ongoing research promises further advancements, including retinal transplantation and neuroregeneration, offering hope for improved outcomes and quality of life for patients with macular diseases.

Keywords Macular surgery · Pars plana vitrectomy · Macular hole surgery · Internal limiting membrane (ILM) peeling · Myopic foveoschisis · Lamellar macular hole · Electronic retinal prostheses · Retinal gene therapy · Retinal transplantation · Neuroregeneration

An overview of the remarkable history of macular surgery must begin with a definition. Although macular photocoagulation has been used to improve central vision for many decades, retina surgeons have been reattaching the macula for over a century, and while cataract surgeons have restored vision by reilluminating the macula for centuries more, true macular surgery may be defined as the direct manipulation of the central retina by invasive surgery. Given this definition, the beginning of macular surgery is closely linked to the very introduction of pars plana vitrectomy itself by Dr. Robert Machemer in 1970. The earliest direct manipulation of the macula occurred in the context of his transformative approaches to repair the retinal damage produced

D. J. D'Amico (✉)
Weill Cornell Medicine Ophthalmology, New York, NY, USA
e-mail: djd2003@med.cornell.edu

New York-Presbyterian Hospital, New York, NY, USA

F. Patelli et al. (eds.), *Macular Surgery*, https://doi.org/10.1007/978-3-031-63508-3_1

by proliferative diabetic retinopathy. This quote (emphasis added) from his seminal 1974 article [1] on two instrument techniques is perhaps the first mention of macular surgery in the literature. "With the removal of the preretinal membrane, all tangential traction on the retina is eliminated. A retina that was detached due to this traction can settle down, and the possibility of future contraction of this membrane is eliminated. **This procedure is especially rewarding when membranes overlying the fovea can be removed. This should have an immediate beneficial effect on the resulting visual acuity."** With those short phrases written a half century ago, preceded by his exacting and extensive experimental work with talented collaborators, macular surgery was born.

In the subsequent rich development of macular surgery, it is easier to identify major innovations and inflexion points than to establish clear credit for the individuals who were responsible for every change. Important presentations at conferences may have remained unpublished with credit awarded to others, literature searches may fail due to foreign language publication or older terminology difficulties, and others may disagree with the priorities selected herein. The author regrets—and sincerely apologizes for—any errors or slights in the attributions and timeline presented. The author will also attribute innovations within the text to the senior author, authors, or acknowledged developers while the corresponding references will be displayed in the reference list with all coauthors in their officially cited author order.

Certain major turning points in macular surgery can be offered that dramatically changed the discipline. Similar to historians dividing earth's history into major geologic time periods in the past such as Jurassic versus Cretaceous, it is possible to offer a timeline of major changes in macular surgery with additional contributions placed in between (Fig. 1). The timeline in this macular surgery specific history intentionally omits many other important developments that advanced vitreoretinal surgery in general such as the introduction of the endolaser, air/fluid exchange, tamponades, and perfluorochemicals, etc.; these general developments certainly aided macular surgery but are beyond the scope of the present review.

Given these parameters, it is possible to identify seven major inflection points in macular surgery: (1) the introduction of vitrectomy with specific macular membrane peeling [1]; (2) macular hole surgery [2]; (3) internal limiting membrane peeling for macular hole [3]; (4) membrane dyes[4, 5]; (5) electronic retinal prosthesis [6]; (6) retinal gene therapy [7]; and (7) ILM flap technique [8]. Within the context of these critical turning points, one can unfold the timeline of innovation in macular surgery.

Following the initial interventions for proliferative diabetic membranes, surgery to remove epiretinal membranes in proliferative vitreoretinopathy (termed "massive periretinal proliferation" at the time) in 1976 [9], and macular pucker in 1977 [10] followed quickly. During these years, there was intensive study of the genesis of the various types of membranes encountered, whether derived from liberated retinal pigment epithelial cells, astrocytes, or fibrocytes in penetrating trauma [11]. Macular surgery in this period primarily consisted of macular pucker removal and macular reattachment/membrane peeling in the context of surgery for proliferative diabetic retinopathy and proliferative vitreoretinopathy. The peeling was performed for years

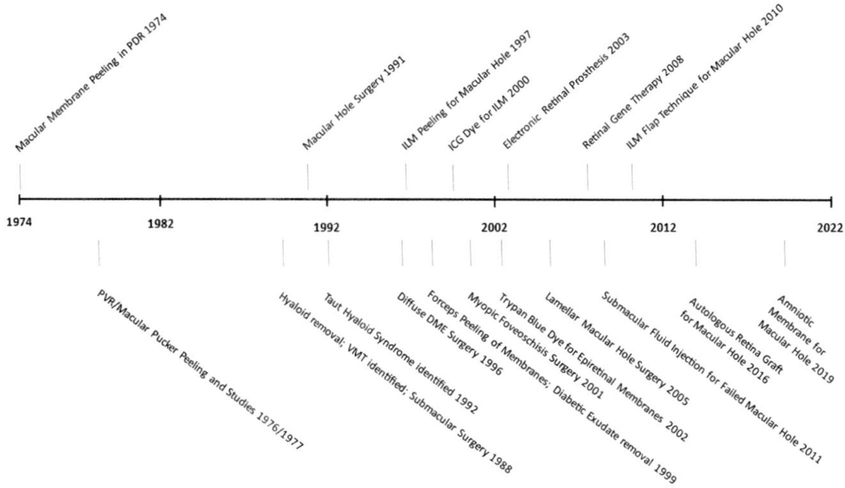

*Attributions are given in text and reference list

Fig. 1 Timeline of developments in macular surgery*

with bent needles, later specialized membrane pics, and ultimately with forceps after the introduction of "pinch peeling" by Dr. Charles [12].

Three important innovations were introduced in the banner year 1988: (1) the direct surgical elevation and removal of the posterior hyaloid by Drs. Han et al. [13]; (2) the recognition of vitreomacular traction syndrome as a cause of visual loss and the use of vitrectomy as a treatment by Dr. Smiddy [14]; and, perhaps most astonishingly, (3) vitreoretinal surgery to remove submacular hemorrhage and disciform membranes in patients with are-related macular degeneration by Drs. de Juan and Machemer [15].

Posterior hyaloid removal would become a foundational maneuver in vitreoretinal surgery of all types, and numerous techniques and instrument approaches are now available and employed on thousands of cases every year. The identification of vitreomacular traction as a distinct cause of visual loss was a remarkable insight under any circumstances, but in a world before optical coherence tomography, it was nothing less than a triumph; indeed, it brought an entirely new and treatable entity into the field. Subsequent developments would include the use of triamcinolone to better identify vitreous attachments, the injection of intravitreal air to relieve the macular traction, and the use of enzymatic vitreolysis to treat the condition without vitrectomy. Finally, the submacular surgical approaches for hemorrhage and disciform membranes presented are extraordinary for several features. While the subretinal space had previously been approached intentionally in the context of membrane removal in proliferative vitreoretinopathy, foreign body removal, suprachoroidal hemorrhage, and other conditions, the procedures described in 1988 are perhaps the very first time an attached macula was intentionally detached as a distinct maneuver. Later macular surgeries would build on this approach to refine subretinal hemorrhage and membrane removal, irrigate retained perfluorochemical from the subfoveal area, and most notably, introduce vectors for gene therapy for an ever-increasing array of inherited retinal degenerations.

Although these three innovations energized the field, virtually no one could have been prepared for the supernova event in 1991: the first report of macular hole surgery by Drs. Kelly and Wendel [2]. Their statement of purpose merits repeating: "Our study was a pragmatic, clinical approach toward treating a condition previously considered untreatable." They achieved an anatomic success in 58% of eyes with visual improvement in 42%, taking one of the most hopeless retina conditions and turning it overnight into a successful mainstay of retinal practice. The effectiveness of the initial procedure was subsequently amplified by many additional innovations detailed below, and the pace of innovations around this procedure continues without pause.

The following year, 1992, would bring the identification of taut hyaloid syndrome with macular edema in diabetic retinopathy and demonstration of improvement with vitrectomy and hyaloid removal [16]. Others would later attempt macular surgery for more common forms of diabetic macular edema: Drs. Tachi and Ogino performed hyaloid removal for diffuse diabetic macular edema in 1996 [17], and Dr. Takagi et al. removed hard exudates in 1999 [18]. Although the elimination of taut hyaloid (later identified by Dr. Kaiser et al. as a mini traction retinal detachment [19]) is convincingly joined to visual improvement, the role of surgery for other forms of diabetic macular edema continues to be debated to this day. Modifications have included internal limited membrane peeling, patient selection to enroll patients prior to laser or drug treatment and without chronic features, but the results remain variable and inconclusive. In the face of increasingly successful pharmacotherapy, vitrectomy for diabetic macular edema remains limited or perhaps decreasing in many centers; a much more dramatic decline has already befallen the surgical removal of subretinal neovascular membranes in age-related macular degeneration, also a result of spectacular improvements in drug treatment.

Internal limiting membrane (ILM) peeling has a history that is difficult to ascertain with precision. Dr. Eckardt applied ILM peeling to macular hole surgery in 1997 [3], demonstrating an improvement in closure rates, and this procedure became widespread with the introduction of indocyanine green (ICG) as an ILM stain by Drs. Kadonosono [4] and also by Dr. Burk [5] in 2000. Contributions rapidly followed by Drs. Gandorfer, Kampik, and others in which the potential toxicity of ICG was explored, the alteration of cleavage plane after ICG staining was demonstrated by ultrastructural studies [20], and the multimonth persistence of ICG staining of the optic disc was demonstrated by Dr. Tadayoni [21]. Trypan blue [22] was introduced by Dr. Feron et al. in 2002; other blue dyes introduced subsequently for staining of epiretinal membranes along with ILM (as opposed to ICG which does not stain epiretinal membranes) facilitated their current widespread use in membrane peeling for macular pucker and proliferative vitreoretinopathy. Indeed, the available dyes for vitreoretinal surgery, most recently including lutein, have become a rich palette that permits differential identification of membranes and tissues and facilitates their complete removal.

Macular surgery for myopic foveoschisis and lamellar macular hole, both very common and important conditions, may be considered parallel stories to the developments already mentioned. Drs. Ishikawa and Ogino performed successful vitreoretinal surgery in 2001 for myopic foveoschisis [23], and shortly thereafter, in 2005 Dr. Hirakawa reported successful results in two cases of lamellar macular hole with the use of vitrectomy, ILM peeling, and gas tamponade [24]. Despite these early successes, both conditions remain unpredictable in their outcomes after treatment, and the precise indications for surgery remain unclear to this day. Foveal-sparing ILM or membrane peeling has been recommended for both, and Dr. Shiraga has reported positive results with an ILM inversion technique with embedding of the epiretinal proliferation for repair of lamellar macular holes [25].

Returning to full thickness macular hole, a major innovation was the demonstration of improved closure rates with the use of an inverted ILM flap by Drs. Michalewska (Nawrocka) and Nawrocki in 2010 [8]. The technique was quickly adopted and modified, and the original developers demonstrated that the "taco-like" or folded over temporal flap had equal effectiveness and is now the technique most widely performed [26]. This successes of both ILM peeling and later ILM flap techniques have surprisingly led to several controversies. First, although Dr. Tadayoni demonstrated that ILM peeling is not necessary in surgery for macular holes smaller than 400 microns [27], it is now widely performed in full thickness holes of virtually any size [28]. Second, given the high success with ILM peeling for all macular holes 400 microns or less, most surgeons still peel and discard the ILM for primary cases despite the fact that performing a flap procedure instead would preserve the ILM for use in the rare case that requires reoperation. The first controversy has probably been settled by, unfortunately, ignoring Dr. Tadayoni's data for the smallest macular holes, and the potential negative consequences of unnecessary ILM peeling await further study. The second controversy is only now coming into active discussion and will require additional comparative trials to establish the preferred approach for typical primary cases.

Larger (>400 microns), failed, and recalcitrant macular holes are important categories that have seen numerous innovations for closure, though visual success becomes increasingly uncertain in proportion to macular hole size, duration, and number of unsuccessful interventions. For these difficult cases, Dr. Mahmoud developed an autologous retinal patch technique in 2016 in which a peripheral piece of retina was first delimited by surrounding laser and then slid (most commonly under perfluorochemical) into position under the hole [29]. Later modifications include placement over the retina with maintenance in position by two-week perfluorochemical tamponade. While the anatomic integration of the retinal tissue is impressive and closure of large holes has been demonstrated, the neural functioning of the graft remains conjectural; nevertheless, this work is foundational to several important themes in macular surgery and requires continued careful study.

Realizing the advantages of utilizing a readily available and biocompatible material, submacular insertion of amniotic membrane across the hole was used successfully by Dr. Rizzo et al. [30]. This technique can achieve closure in even the largest holes, though visual results will be progressively limited as the hole size increases.

This innovative approach may also be adapted to macular breaks with retinal detachment in myopia and other difficult situations. Other approaches for failed or difficult macular holes, including stretching the macular tissue by (1) remote subretinal fluid injection by Drs. Oliver and Wojcik [31], or (2) directly injecting viscoelastic across the hole by Dr. Kovacs and D'Amico, have salvaged visual success in mid-large size holes [32], but the largest macular holes (typically greater than 600 or 800 microns) typically require the implantation of a material plug or graft to secure closure.

The final two areas presented in this brief history of macular surgery are so revolutionary they have impact far beyond the confines of the eye. The initial implantation by Dr. Humayun in 2003 with FDA approval in 2103 of the Argus™ II Retinal Prosthesis System offered the first possibility for visual improvement in patients with severe to profound retinitis pigmentosa [6]. This remarkable device was most appropriately lauded for being a breakthrough technology, and a substantial percentage of patients who received the device valued the improvement in visual function it offered. Despite these benefits, difficulties including the need for extensive training to properly interpret the visual signals, the limited and impermanent visual function gained, the exceptionally costly nature of the device, and the failure to develop a financially sustainable model for the company led to its withdrawal from the market in 2020. Other research groups and companies remain highly active with other devices, including epiretinal, subretinal, and cortical, and continued advances in these astonishing technologies may be expected to accompany the parallel progress in microelectronics and vitreoretinal surgery in general. Indeed, though currently unavailable, the Argus™ II program has greatly advanced our understanding of residual retinal function in retinitis pigmentosa, visual processing, and the challenges involved in an electronic neural replacement—the latter two subjects being of great interest to the development of other chip-based prosthetics.

The final area has brought a first in human medicine—the successful, safe, and approved use of gene therapy to treat an inherited condition. The treatment of patients with Leber's congenital amaurosis by Drs. Maguire and Bennett in 2008 is nothing less than a tour de force of focused basic, translational, and clinical research [7]. After carefully targetted basic research, followed by extensive testing in animal models, and culminating in a clinical trial that required construction of a unique "obstacle course" to evaluate the results, the subretinal injection of Luxturna® has restored useful vision to an increasing number of patients. Spurred by this success, a number of gene therapy trials are ongoing for a variety of inherited and non-inherited retinal conditions, and further approvals may be expected. Substantial difficulties in these programs have been encountered: inflammatory responses to injected vectors, difficulty attaining a sufficient dosing for certain desired constructs, areas of retinal pigment epithelial atrophy that appear and enlarge in the months and years following transfection, and others, but the potential of gene therapy is so vast that, similar to the electronic prosthesis, further progress seems assured.

In conclusion, in the short span of fifty years, macular surgery has gone from stripping membranes from the macular surface with a bent needle to embracing the active development of electronic retinal implants while also demonstrating to the world that transformative gene therapy is possible. Thousands of patients benefit every year from now-routine interventions that did not exist when perhaps one half of currently practicing macular surgeons were born. It is clear that our increasing understanding of macular diseases, coupled with ever more helpful diagnostic tools, will drive continued progress in macular surgery to future refinements and breakthroughs such as partial thickness retinal surgery, true retinal transplantation, retinal revascularization, stem cell replacement therapy, neuroregeneration via biologics or other growth factors, and other approaches as yet unimagined. For the macula, there is certainly much more direct manipulation ahead, and for patients, there will be visual improvement with every innovation.

References

1. Machemer R. A new concept for vitreous surgery. 7. Two instrument techniques in pars plana vitrectomy. Arch Ophthalmol. 1974;92:407–412. https://doi.org/10.1001/archopht.1974.01010010419009
2. Kelly NE, Wendel RT. Vitreous surgery for idiopathic macular holes. Results of a pilot study. Arch Ophthalmol. 1991;109:654–9.
3. Eckardt C, Eckardt U, Groos S, Luciano L, Reale E. Removal of the internal limiting membrane in macular holes: clinical and morphological findings. Ophthalmologe 1997;94545-51
4. Kadonosono K, Itoh N, Uchio E, Nakamura S, Ohno S. Staining of internal limiting membrane in macular hole surgery. Arch Ophthalmol. 2000;118:1116–8.
5. Burk SE, Da Mata AP, Snyder ME, Rosa RH Jr, Foster RE. Indocyanine green-assisted peeling of the retinal internal limiting membrane. Ophthalmology. 2000;107:2010–4. https://doi.org/10.1016/s0161-6420(00)00375-4.
6. Humayun MS, Weiland JD, Fujii GY, et al. Visual perception in a blind subject with a chronic microelectronic retinal prosthesis. Vision Res. 2003;43:2573–81. https://doi.org/10.1016/s0042-6989(03)00457-7.
7. Maguire AM, Simonelli F, Pierce EA, et al. Safety and efficacy of gene transfer for Leber's congenital amaurosis. N Engl J Med. 2008;358:2240–8. https://doi.org/10.1056/NEJMoa0802315.
8. Michalewska Z, Michalewski J, Adelman RA, Nawrocki J. Inverted internal limiting membrane flap technique for large macular holes. Ophthalmology. 2010;117:2018–25.
9. Machemer R. Pars plana vitrectomy. Removal of preretinal membranes. Trans Sect Ophthalmol Am Acad Ophthalmol Otolaryngol. 1976;81:420–425
10. Kenyon KR, Michels RG. Ultrastructure of epiretinal membrane removed by pars plana vitreoretinal surgery. Am J Ophthalmol. 1977;83:815–23. https://doi.org/10.1016/0002-9394(77)90908-4.
11. Van Horn DL, Aaberg TM, Machemer R, Fenzl R. Glial cell proliferation in human retinal detachment with massive periretinal proliferation. Am J Ophthalmol. 1977;84:383–93. https://doi.org/10.1016/0002-9394(77)90684-5.
12. Charles S, Calzada J, Wood B. Epimacular membranes. In: Guyer DR, Yannuzzi LA, Chang S, et al., editors. Retina-Vitreous-Macula; 1999, vol 2, pp 230–7
13. Han DP, Abrams GW, Aaberg TM. Surgical excision of the attached posterior hyaloid. Arch Ophthalmol. 1988;106:998–1000. https://doi.org/10.1001/archopht.1988.01060140144042.
14. Smiddy WE, Michels RG, Glaser BM, deBustros S. Vitrectomy for macular traction caused by incomplete vitreous separation. Arch Ophthalmol. 1988;106:624–8. https://doi.org/10.1001/archopht.1988.01060130678025.
15. de Juan Jr E, Machemer R. Vitreous surgery for hemorrhagic and fibrous complications of age-related macular degeneration. Am J Ophthalmol. 1988;105:25–9. https://doi.org/10.1016/0002-9394(88)90116-x.

16. Lewis H, Abrams GW, Blumenkranz MS, Campo RV. Vitrectomy for diabetic macular traction and edema associated with posterior hyaloidal traction. Ophthalmology. 1992;99:753–9. https://doi.org/10.1016/s0161-6420(92)31901-3.
17. Tachi N, Ogino N. Vitrectomy for diffuse macular edema in cases of diabetic retinopathy. Am J Ophthalmol. 1996;122:258–60. https://doi.org/10.1016/s0002-9394(14)72018-5.
18. Takagi H, Otani A, Kiryu J, Ogura Y. New surgical approach for removing massive foveal hard exudates in diabetic macular edema. Ophthalmology. 1999;106:249–57. https://doi.org/10.1016/S0161-6420(99)90054-4.
19. Kaiser PK, Riemann CD, Sears JE, Lewis H. Macular traction detachment and diabetic macular edema associated with posterior hyaloidal traction. Am J Ophthalmol. 2001;131:44–9. https://doi.org/10.1016/s0002-9394(00)00872-2. PMID: 11162978.
20. Haritoglou C, Gandorfer A, Gass CA, Schaumberger M, Ulbig MW, Kampik A. Indocyanine green-assisted peeling of the internal limiting membrane in macular hole surgery affects visual outcome: a clinicopathologic correlation. Am J Ophthalmol. 2002;134:836–41. https://doi.org/10.1016/s0002-9394(02)01816-0.
21. Tadayoni R, Paques M, Girmens JF, Massin P, Gaudric A. Persistence of fundus fluorescence after use of indocyanine green for macular surgery. Ophthalmology. 2003;110:604–8. https://doi.org/10.1016/S0161-6420(02)01761-X. PMID: 12623830.
22. Feron EJ, Veckeneer M, Parys-Van Ginderdeuren R, Van Lommel A, Melles GR, Stalmans P. Trypan blue staining of epiretinal membranes in proliferative vitreoretinopathy. Arch Ophthalmol. 2002;120:141–4. https://doi.org/10.1001/archopht.120.2.141.
23. Ishikawa F, Ogino N, Okita K, et al. Vitrectomy for macular detachment without macular hole in highly myopic eyes. At-arashii Ganka. 2001;18:953–6.
24. Hirakawa M, Uemura A, Nakano T, Sakamoto T. Pars plana vitrectomy with gas tamponade for lamellar macular holes. Am J Ophthalmol. 2005;140:1154–5. https://doi.org/10.1016/j.ajo.2005.07.022.
25. Shiraga F, Takasu I, Fukuda K, Fujita T, Yamashita A, Hirooka K, Shirakata Y, Morizane Y, Fujiwara A. Modified vitreous surgery for symptomatic lamellar macular hole with epiretinal membrane containing macular pigment. Retina. 2013;33:1263–9. https://doi.org/10.1097/IAE.0b013e31828bcb61. PMID: 23594723.
26. Michalewska Z, Michalewski J, Dulczewska-Cichecka K, Adelman RA, Nawrocki J. Temporal inverted internal limiting membrane flap technique versus classic inverted internal limiting membrane flap technique: a comparative study. Retina. 2015;35:1844–50. https://doi.org/10.1097/IAE.0000000000000555.
27. Tadayoni R, Gaudric A, Haouchine B, Massin P. Relationship between macular hole size and the potential benefit of internal limiting membrane peeling. Br J Ophthalmol. 2006;90:1239–41. https://doi.org/10.1136/bjo.2006.091777.
28. Rossi T, Bacherini D, Caporossi T, Telani S, Iannetta D, Rizzo S, Moysidis SN, Koulisis N, Mahmoud TH, Ripandelli G. Macular hole closure patterns: an updated classification. Graefes Arch Clin Exp Ophthalmol. 2020;258:2629–38. Epub 2020 Sep 10. https://doi.org/10.1007/s00417-020-04920-4.
29. Grewal DS, Mahmoud TH. Autologous neurosensory retinal free flap for closure of refractory myopic macular holes. JAMA Ophthalmol. 2016;134:229–30. https://doi.org/10.1001/jamaophthalmol.2015.5237.
30. Rizzo S, Caporossi T, Tartaro R, et al. A human amniotic membrane plug to promote retinal breaks repair and recurrent macular hole closure. Retina. 2019;39(1):S95–103. https://doi.org/10.1097/IAE.0000000000002320.
31. Oliver A, Wojcik EJ. Macular detachment for treatment of persistent macular hole. Ophthal Surg Lasers Imag. 2011;42:516–8. Epub 2011 Sep 1. https://doi.org/10.3928/15428877-20110825-01.
32. Kovacs KD, Gonzalez LA, Mahrous A, D'Amico DJ. Viscostretch: a novel surgical technique for refractory macular holes. J Vitreoretin Dis. 2020;4:239–42. https://doi.org/10.1177/2474126420910914.

History of Dye

Kazuaki Kadonosono

Abstract Dye is an essential element for visualization of structures in the human eye. Vital staining utilized in ophthalmology is one of the most useful examinations to check for any abnormalities, including corneal staining. However, as vitrectomy progressed and began to include the macular region, indocyanine green was used for macular hole surgery by assisting in visualization of the internal limiting membrane (ILM). The ILM has a biochemical composition similar to other basement membranes. A proteomic study demonstrated that collagen IV is the major component of the ILM. Various vital dyes are used to visualize the ILM, and both visualization and toxicity varies depending on the properties of each dye. Digital technology has also recently seen huge progression, enabling surgeons to enhance the ILM with lower concentrations of dye, and even visualize the ILM without additional injections of dye.

Keywords Intravitreal dye · Corneal staining · Vital dyes · Macular hole surgery · Indocyanine green dye · Internal limiting membrane (ILM) · Brilliant blue G · Trypan blue · Triamcinolone

1 Introduction on First Vitrectomy with Vital Dye

1.1 The Era Before Intravitreal Dye

Dye is a crucial element for visualization of structures in the human eye. There are 3 typical methods of injection- general route, vital staining and intra vital staining. Fluorescein angiography (FA) was first used to highlight retinal vessels around 1960 [1–3], using a procedure in which dye was injected intravenously. FA is one of the

K. Kadonosono (✉)
Department of Ophthalmology and Microtechnology, School of Medicine, Yokohama City University, Yokohama, Japan
e-mail: kado@med.yokohama-cu.ac.jp

F. Patelli et al. (eds.), *Macular Surgery*, https://doi.org/10.1007/978-3-031-63508-3_2

most important examinations using dye and has been widely adopted in clinics worldwide. Corneal staining [4] is a key method of vital staining utilized in ophthalmology and one of the most useful examinations to check for any abnormalities.

As eye surgery has progressed, there has been increasing interest in methods of improving visualization of transparent eye structures. Research and development of equipment, such as operating microscopes and illumination probes, has allowed surgeons to observe these structures more clearly during surgery. Microscopes have progressed significantly with improved objective lenses, apochromat lenses and contact lenses with surface coatings. Xenon replaced halogen as the primary light source in illumination, allowing for brighter images. However, visualization of the transparent membranes remained elusive to Retinal Surgeons.

The first vitrectomy was done by Machemer for epiretinal membrane in the 1960s [5]. In those days, it was extremely complicated for surgeons to perform vitrectomies, especially macular surgery. We can imagine how challenging the first macular surgery was due to poor visualization, however pioneers must have also been excited at the opportunity of discovering a new therapy.

Macular hole surgery was first performed with separation of the posterior hyaloid membrane and injection of gas in the 1980s. That was a turning point in macular surgery, and it soon gained widespread acceptance among Retinal Surgeons. This innovative surgical technique was performed by two young retinal fellows named Kelly and Wendel [6] based on the pathogenesis of macular hole from Gass's theory [7]. The retina community was enthused at the idea of improving the success rate of macular hole surgery, which was approximately 80% at the time.

About one decade after Gass reported classification of macular holes [7], research on macular hole surgery was performed to look for effective alternatives to posterior hyaloid membrane removal. There was a paper which advocated the importance of the internal limiting membrane in macular hole surgery. Yooh et al. [8] noted that the internal limiting membrane might be an essential element in the treatment of macular holes. This idea was thought to be reasonable based on pathological examinations in which a macular hole was closed by intentionally removing surface tissues, including the ILM, glial cells, and fibrovascular membrane, from around the macular hole.

A small number of Retinal Surgeons who believed in the concept tried to use special instruments such as diamond dusted membrane scrapers to assist in removal of membranes. The diamond-dusted membrane scraper is made from flexible silicone tubing, allowing immature membranes and pigmented cells to be removed from the surface of the retina [9]. Residual cortex vitreous or epiretinal membrane at the edge of a macular hole was thought to be the main cause of macular hole formation, and Retinal Surgeons increasingly came to understand the importance of removing these membranes in macular hole surgery.

However, removal of the ILM without any surgical damage to the retina was still a huge challenge, as the membrane is transparent and can be as thin as 10 μ [10]. Surgeons continued to believe that removal of the perifoveal cortical vitreous, internal limiting membrane, and adherent contractile cells was the best surgical approach to relieving tangential traction and closing idiopathic macula hole and continued researching surgical approaches to gently removing the internal limiting membrane [11].

2 Internal Limiting Membrane

The internal limiting membrane (ILM) is a vital component of the vitreoretinal interface, exerting a major influence on the development of various eye conditions such as epiretinal membrane (ERM), macular hole, and macular edema [12, 13]. This interface consists of three essential elements: the posterior vitreous cortex, the ILM, and an intervening extracellular matrix. Due to their close interconnection, achieving complete separation is often unfeasible in pathological conditions, leading to complete relief of vitreo-macular traction. Consequently, the standard approach involves the comprehensive removal of the ILM. A profound understanding of the ILM's anatomy is paramount for enhancing the outcomes of ILM removal in macular surgery.

2.1 Biochemical Composition

The ILM has a biochemical composition similar to other basement membranes. The proteomic study demonstrated that collagen IV is the major component of the ILM and the other basement membranes in the eye [14] (Fig. 1).

The origin of the ILM is not clear. The Müller cells are thought to be the major source of ILM proteins, as the ILM is adjacent to the end feet of the Müller cells. It is thought that the ILM proteins are secreted from the lens, ciliary body, and optic disc into the vitreous and then are assembled into the ILM at the retinal surface.

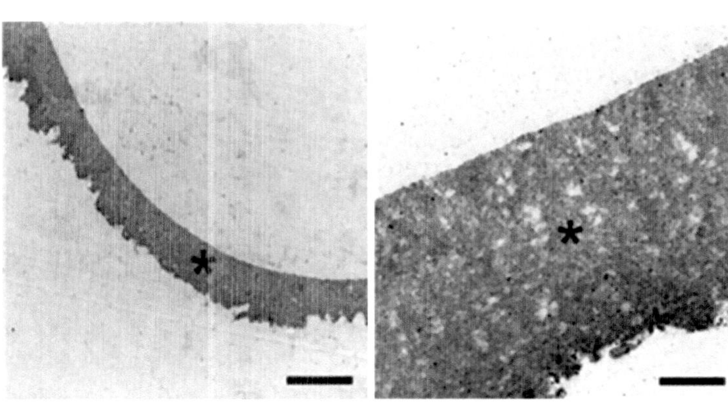

Fig. 1 Transmission electron microscope of ILM. The ILM is 4–10 μ and basement membrane of ILM

There is some debate about whether the ILM regenerates after surgical removal. The expression of the ILM proteins decreased after the developmental process, and most ILM proteins were not detectable in adults [15]. Considering the above findings, ILM regeneration is not likely to occur. No apparent ILM regeneration was noted within 12 months after experimental removal of the ILM using indocyanine green in primate eyes. On the other hand, cultured Müller cells were capable of synthesizing collagen proteins in vitro [16]. Remodeling of the extracellular matrix at the vitreoretinal interface may occur in some pathologic conditions, although the ILM cannot be regenerated completely.

2.2 Role of Internal Limiting Membrane in Macular Surgery

The internal limiting membrane (ILM) plays a key role in the pathogenesis of proliferative diseases, necessitating cell migration, adhesion, and proliferation on the retinal surface. Cell adhesion is facilitated by specific proteins, such as laminin and fibronectin. Interestingly, laminin is primarily situated on the retinal side of the ILM rather than the vitreal side [17]. Furthermore, fibronectin, which is not typically part of the normal ILM composition, is detected in eyes afflicted with conditions like diabetes or proliferative vitreoretinopathy (PVR) [18, 19]. These observations suggest that alterations occur on the vitreal side of the ILM to promote cell adhesion in proliferative conditions, underscoring the importance of removing the pathological ILM to prevent membrane formation. Notably, peeling of the ILM has been reported to reduce postoperative macular pucker following retinal detachment surgery. and to decrease the recurrence of epiretinal membranes (ERM) [20, 21]. In a clinical setting there are advantages including acquired flexibility of the ILM, prevention of reproliferation, and regeneration of muller cells. Drawbacks include damage to ganglion cells, and harm to the neurofiber layer resulting in visual field defects. Intraoperative pictures of ILM removal in macular surgery show a meshwork appearance which does not appear to harm retinal function. These days ILM removal during macular hole surgery has become widely accepted in the retina community.

3 Era of Vital Dye for Vitrectomy

3.1 Safe Use of Indocyanine Green Dye in the Human Body

Indocyanine green (ICG) is a relatively nontoxic Tricarbocyanine dye and has been used in humans for many years [22, 23]. We use ICG dye in angiography examination for macular diseases related to choroidal abnormalities such as PCV, exudative age-related macular degeneration and pachychoroid spectrum since Yannuzzi introduced his unique analysis method of vascularized pigment epithelial detachments using indocyanine green video angiography [24]. There have been no reports of patients who suffered severe issues such as anaphylactic shock.

The evaluation of hepatic function and functional capacity of the liver are essential tasks in hepatology as well as in hepatobiliary surgery. Indocyanine green (ICG) is a widely applied test compound that is routinely used in clinical settings to evaluate hepatic function. After intravenous administration, ICG is taken up exclusively by the liver and excreted unchanged into the bile [25]. It is not reabsorbed by the intestine and does not undergo enterohepatic circulation. As a result, ICG is an ideal test compound to test hepatic uptake and biliary excretion.

Furthermore, ICG was used to stain the anterior capsule membrane in white mature cataracts [26]. This history of clinical applications of ICG to the human body, and especially the eye, made it a safe and reliable choice for use in retinal surgery.

3.2 Selective Staining of the ILM with ICG

ICG was first used for macular hole surgery in 2000 [27] (Fig. 2). There had been no way for Retinal Surgeons to resolve the issue of visualizing the ILM, until the intra-operative vital dye ICG was first used for idiopathic macular hole surgery, leading to a dramatic change in approaches to macular surgery (Fig. 3).

ILM removal has become an essential procedure in the field because ICG dye can not only visualize the ILM, but negatively visualize other components such as the ERM, and fibrovascular tissues (Fig. 4). This selective staining property of ICG was an essential factor in it becoming widely accepted as a necessary surgical procedure in macular surgery. The ILM consists of collagen IV, along with other basement membrane proteins including the laminin family, nidogen, agrin, perlecan, and collagen XVIII [20]. The ILM has a lower concentration of collagen IV compared to other basement membranes, and the most prominent proteoglycan is perlecan, which is responsible for the high-water content of the ILM [21]. These characteristics are the main reason that ICG can be used to stain the ILM selectively.

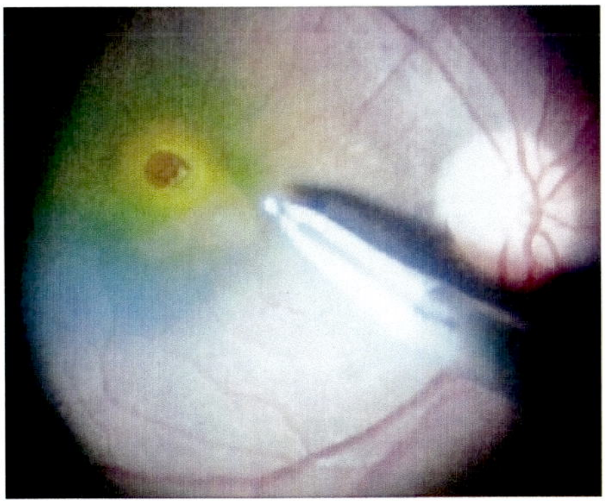

Fig. 2 An intraoperative picture of ILM staining in macular hole surgery from a journal. The first report on ILM peeling with ICG was published in 2000

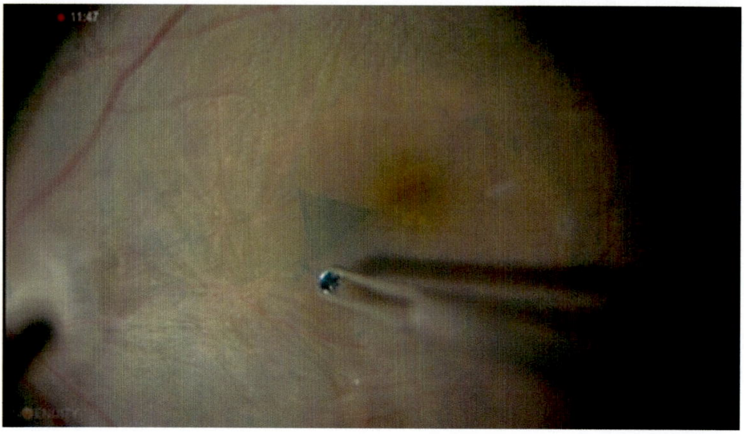

Fig. 3 An intraoperative image of recent surgical technique for ILM peeling with ICG. The concentration of ICG is 0.03% mixed with low molecule weight visco-elastic material

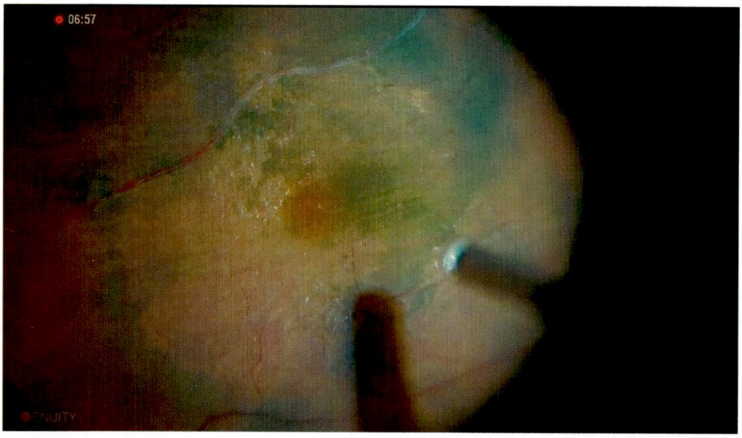

Fig. 4 An intraoperative image of an eye with ERM stained with ICG. Parts both negatively and positively stained with ICG, allow surgeons to identify the location of the ERM

Therefore, ICG which previously could only be utilized through injections into the body for liver examination, was selected as an ideal dye for use in staining the posterior segment. The first report of ILM staining with ICG encouraged Retinal Surgeons to perform macular hole surgery leading to improvements in anatomical and functional results.

3.3 *Clinical Setting of Indocyanine Green to Macular Surgery*

A procedure of intravitreal indocyanine green that we developed is that 25 mg of ICG was distributed into 10 cc balanced saline solution, and 0.2 cc of which was mixed with viscoelastic material with low molecule. The concentration of that is 0.03% and ICG is unlikely to be dispersed.

There are different methods used for injection of vital dyes from injections into the body, to irradiation using light as a photosensitizer. The shift of absorption wavelength occurs in the absorption spectrum of ICG when albumin is present in solution and the dye is bound to albumin [28]. The similarity of the absorption spectrum of the dye in human plasma and in albumin solution, and the identity of the absorption maxima suggest that plasma proteins other than albumin are not important in the binding of ICG. These data are supported by the results of starch block electrophoresis.

The absorption of light by indocyanine green (ICG) can trigger retinal phototoxicity. While it is commonly understood that ultraviolet and blue light radiation pose risks to the retina, there is also concern that the light emitted by ICG in the range of 780–810 nm wavelength might have a photochemical impact on the retina. Some studies have suggested a potential photosensitizing effect when the stained retina is exposed to intraoperative illumination within the 380–760 nm wavelength range, emitted by commonly used vitrectomy light sources, which could lead to morphological damage in the inner retina. However, it is important to note that these findings have not been consistently confirmed by other investigations. When performing macular surgery with endoillumination that includes longer wavelengths, such as 810 nm, there could be a possibility of irradiation effects on the retina.

Additionally, recent research has focused on assessing retinal light hazards during macular surgery using digital three-dimensional visualization systems (3D) in comparison to conventional microscopes (CM). It has been found that the 3D digitally assisted visualization system offers a significantly safer approach to macular surgery when considering potential retinal hazards.

In in vivo studies, RPE cells were susceptible to damage with high concentrations of ICG and/or longer exposure times. Enaida et al. reported that RPE-19 cells showed significantly decreased survival rates with an exposure time of more than 24 h and at higher concentrations of ICG than the normal range which is between 0.05 and 0.5%. The method of injecting ICG into the vitreous is a key factor in avoiding direct mechanical injury to the RPE cells in a macular hole. These clinical findings changed the clinical settings in which ICG vital dyes were used, leading to safer methods approved by the majority of Surgeons.

4 Other Dyes

4.1 Brilliant Blue G

In the early 2000s several new dyes were researched and developed, and there was some controversy over which vital dye was the best for application to macular surgery. Trypan Blue was introduced to stain the membrane blue; however, it didn't seem to selectively stain the ILM as well as ICG. Brilliant blue G (BBG) was another dye that had been used to stain micro-organs inside cells in the laboratory [29]. According to the first laboratory examination of BBG, it proved to have lower toxicity than other dyes such as ICG and Trypan Blue. Clinical studies of BBG application reported acceptable results without any related issues. As a result, BBG became widely accepted among Retinal Specialists hoping to avoid unexpected complications [30].

BBG was introduced as a surgical adjuvant for chromovitrectomy in 2006 and, this dye was purported to stain the ILM and to have no significant in vivo toxicity. After other dyes such as BBG were introduced, the technique of using vital dye became known as chromovitrectomy.

BBG is more hydro soluble than ICG and IfCG; it would thus penetrate less into the cells and be more easily washed away, leaving less residues after surgery. For this reason, BBG represents a viable alternative to ICG and IfCG in chromovitrectomy due to its suitable affinity for the ILM.

4.2 Trypan Blue

Trypan blue (TB) usage mostly extends to blue dye application for ERM staining [31]. TB exhibits outstanding affinity for the ERM because of the strong presence of dead glial cells within those membranes. I personally use it for immature PVR which may minimize mechanical trauma to the retina during ERM removal and allows me to determine the full extent of the ERM. TB in various doses may enhance the ability to detect both the prolapsed vitreous in the anterior chamber and the posterior vitreous remaining in the vitreous cavity, but it is inferior to triamcinolone acetonide. Regarding the chronic toxicity of TB, it has been reported that it induces arrest of the cell cycle at G0–G1 via increased expression of p21.

4.3 Triamcinolone Acetonide

Triamcinolone acetonide improves visualization as well as other dyes [32]. The crystals of the steroid adhere to the acellular tissue, thereby enabling a clear contrast between the empty vitreous cavity compared to areas with the vitreous fibers remaining. The surgical technique for TA application consists of a direct injection of the agent into the vitreous cavity toward the area of interest. TA-assisted removal of the internal limiting membrane was used in many cases since the white specks and crystals may deposit over the ILM, thereby facilitating ILM removal. For this reason, some authors suggest that postoperative residual TA could enhance surgical results. Injecting this steroid during vitrectomy for the management of retinal detachment may prevent fibrin reaction and PVR postoperatively. The commonly used formulation of TA, kenalog, is not formulated for the eye, for this reason, there is a risk of pseudoendophthalmitis and retina toxicity when injected intravitreally. There have been reports on the toxicity of TA on retinal pigment epithelial cells (RPE) in vitro whereas ex vivo and in vivo studies have not shown any significant toxicity to the retina.

5 Use of Retinal Vital Dyes and Issues with Toxicity

In the first report on clinical application of ICG, ICG was prepared as a vital dye for macular hole surgery at a concentration of 0.06% ICG mixed with a low molecular weight viscoelastic material [27]. The study reported a success rate of macular hole closure of 82.4% among the 12 eyes studied, and mean visual improvement was 0.34 logMAR (from 20/200 to 20/25) at 6 months postoperatively. In this study there were no eyes with decreased visual acuity, and there were not any intra or postoperative complications such as endophthalmitis, or retinal detachment seen.

After ICG dye application was introduced in macular hole surgery, a number of reports surfaced describing issues related to ICG use such as macular atrophy, disc atrophy and other serious issues [33, 34]. Some pathological examinations with in vivo studies showed that RPE cells were negatively affected by ICG depending on the concentration of dyes exposure time of ICG to the retina and the method of injection [35]. Other experimental studies showed cell damage such as shortened survival time in ganglion cells [36–38]. These findings led to updated techniques for ICG vital dye staining as well as the development of new dyes.

6 Differences in Visualization of Each Dye

Visualization is influenced by several factors such as brightness, color contrast, huc, gamma and saturation, and a good combination of these elements makes it possible to enhance visualization. The color of dyes is a key factor which varies depending on the dye (Fig. 5).

Vital dyes are used to visualize the ILM, and visualization of the ILM varies depending on the property of each dye. In certain conditions, and at safe concentrations, visualization depends heavily on color contrast. Studies indicated that a green color such as ICG can provide higher contrast than either the blue or light blue colors

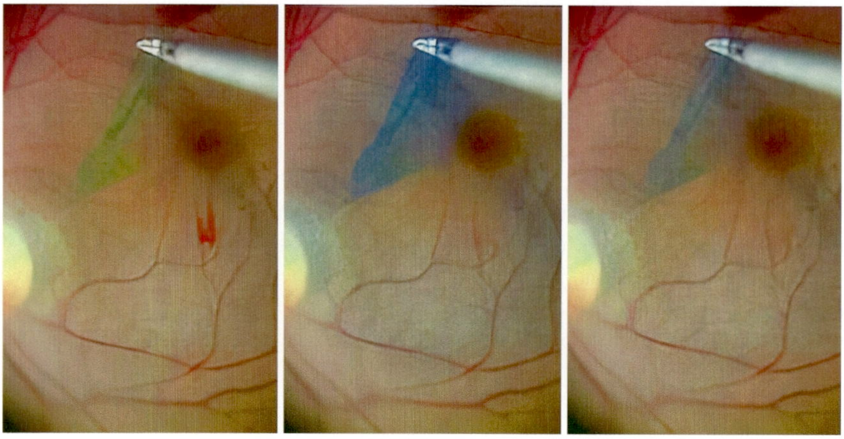

Fig. 5 Images showing differences in visualization between ICG, BBG and Trypan blue. There are clear differences in visibility with different dyes

typically seen with BBG. It has also become apparent that visualization of the ILM changes in Caucasian, Asian and African populations due to differences in choroidal color [39].

In highly myopic eyes displaying macular atrophy, the green color allows us to observe the ILM more clearly than with blue colors, resulting in ICG being more widely used in eyes with myopic traction maculopathy (Fig. 6).

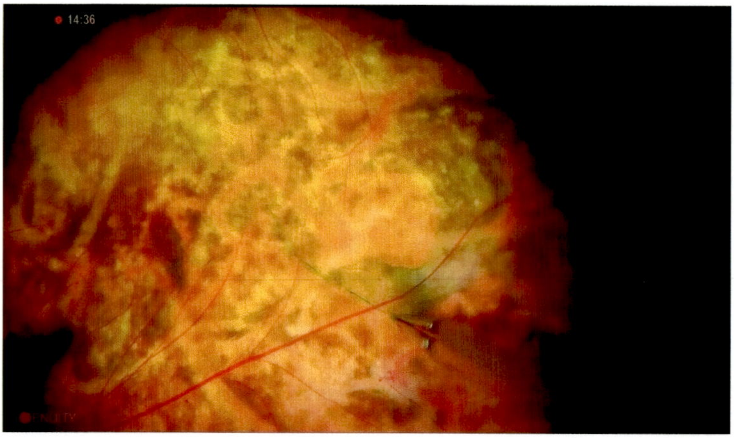

Fig. 6 An intraoperative image of ILM peeling using ICG. The ILM is more clearly stained with ICG than other dyes in a highly myopic eye

7 Current Trends in Use of Vital Dyes for Vitrectomy

Many Surgeons have preferences based not only on scientific facts, but also their own experience and feelings. The PAT survey conducted by the ASRS allows us to see trends in the preference of dyes currently used in surgery [40]. The results indicated that the kind of dyes used varies depending on geographical region, showing BBG is used mostly in Europe, while ICG is preferred in the US. Overall, BBG is the most widely used at about 64.8%, with ICG used by 56.0% of surgeons, and other dyes making up the rest.

Vital dyes are widely used for retinal diseases other than macula hole requiring ILM removal. Epiretinal membrane (ERM) is the most common retinal disorder. Vital dye is also effective for use in negatively staining the ERM, allowing surgeons to choose to remove only the ERM, or both the ERM and ILM simultaneously. In eyes with proliferative diabetic retinopathy (PDR), ILM peeling has become commonplace to avoid postoperative proliferation. In addition, ILM removal using vital dyes is useful in eyes with PVR to stretch the retina, while avoiding any occurrence of tissue proliferation.

8 The Future

Digital technology has recently seen huge progression, enabling surgeons to enhance the ILM with lower concentrations of dye, and even visualize the ILM without additional injections of dye (Fig. 7). The use of algorithms and AI have contributed to improved visualization of the ILM without any additional vital dye [41, 42]. This technology will surely continue to contribute to much safer and effective use of vital dyes, and eventually digital staining techniques. The progress in ILM staining has far exceeded what we could have imagined two decades ago, ushering in a new era of ophthalmic procedures.

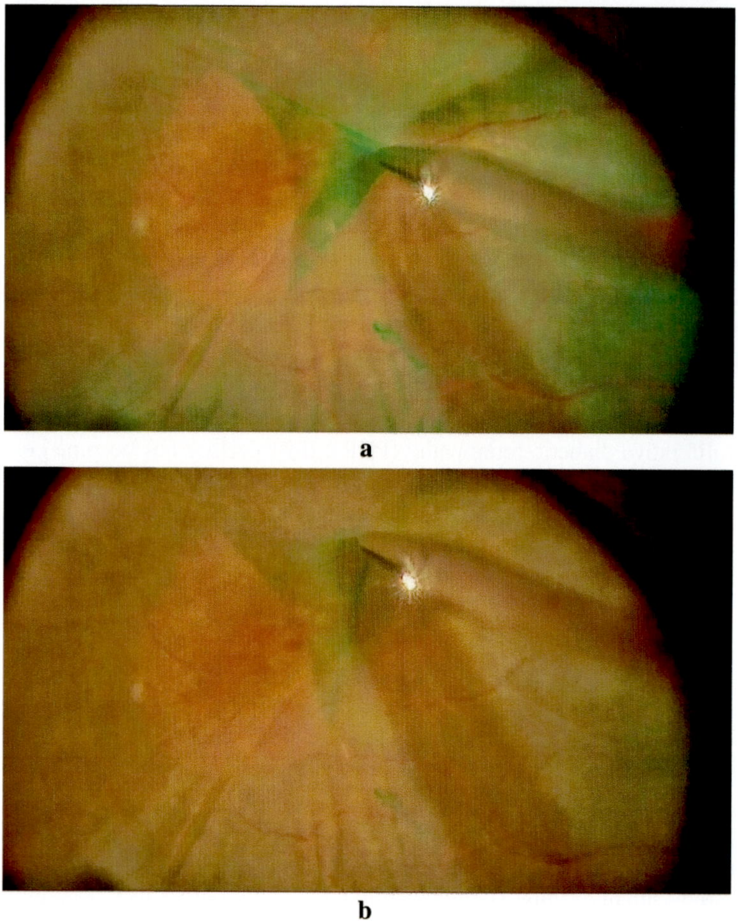

Fig. 7 ILM enhanced with algorithm. Digitally enhanced ILM stained with ICG (**a**) is much clearer than normal ILM (**b**)

References

1. Norton EW, Gutman F. Diabetic retinopathy studied by fluorescein angiography. Ophthalmologica. 1965;150(1):5–17.
2. Ehrlich P. Uber provilirte fluoresceinzerscheinungen. Am Aug Dtsch Med Wochenschr. 1882;1884:8–21.
3. Gass JDM, Sever RJ, Sparks D, et al. A combined technique of fluorescein fundoscopy and angiography of the eye. Arch Ophthalmol. 1967;78:455–61.
4. Joyce PD. Corneal vital staining. Ir J Med Sci. 1967;6(500):359–67. https://doi.org/10.1007/BF02954080.
5. Machemer R. The surgical removal of epiretinal macular membranes (macular puckers) (author's trans.). Klin Monbl Augenheilkd. 1978;173(1):36–42.
6. Kelly NE, Wendel RT. Vitreous surgery for idiopathic macular holes. Results of a pilot study. Arch Ophthalmol. 1991;109(5):654–9.

7. Johnson RN, Gass JD. Idiopathic macular holes. Observations, stages of formation, and implications for surgical intervention. Ophthalmology. 1988;95(7):917–24.
8. Yooh HS, Brooks HL Jr, Capone A Jr, L'Hernault NL, Grossniklaus HE. Ultrastructural features of tissue removed during idiopathic macular hole surgery. Am J Ophthalmol. 1996;122(1):67–75. https://doi.org/10.1016/s0002-9394(14)71965-8.
9. Lewis JM, Park I, Ohji M, Sato Y, Tano Y. Diamond-dusted silicone cannula for epiretinal membrane separation during vitreous surgery. Am J Ophthalmol. 1997;552–4.
10. Zhang KY, Johnson TV. The internal limiting membrane: roles in retinal development and implications for emerging ocular therapies. Exp Eye Res. 2021;206:108545. https://doi.org/10.1016/j.exer.2021.108545. Epub 2021 Mar 2
11. Wolter JR. Pores in the internal limiting membrane of the human retina. Acta Ophthalmol (Copenh). 1964;42:971–4. https://doi.org/10.1111/j.1755-3768.1964.tb03664
12. Uechi G, Sun Z, Schreiber EM, Halfter W, Balasubramani M. Proteomic view of basement membranes from human retinal blood vessels, inner limiting membranes, and lens capsules. J Proteome Res. 2014;13:3693–705. https://doi.org/10.1021/pr5002065.5.
13. Koo GH, Lee JE, Choi HY, Oum BS. Ultrastructure of the internal limiting membrane removed during macular hole and diabetic macular edema surgery. J Korean Ophthalmol Soc. 2010;51:42. https://doi.org/10.3341/jkos.2010.51.1.42
14. Henrich PB, Monnier CA, Halfter W, Haritoglou C, Strauss RW, Lim RYH, Loparic M. Nanoscale topographic and biomechanical studies of the human internal limiting membrane. Invest Ophthalmol Vis Sci. 2012;53:2561–70. https://doi.org/10.1167/iovs.11-8502.7.
15. Nakamura T, Murata T, Hisatomi T, Enaida H, Sassa Y, Ueno A, Sakamoto T, Ishibashi T. Ultrastructure of the vitreoretinal interface following the removal of the internal limiting membrane using indocyanine green. Cur Eye Res. 2003;27:395–9. https://doi.org/10.1076/ceyr.27.6.395.18189.10.
16. Ponsioen TL, van Luyn MJA, van der Worp RJ, Pas HH, Hooymans JMM, Los LI. Human retinal Müller cells synthesize collagens of the vitreous and vitreoretinal interface in vitro. Mol Vis. 2008;14:652–6.
17. Halfter W, Monnier C, Müller D, Oertle P, Uechi G, Balasubramani M, Saf F, Lim R, Loparic M, Henrich PB. The bi-functional organization of human basement membranes. PLoS One. 2013;8:e67660. https://doi.org/10.1371/journal.pone.0067660
18. Foveau P, Leroy B, Berrod JP, Conart JB. Internal limiting membrane peeling in macula-off retinal detachment complicated by grade b proliferative vitreoretinopathy. Am J Ophthalmol. 2018;191:1–6. https://doi.org/10.1016/j.ajo.2018.03.037.
19. Díaz-Valverde A, Wu L. To peel or not to peel the internal limiting membrane in idiopathic epiretinal membranes. Retina. 2018;38:S5–11. https://doi.org/10.1097/IAE.0000000000001906
20. Feist RM, King JL, Morris R, Witherspoon CD, Guidry C. Myofibroblast and extracellular matrix origins in proliferative vitreoretinopathy. Graefes Arch Clin Exp Ophthalmol. 2014;252:347–57. https://doi.org/10.1007/s00417-013-2531-0
21. Gupta P, Yee KMP, Garcia P, Rosen RB, Parikh J, Hageman GS, Sadun AA, Sebag J. Vitreoschisis in macular diseases. Br J Ophthalmol. 2011;95:376–80. https://doi.org/10.1136/bjo.2009.175109.
22. Fox IJ, Brooker LGS, Heseltine DW, Essex HE, Wood EH. A tricarbocyanine dye for continuous recording of dilution curves in whole blood independent of variations in blood oxygen saturation. Proc Mayo Clin. 1957;32:478.
23. Fox IJ, Wood EH. Applications of dilution curves recorded from the right side of the heart or venous circulation with the aid of a new indicator dye. Proc Mayo Clin. 1957;32:541.
24. Yannuzzi LA, Hope-Ross M, Slakter JS, Guyer DR, Sorenson JA, Ho AC, Sperber DE, Freund KB, Orlock DA. Analysis of vascularized pigment epithelial detachments using indocyanine green videoangiography. Retina. 15(1):76. https://doi.org/10.1097/00006982-1994
25. Sharma P. Value of liver function tests in cirrhosis. J Clin Exp Hepatol. 2022;12(3):948–64. https://doi.org/10.1016/j.jceh.2021.11.004. Epub 2021 Nov 14.

26. Horiguchi M, Nagata S, Yamamoto N, Kojima Y, Shimada Y. Kinetics of indocyanine green dye after intraocular surgeries using indocyanine green staining. Arch Ophthalmol. 2003;121(3):327–31. https://doi.org/10.1001/archopht.121.3.327.
27. Kadonosono K, Itoh N, Uchio E, Nakamura S, Ohno S. Staining of internal limiting membrane in macular hole surgery. Arch Ophthalmol. 2000;118(8):1116–8. https://doi.org/10.1001/archopht.118.8.1116.
28. Cherrick GR, Stein SW, Leevy CM, Davidson CS. Indocyanine green: observations on its physical properties, plasma decay, and hepatic extraction. J Clin Invest. 1960;39(4):592–600. https://doi.org/10.1172/JCI104072.
29. Enaida H, Hisatomi T, Goto Y, Hata Y, Ueno A, Miura M, Kubota T, Ishibashi T. Preclinical investigation of internal limiting membrane staining and peeling using intravitreal brilliant blue G. Retina. 2006;26(6):623–30. https://doi.org/10.1097/01.iae.0000236470.71443.7c
30. Enaida H, Ishibashi T. Brilliant blue in vitreoretinal surgery. Dev Ophthalmol. 2008;42:115–25. https://doi.org/10.1159/000138989.
31. Teba FA, Mohr A, Eckardt C, Wong D, Kusaka S, Joondeph BC, Feron EJ, Stalmans P, Van Overdam K, Melles GR. Trypan blue staining in vitreoretinal surgery. Ophthalmology. 2003;110(12):2409–12. https://doi.org/10.1016/s0161-6420(03)00716-4.
32. Sakamoto T, Ishibashi T. Visualizing vitreous in vitrectomy by triamcinolone. Graefes Arch Clin Exp Ophthalmol. 2009;247(9):1153–63. https://doi.org/10.1007/s00417-009-1118-2. Epub
33. Gass CA, Haritoglou C, Schaumberger M, Kampik A. Functional outcome of macular hole surgery with and without indocyanine green-assisted peeling of the internal limiting membrane. Graefes Arch Clin Exp Ophthalmol. 2003;241(9):716–20. https://doi.org/10.1007/s00417-003-0710-0. Epub 2003 Aug 13
34. Rodrigues EB, Meyer CH, Mennel S, Farah ME. Mechanisms of intravitreal toxicity of indocyanine green dye: implications for chromovitrectomy. Retina. 2007;27(7):958–70. https://doi.org/10.1097/01.iae.0000253051.01194.ab.
35. Enaida H, Sakamoto T, Hisatomi T, et al. Morphological and functional damage of the retina caused by intravitreous indocyanine green in rat eyes. Graefes Arch Clin Exp Ophthalmol. 2002;240:209–13.
36. Kwok AK, Lai TY, Man-Chan W, et al. Indocyanine green assisted retinal internal limiting membrane removal in stage 3 or 4 macular hole surgery. Br J Ophthalmol. 2003;87:71–4.
37. Yip HK, Lai TY, So KF, Kwok AK. Retinal ganglion cells toxicity caused by photosensitising effects of intravitreal indocyanine green with illumination in rat eyes. Br J Ophthalmol. 2006;90(1):99–102. https://doi.org/10.1136/bjo.2005.076042.
38. Lai C-C, Wu W-C, Chuang L-H, Yeung L, Chen T-L, Lin K-K. Prevention of indocyanine green toxicity on retinal pigment epithelium with whole blood in stain-assisted macular hole surgery. Ophthalmology. 2005;112(8):1409–14. https://doi.org/10.1016/j.ophtha
39. Kadonosono K, Arakawa A, Inoue M, Yamane S, Uchio E, Yamakawa T, Taguri M, Morita S, Ridgeley JR, Yanagi Y. Internal limiting membrane contrast after staining with indocyanine green and brilliant blue G during macular surgery. Retina. 2013;33(4):812–7. https://doi.org/10.1097/IAE.0b013e3182807629.
40. https://www.asrs.org/publications/retina-times/details/6261/asrs-preferences-and-trends-survey-celebrates-25th-anniversary2
41. Akiyama K, Watanabe K, Fukui M, Higuchi H, Noda T. Quantitative evaluation of digital-image enhancement during heads-up surgery. Sci Rep. 2019;9(1):15931. https://doi.org/10.1038/s41598-019-52492-z
42. Horigome Y, Iwashita Y, Hirono K, Inoue T, Konno A, Kadonosono K, Yanagi Y. Evaluation of the retinal hazard with 3d digitally assisted visualization system and conventional microscope in macular surgeries*. Retina. 2022;42(12):2301–6.

Efficacy and Safety Profile of Vital Dyes

Mario R. Romano, Daniele Criscuolo, and Mariantonia Ferrara

Abstract Vital dyes represent important intraoperative tools in vitreoretinal surgery due to their ability to stain different intraocular structures and, thus, facilitate several surgical maneuvers, including removal of the vitreous and peeling of epiretinal membrane and internal limiting membrane. The chemical structure of these compounds determines their protein binding affinity and, thus, the staining properties. From a surgical point of view, vital dyes are commonly divided in dyes for the vitreous (triamcinolone acetonide and lutein-based vitreous dye) and dyes for the vitreoretinal interface (cyanine dyes, blue dyes and lutein-based dyes). Despite the established advantages deriving from performing pars plana vitrectomy with the aid of vital dyes (chromovitrectomy), several reports documented the potential intraocular toxicity of these compounds, mainly in form of progressive outer retinal layers disruption and atrophic changes of the retinal pigment epithelium. Multiple regulations are currently aimed to ensure the safety of intraocular medical devices, including vital dyes, and, in this regard, *in vitro* cytotoxicity tests play a crucial role in assessing the biocompatibility of these compounds. The aim of this chapter is to provide an overview of the main vital dyes currently available in terms of physicochemical characteristics, staining properties, clinical use and outcomes, evidence of safety from experimental studies and potential intraocular toxicity. In particular, with regard to the dye-related retinal toxicity, we will focus on the common clinical findings and surgical details of the cases reported.

Keywords Blue dyes · Chromovitrectomy · Dye toxicity · Medical devices · Lutein-based dyes · Vitreous staining

M. R. Romano (✉) · D. Criscuolo
Department of Biomedical Sciences, Humanitas University, Pieve Emanuele - Milan, Italy
e-mail: mario.romano@hunimed.eu

M. Ferrara
Department of Medical and Surgical Specialties, Radiological Sciences, and Public Health, University of Brescia, Brescia, Italy

F. Patelli et al. (eds.), *Macular Surgery*, https://doi.org/10.1007/978-3-031-63508-3_3

1 Introduction

The term "chromovitrectomy" is used to indicate a pars plana vitrectomy (PPV) performed with the aid of vital dyes, chemical substances, able to bind living tissues or cells, leading to a colored appearance (staining) [1]. The aim is to enhance the visualization of specific intraocular structures, such as vitreous, epiretinal membranes (ERM) and internal limiting membrane (ILM), and, thus, facilitate surgical maneuvers, such as vitreous removal, ERM and/or ILM peeling, potentially reducing the risk of mechanical retinal trauma [2, 3].

According to the Medical Device Regulation (EU) 2017/745, vital dyes are classified as medical devices class IIa, 'surgically invasive devices intended for transient use' (continuous use for less than 60 min). In addition to the general safety and performance requirements of the MDR 2017/745 and of the U.S. Food and Drug Administration, medical devices need to conform to specific International Organisation for Standardization (ISO) standards in order to be approved for surgical use [4].

2 Dye Characteristics

From surgical point of view, vital dyes can be divided in dyes for the vitreous and dyes for the vitreoretinal interface, based on their main binding affinity. Relevant properties for the intraoperative use and the biocompatibility of these compounds are chemical group, solubility, staining properties, pH, osmolarity and purity of the final formulation. Table 1 provides a brief overview of the properties of the main vital dyes currently used in surgical practice.

2.1 Vital Dyes for Vitreous Staining

Dyes for vitreous staining are used to facilitate maneuvers like posterior vitreous detachment induction, vitreous base trimming, and removal of vitreous cortex remnants. The main dyes currently used for vitreous staining are:

- *Triamcinolone acetonide (TA)*: synthetic water-insoluble corticosteroid crystals dispersed in water. The crystals can adhere to the acellular vitreous fibers and deposit onto the layers of vitreous cortex, enhancing the visualization of residual vitreous in contrast with the empty vitreous cavity [5]. Preserved TA formulation, containing benzyl alcohol (BA), have been traditionally used off label in vitreoretinal surgery. Due to the concerns related to the potential toxicity of this preservative (see Sect. 4.1), several strategies have been introduced to reduce the exposure of intraocular tissues to the preserved compound, including the use of TA diluted with balanced salt solution (BSS), the removal of preservatives by a

Table 1 Properties of the main vital dyes currently in use

Dye	Chemical group	Chemical formula	Main intraocular structure affinity	More commonly used concentration(s) (%)
Triamcinolone acetonide	Corticosteroid	$C_{24}H_{31}FO_6$	Vitreous	4
Indocyanine green	Cyanine dye	$C_{43}H_{47}N_2NaO_6S_2$	ILM	$\leq$0.05
Infracyanine green	Cyanine dye	$C_{43}H_{47}N_2NaO_6S_2$	ILM	0.05
Trypan blue	Azo-dye	$C_{34}H_{24}N_6Na_4O_{14}S_4$	ERM	0.09, 0.15, 0.18
Bromphenol blue	Arylmethane	$C_{19}H_{10}Br_4O_5S$	ERM	0.13
Brillian blue G	Arylmethane	$C_{47}H_{48}N_3S_2O_7Na$	ILM	0.025
Pure Benzyl-BBG	Arylmethane	$C_{54}H_{54}N_3NaO_7S_2$	ILM	0.05
Bluelife	Arylmethane	$C_{48}H_{50}N_3NaO_7S_2$	ILM	0.03
DDG	Arylmethane	$C_{46}H_{46}N_3NaO_7S_2$	ILM	0.025
Lutein	Hydride of a (6′R)-beta, epsilon-carotene	$C_{40}H_{56}O_2$	Vitreous	2

compounding pharmacy [6] or the manual aspiration of the TA without vehicle [7]. More recently, preservative-free TA (PF-TA) formulations containing 4% TA have been developed, registered as medical device, and licensed for intraocular use [7].

- *Lutein-based vitreous dye (LB-VD)*: 2% soluble micronized crystalline lutein. Lutein is a natural orange lipophilic pigment, also present in the retina. This pigment is certified as "Generally Recognized As Safe" (GRAS) from the U.S. Food and Drug Administration. Compared to the original pigment, the lutein crystals in the lutein-based vitreous dye consist of a "water-soluble" polar form of lutein, developed to increase the affinity with the vitreous. Several properties of this molecule have been advocated as advantageous for its intraocular use, including the blue-light filtering and antioxidant properties that could protect against the potential phototoxicity, and retinal neuroprotective properties [8, 9].

2.2 *Vital Dyes for Vitreoretinal Interface Staining*

Vital dyes for vitreoretinal interface staining are hydrophilic anionic salts of sulphonic aromatic acids [1]. Different functional groups are responsible for the properties of the dye [1], in particular:

- chromogens determine the color of the molecule;
- auxochrome groups determine wavelength and light absorption intensity;

- hydrophobic groups (alkyl or aromatic groups) determine the binding properties and, thus, the intensity of staining [10].

A common strategy adopted for the intraocular formulations of vital dyes is the combination of the dye with a density-increasing additive (e.g. polyethylene glycol (PEG), diglycerol, deuterium oxide, etc.) to obtain a final compound heavier than water that sink itself, with the aim to minimize its dispersion into the vitreous cavity and to improve the settling on the target tissue, avoiding the need of prolonged staining or staining under air (see Sect. 5.3). Ideally, a vital dye should have high affinity and selectivity for the target structures (ERM or ILM) and low affinity for underlaying retinal layers to maximize the staining and minimize the retinal penetration and, thus, potential retinal toxicity [10].

The main dyes for vitreoretinal interface currently used are:

- *Indocyanine green (ICG)*: green tricarbocyanine dye containing iodine, highly coloured. ICG exhibits a strong affinity for ILM components, including collagen type 4, laminin, and fibronectin [11]. It has also been demonstrated that this dye induces an increase of ILM stiffness, providing an advantage during peeling manoeuvres, but also potentially increasing the risk of iatrogenic retinal damage (see Sect. 4.3) [12–14]. The dye is commercialized as a power to be diluted and is commonly diluted first in distilled water and then in saline solution, due to the risk of precipitation in the latter [1]. The dilution in water results in a hypo-osmotic solution (248–275 mmol/kg) [1], with consequent potential harmful effect on retinal tissue (see Sect. 4.3) [15].
- *Infracyanine green (IfCG)*: green tricarbocyanine dye, proposed as safer alternative to ICG [1]. Indeed, compared to ICG, IfCG has the same chemical formula, but does not contain sodium iodine avoiding the exposure of the retina to iodine and allowing a dilution in glucose 5% to obtain an iso-osmotic solution (294–314 mmol/kg). As osmolarity alterations at epiretinal or subretinal level can exert toxic effects on the retina [15], the injection of an iso-osmotic solution reduces the risk of potential hypoosmotic-induced toxicity [1]. Finally, the longer wavelengths of the absorption spectrum of IfCG compared to ICG determine a decreased absorption using a Xenon endoillumination and, thus, decreased risk of phototoxicity [16].
- *Trypan blue (TB)*: hydrophilic azo-dye, characterized by a nitrogen linkage [11]. Traditionally used in cataract surgery for the staining of the anterior capsule [17], TB exhibits a strong affinity for ERM [1]. Its binding is not allowed in live cells because of size and polarity [1].
- *Bromphenol blue (BrB)*: hydroxytriarylmethane, also called tetrabromophenolsulfonephthalein [1]. Currently approved at the concentration of 0.13% and available in combination with brilliant blue G (BBG).
- *Brilliant Blue G*: aminotriarylmethane blue dye. Primarily used to stain the ILM due to its high affinity for this tissue. In this regard, hydrophobic interactions, in addition to electrostatic interactions, appear to play a crucial role in the binding of BBG with ILM components [18]. As ICG, BGG is able to induce an increase

of ILM stiffness, but with less pronounced effect [13]. More commonly used at the concentration of 0.025% in an iso-osmolar solution [1].

- *BBG-derivatives*: BBG-derivatives have been developed to improve the staining properties and the safety profile of BBG. In particular, pure benzyl-BBG (PBB), blulife and DDG are currently used in commercially available vital dye formulations.
  - PBB is a benzyl-BBG derivate, characterized by the addition of a benzyl moiety at the diphenylic nitrogen of BBG [10]. Compared to BBG, PBB exhibits higher lipophilicity (defined as the enhanced ability of the ionized substance to prefer the oily phase over the aqueous phase in a two-phase system) [10]. Based on the assumption that higher lipophilicity can increase ILM protein binding/affinity, PBB would be expected to have greater selectivity for ILM avoiding the diffusion of the dye into the adjacent neurosensory retina [10]. In this regard, a recent experimental study confirmed that hydrophobic interactions appeared crucial for the binding affinity for proteins, including fibronectin, of PBB *in vitro* and *in silico* [10]. Moreover, compared to BBG, PBB demonstrated greater ILM protein binding/staining, greater ILM selectivity, increased distribution of the dye on the ILM and reduced distribution in neurosensory retina in an *ex vivo* porcine eye model [10].
  - Blulife is a patented BBG-derivative with affinity for ILM.
  - DDG is also patented and characterized by the replacement of the ethoxy substituent of BBG with a methoxy substituent. DDG in combination with TB 0.09%, demonstrated good staining properties on different membrane models, namely polyvinylidene difluoride filter mimicking ILM, a collagen type I membrane mimicking ERM and a plastic surface with proteins adsorbed mimicking ILM components [19].

- *Combined blue dyes*: combined formulations of blue dyes have been developed to improve the staining properties (both ERM and ILM are targeted) and the safety profile of the final compound. Among those currently available, there are the following:
  - TB 0.15% + BBG 0.025% + 4% PEG;
  - BrB 0.13% + BBG 0.025%;
  - TB 0.09% + DDG 0.025%;
  - TB 0.18% + Blulife 0.03%;
  - Soluble lutein 1% + PBB 0.05%;
  - Soluble lutein 2% + TB 0.15% + PBB 0.05%.

3 Clinical Use and Outcomes

3.1 *Triamcinolone Acetonide*

The efficacy of TA for vitreous staining has been widely documented [1, 20–23]. The persistence of preserved TA into the vitreous cavity has been demonstrated up to 40 days after PPV [24, 25], representing a significant concern in view of the documented time-dependency of preserved TA-associated cytotoxicity (see Sect. 4.1). Shorter intraocular retention time has been documented for PF-TA formulations compared to preserved TA [26].

3.2 *Indocyanine Green*

ICG has been widely used for ILM staining, although still off label. Despite satisfactory anatomical results have been reported using ICG in PPV for both ERM and full-thickness macular hole (FTMH) repair [1], its clinical use has been gradually limited due to the concerns related to its potential intraocular toxicity (see Sects. 4.3 and 5.2). A meta-analysis, including 837 eyes treated with ILM peeling with or without ICG for FTMH repair, showed comparable anatomical outcomes but significantly worse functional results and higher incidence of retinal pigment epithelium (RPE) alterations in ICG group [27]. It has to be noted that most of the studies used high ICG concentrations and/or volumes, and it is now established that ICG concentration correlates strongly with the incidence of complications [27]. In FTMH surgery with ILM peeling, better anatomical outcomes have been associated with a low concentration of ICG at 0.05%, compared to higher concentrations of 0.5, 0.1, 0.25, 0.125% [28]. Recently, the use of ICG for ILM peeling has been also identified as risk factor for macular hole formation after PPV for myopic traction maculopathy [29].

In case ICG is used, it has been recommended a concentration $\leq 0.05\%$ to be injected not directly over bared RPE and promptly removed to minimize the contact of the dye with the retinal tissue [30].

3.3 *Infracyanine Green*

As ICG, it is currently used off label and, compared to the latter, appear to have a better safety profile [1]. Good anatomical and functional results have been reported for IfCG-assisted PPV in case of both ERM and FTMH, also using low concentrations at 0.05%, with lower incidence of retinal toxicity compared to ICG [31, 32].

3.4 Trypan Blue

Due to its strong affinity for EMR, TB is generally considered the preferred dye to identify the precise extent of ERM [1]. However, due to the poor affinity for ILM, TB is mainly used in combination with BBG at concentrations from 0.09 to 0.018%, more commonly 0.15%. The use of TB for ERM peeling has been associated with favourable results in terms of visual function, also supported by electrophysiological and histopathological findings [33–36]. Better visual outcomes have been reported comparing TB- and ICG-assisted PPV for both ILM and EMR peeling in TB group [37–39]. A recent meta-analysis identified TB 0.15%, along with BBG 0.025%, as the more efficient dyes for ILM peeling in FTMH [28]. However, experimental studies raised some concerns regarding the potential neurotoxicity of TB (see Sect. 4.4).

3.5 Brilliant Blue G

Due to its strong affinity for ILM, BBG has been proposed as alternative to ICG with better safety profile [1]. Two meta-analyses reported that BBG-assisted ILM peeling for FTMH repair may be beneficial in terms of functional outcomes, compared to ICG, TA, TB and no dye [40, 41]. A recent meta-analysis including 1492 patients treated with ILM peeling for FTMH recommended TB 0.15% and BBG 0.05% as the more efficient dyes for ILM peeling in FTMH [28]. Several case series supported the clinical safety profile of BBG in chromo-PPV, also supported by electrophysiological findings [42, 43]. Better electrophysiological outcomes [44] and greater long-term visual gain [45] have been reported comparing BBG-assisted versus ICG-assisted ILM peeling.

In addition, due to the concerns related to the potential neurotoxic effects of TB (see Sect. 4.4), BBG has been proposed also as potential alternative to the TB for ERM through the technique of the "negative staining" [46].

3.6 Lutein-Based Blue dyes

Good anatomical and functional results have been reported in eyes treated with PPV and ERM/ILM peeling with the aid of lutein-based blue dyes for FTMH and ERM [47–49].

A prospective randomized study compared eyes with idiopathic ERM treated with PPV + ERM/ILM peeling using TB 0.15% + BBG 0.05% + lutein 2% (15 eyes), TB 0.15% + BBG 0.025% + PEG 4% (15 eyes), and ICG 0.05% (15 eyes), in terms of functional results (visual acuity and macular sensitivity) and histopathological findings [49]. Despite comparable functional results at 6-month follow-up, the lutein-based dye group was characterized by significantly better visual acuity and macular sensitivity at 1- and 3-month follow-up and significantly lower expression of glial fibrillary acidic protein (GFAP) and neurofilament protein (NF) on ILM specimens [49]. The faster functional recovery and the histopathological findings associated with the use of the lutein-based blue dye may suggest a role of lutein in reducing the adhesion to the retinal tissue and, thus, the iatrogenic stress and damage during peeling manoeuvres [49]. The demonstration of a different interaction of lutein-based dyes with ILM and ERM membrane models, compared with other vital dyes, may support these results (see Sect. 4.7).

3.7 Combine Blue dyes

Satisfactory anatomical and functional outcomes have been reported following PPV + ERM and/or ILM peeling using TB 0.15% + BBG 0.025% + 4% PEG [50–53].

A recent cross-sectional study compared eyes with idiopathic ERM treated with ERM/ILM peeling using two different combined blue dyes, namely TB 0.15% + BBG 0.025% + 4% PEG versus TB 0.18% + Blulife 0.03% [54]. Comparable anatomical and functional results have been found; however, TB 0.18% + Blulife 0.03% was judged superior in terms of staining efficacy by the only surgeon involved [54].

4 Experimental Evidence of Safety

Physico-chemical and biological analytical methods can be used to assess the potential toxicity and, thus, the safety profile of medical devices, such as vital dyes [4]. Among physico-chemical methods, liquid chromatography is a fundamental step in the assessment of the purity of the vital dye formulations. Indeed, after the synthesis, several impurities can be present and specific subsequent purification processes are aimed to increase the purity of the final compound. Biological methods include *in vitro*, *ex vivo* and *in vivo* analyses aimed to effectively assess the biocompatibility of a given compound testing the ability of specific concentrations to exert toxic effects on biological cells and tissues [4, 55]. *In vitro* cytotoxicity tests represent an established method for the safety evaluation of medical devices [4]. In particular, the reduction of cell viability after the exposure to a given compound is a main parameter to assess its cytotoxicity and, according to ISO 10993-5, a cytotoxic effect is defined by the reduction of cell viability >30% (thus, cell viability <70%) [56].

Moreover, recent experimental *in vitro* and *ex vivo* studies supported the potential role of interactions between different intraocular medical devices in inducing additive and/or cumulative cytotoxic effect [7, 57].

4.1 Triamcinolone Acetonide

A cytotoxic effect of TA, with or without preservatives, on both RPE and neurosensory retinal cells *in vitro* has been demonstrated in various experimental studies [7, 58–64]. Although both the vehicle and, more specifically, the preservative benzyl alcohol have been proposed as the factors primarily responsible for the detected cytotoxicity, the experimental results are still controversial [26, 58, 64, 65]. The mechanisms suggested as causative of retinal toxicity are non-physiologic changes of vitreous pH and the enhancement of TA-induces cytotoxicity for the vehicle and induction RPE necrosis and mitochondrial apoptosis for benzyl alcohol [62, 63].

A time-dependent cytotoxic effect has been demonstrated *in vitro* for both diluted and undiluted preserved TA [7]. Moreover, the sequential exposure of ARPE-19 cells to preserved and PF-TA formulations and perfluorodecalin (PFD) induced a significantly greater reduction of cell viability, compared to PFD alone [7].

In a recent *in vitro* study, significant morphological changes and decreased cell adhesion have been detected after the exposure of ARPE-19 cells to both diluted and undiluted preserved TA [7]; whereas PF-TA formulations appeared to form larger aggregates on cell layer [7], whose size may correlate with induced cellular damage and death [58, 66]. Finally, it has been demonstrated that the toxic effect of TA may be greater when the compound is in direct contact with the retina in absence of the vitreous [58].

4.2 Lutein-Based Vitreous Dye

So far, only one experimental study investigated the safety profile of the LB-VD demonstrating that the latter showed a more favorable safety profile compared to both preserved TA and PF-TA formulations [7]. Indeed, LB-VD was associated with no significant cellular damage and no cytotoxic effect on ARPE-19 cells after 1-, 5- and 30-min exposure [7]. In addition, a limited impact of LB-VD on cell viability was supported by the detection of a non-significant decrease of cell survival after the sequential exposure to LB-VD and PFD, compared to PFD alone [7].

4.3 Indocyanine Green

Dose-and time-dependent cytotoxicity of ICG has been demonstrated *in vitro* on ARPE-19 cells, retinal ganglion cells (RGC) and Müller cells [15, 67–69]. Several *in vivo* studies in animal eye models demonstrated the concentration-dependent retinal toxicity of ICG, in terms of structural retinal damage, RPE atrophy and significant reduction of photopic and scotopic ERG amplitudes [70–74]. Low doses of intravitreal ICG at 0.25 or 0.025 mg/ml have been associated with delayed alterations on electroretinogram (ERG) in rat eyes [70].

Multiple mechanisms are supposed to contribute to ICG-related toxicity [75], including:

- Induction of apoptosis in retinal cells: *in vitro* experiments demonstrated that the exposure of ARPE-19 cells to ICG induced the downregulation of the anti-apoptotic protein Bcl-2 and the upregulation of the pro-apoptotic protein Bax [76, 77].
- Light-mediated damage: ICG absorption spectra overlap with the emission light wavelengths of commercial light sources (380–830 nm), potentially causing phototoxicity [1]. ICG may alter the retinal absorption spectra in a dose-dependent manner [78, 79]. The influence of light types, wavelengths and duration on ICG-induced retinal damage have been documented *ex vivo* [75, 79, 80].
- Iodine- and Sodium-mediated toxicity: Iodine and related derivative compounds exert highly toxic effects on the retina [1]. Diluting ICG from the solvent may reduce the uptake by RPE cells [81]; consistently, less morphological changes and increased viability have been detected in ARPE-19 cells exposed to ICG reconstituted with Na(+) free BSS [81].
- Osmolarity-induced toxicity: Osmolarity changes at epiretinal or subretinal level can induce structural retinal damage [12]. The injection of hypo-osmolar ICG solution may induce a rapid change in intravitreal osmolarity with consequent harmful effects, potentially exacerbated by endoillumination [1]. In particular, the increase of calcium influx and the secondarily reduced RPE enzymatic activity may be involved in hypo-osmolarity-induced retinal damage [82]. A correlation between ICG osmolarity and RPE damage and functional outcomes has been documented [83, 84].
- ICG solution decomposition: after light exposure, intravitreal ICG may undergo self-sensitized oxidation [85].
- Peeling-related damage: ICG induce the increase of ILM stiffness and adhesion to the Müller cells and neurofilaments, and this may contribute to the iatrogenic retinal damage during ILM peeling. A light-dependent photosensitizing effect of ICG leading to the formation of reactive oxygen species and a spin triplet state of the dye molecule has been proposed as the mechanism leading to the increased ILM stiffness [12, 86]; however, Haritoglou et al. [13] subsequently demonstrated that the illumination had a limited non-significant additional impact on membrane rigidity. In addition, the analysis of the mode of interaction of different vital dyes with surrogate membrane models of ERM and ILM showed that the use of ICG resulted in strong chemical interaction and adhesion, as well as structural alteration of membrane model [87].

4.4 Trypan Blue

The evidence on the safety profile of TB is controversial. *In vitro*, TB exhibited chronic cytotoxicity at different tested concentrations, including 0.05, 0.06, 0.1 and 0.15%, on human RPE cells after 6-day exposure, but no cytotoxic effect after acute exposure (5 min) [67]; whereas, a dose- and time-dependent neurotoxic effect of TB has been demonstrated on retinal ganglion cells (RGC) after short-term (30 s to 30 min) and long-term (3 days) exposure [88]. In addition, long exposure time (30 min) to TB formulations was associated with significantly greater reduction of ARPE-19 cells viability compared to shorter exposure time (5 min) [89]. As significant remnants of TB have been demonstrated on the retinal surface after washout [90], these experimental results may support the risk of prolonged harmful effects on retinal cells. In addition, a partially irreversible loss of the b-wave on ERG has been documented after 15-s exposure to TB 0.15% in an *ex vivo* model of isolated superfused vertebrate retina [90]. Although both TB 0.15% and BBG 0.025% induced a time-dependent reduction of ERG amplitudes, the full recovery and stability of the b-wave amplitude was reached on average 20–25 min after applying BBG [90].

The intravitreal injection of TB 0.06% and 0.15% did not result in any structural retinal damage at histological examination in animal eye models [91, 92]. In addition, less substantial retinal damage associated with subretinal injection of TB 0.15% compared to that of ICG 0.05% in rabbit eyes [93]. However, a post-mortem study showed inner retina disorganization and absence of the ILM following the application of undiluted TB 0.15% and 0.25% [35].

4.5 Bromphenol Blue

Controversial results on the effect of BrB on RPE and RGC cultures viability have been described for concentrations varying from 0.2 to 0.0005% [94, 95]. Awad et al. [96] investigated the potential cytotoxicity of BrB 0.13%, alone or in combination with BBG 0.025%, on ARPE-19 cells after 30-min exposure with or without 15-min irradiation with Xenon and LED lights. Cells viability <70% was detected in cells exposed to both BrB and BrB + BBG after light exposure, with significantly worse reduction at the assessment 24 h after exposure compared to that performed immediately after [96] In addition, BrB ± BBG induced cells' morphological changes after light exposure [96]. In the light of these results, the Authors described BrB as a dye less suitable for vitreoretinal surgery, compared to the other blue dyes examined (i.e. TB, BBG, TB-BBG, TB-BBG-PEG) [96] Finally, Morales et al. [97] demonstrated that very low concentrations of the dye (0.5 μg/mL) induced a reduced RPE cells viability after 72-h exposure, suggesting long-term harmful effects of potential dye residues after PPV.

4.6 Brilliant Blue G

Compared to other vital dyes, BBG demonstrated significantly less damage on retinal cells and tissue in several animal and *in vitro* studies, in particular when compared to ICG [77, 98, 99]. The comparison *in vitro* of the effects of different dyes on ARPE-19 cells, including ICG, IfCG, BrB and BBG, demonstrated that the latter was the only dye that did not induce apoptosis [76]. In addition, it has also been suggested that BBG may prevent apoptosis in photoreceptors acting as P2RX7 antagonist and inducting the upregulation of Bcl-2 [76, 77, 100].

BBG 0.025% has been associated with greater ARPE-19 cell survival *in vitro*, compared to TB 0.15% [89]. However, BBG 0.025% and 0.05% caused borderline cytotoxicity in ARPE-19 cells and RGC for exposure time >15 min [94].

The good biocompatibility of BBG 0.05% has been demonstrated in rat eyes as absence of structural retinal changes and ERG alterations, but not for high concentrations (BBG 1% and 0.1%) [43, 101].

Although the exposure to BBG 0.025% resulted in a reduction of both a- and b-wave on ERG in an *ex vivo* model of isolated superfused vertebrate retina, these changes were completely reversible [90].

4.7 DDG

DDG demonstrated to be not cytotoxic and to induce similar effect on cell viability compared to BBG [19].

4.8 Lutein-Based Blue Dyes

In an experimental study testing the mode of interaction of different vital dyes (namely TA, ICG, TB, BBG and lutein-based dyes) with surrogate membrane models of ILM and ERM, lutein-based dyes demonstrated a physical interaction with the membranes without significant membrane disorganization, conversely to the others exhibiting a strong chemical interaction [87]. To note, affinity for ILM was revealed for all tested dyes [87].

A recent *in vitro* experimental study suggested that lutein may reduce the cytotoxic effect of ICG and BBG by inducing autophagy in ARPE-19 cells [102].

No ERG alterations and no significant structural abnormalities have been reported in rabbit eyes after the intravitreal injection of various concentrations of lutein/zeaxanthin (0.025–0.5%) in combination with BBG 0.025% or 0.05% [103].

4.9 *Combine Blue dye, TB 0.15% + BBG 0.025% + PEG 4%*

Two combined blue dye formulations consisting of TB 0.15% + BBG 0.025% + 4% PEG, and BBG 0.025% + 4% PEG, have been tested *in vitro* on rat RGCs and isolated perfused bovine retina [104]. Both formulations induced no citotoxicity at different exposure times (30, 60, 120 and 320 s) as well as limited and reversible ERG alterations [104].

To explain the better results of the combined dye compared to the previous results reported testing TB only [67, 105], it has been hypothesized a beneficial effect of a better purified TB or of PEG 4%. Indeed, the latter, may exert a neuroprotective effect related to its fusogenicity, a membrane-stabilizing effect in neuronal cells, and, thus, may reduce the potential negative effect of TB [104]. The potential beneficial role of PEG appears further supported by two experimental *in vitro* studies. Indeed, the addition of PEG to BBG 0.025%, TB 0.15%, and combination of BBG 0.025% + TB 0.15%, resulted in decreased cytotoxic effect detected testing the same concentration of TB alone or in association with BBG [89].

Moreover, the comparison TB 0.15% + BBG 0.025% with or without PEG on ARPE-19 and RGC-5 cells, and demonstrated greater positive effect on mitochondria function, cell viability and apoptosis in presence of PEG [106].

5 Clinical Signs of Dye toxicity

5.1 *Triamcinolone Acetonide*

Clinically detectable functional or anatomical complications appear to be rare after the intraoperative use of TA [1, 23, 107, 108]. The intraocular persistence for TA, in particular over the fovea, may slow MH healing process [24, 108]. Sterile endophthalmitis has been documented as complication after TA intravitreal injection for therapeutic purposes [109, 110].

5.2 *Indocyanine Green*

Multiple complications have been associated with ICG-assisted PPV, including deterioration of visual acuity, RPE alterations and atrophy, optic nerve atrophy, and perimetric defects [1, 30, 111–116]. In addition, the documented long-term persistence of ICG intravitreally (up to 36 months) and persistent deposition on the optic disc after chromo-PPV, along with its ability to migrate subretinally through the FTMH may contribute to its iatrogenic and toxic potential [111, 115–117]. In this regard, the use of hypo-osmolar ICG solution (< 270 mOsm) and of concentration >0.5% has been more commonly associated with RPE toxicity [1].

5.3 Blue Dyes

Table 2 summarizes the main surgical details and clinical findings in reported cases of blue dye-associated retinal toxicity.

Regarding clinical findings, atrophic changes have been more commonly reported in the peeling area, in particular in the areas where ILM was already peeled at the time of repeated dye injection (Table 1); however, extensive atrophic changes, beyond the area of peeling have also been described [127]. Atrophic RPE changes have also been documented in the area of subretinal migration of BBG (Table 1). In case of subretinal migration of the vital dye, the mechanisms involved in retinal damage may be multiple, including the direct toxicity of the dye on RPE cells, the mechanical trauma related to the jet stream of injection itself, and the induction of a localized retinal elevation [119]. It has been suggested that the presence of a thin choroid preoperatively may exacerbate the potential dye-related toxicity and contribute to the development of extensive damage of the RPE [124].

Regarding the surgical procedure, surgical factors that may contribute to the increased risk of vital dye-associated retinal toxicity are prolonged operative time and specific aspects of the staining technique, such as injection of the dye under air, repeated dye application, mainly after an initial ILM peeling, prolonged staining time (Table 1). The injection of the dye under air ("dry method of dye injection") has been previously suggested to improve the staining of the target tissue due to the resulting higher concentration of the dye over the macula, avoiding the potential contact of the dispersed dye with the posterior lens capsule; however, the consequent exposure of the retina to increased dye concentration might be responsible for the retinal toxicity [1]. A higher rate of ORL degeneration and RPE atrophic changes after "dry" dye injection compared to the "wet method" (injection in fluid-filled eye) has been demonstrated in porcine eyes [131]. The re-staining once the ILM has been already partially peeled, results in the direct exposure of the inner retina to the dye. This can increase the risk of intraretinal penetration of the dye and, consequently, the risk of retinal toxicity. Conversely, a second injection of the dye immediately after the first one before starting the peeling manoeuvre, in case of uneven macular staining, may be a safer and more efficient option because of stacking arrangement of chromophores on the coloured interface [132].

It is worth noting that the instructions for use (IFU) of several commercialized blue dyes provide instructions on the staining technique, including a limited time of application of the dye (usually <30 s) and the prohibition/advice to inject the dyes if the ILM has been already peeled.

5.4 The Role of Phototoxicity

Retinal phototoxicity may significantly contribute to the dye-related retinal toxicity and RPE damage. Surgical illumination can be responsible of retinal phototoxic

Table 2 Case reports of blue dye-related toxicity

Authors, country	Eyes (n)	Preop VA	Surgery (baseline diagnosis)	Dye used	Operative time (min)	Staining (n)	Staining time	Eye filling at the time of staining	Final VA	Final FU (months)	Fundus signs	OCT signs	Other
Saeed and Heiman [118], UK	1	20/200	PPV + ILM peeling + C_3F_8 (FTMH)	TB 0.06%	NS	1	3 min	air	20/200	3	Pigmented lesion 1 DD temporally to the fovea	NS	FFA: hyperfluorescent area with surrounding hypofluorescence
Malerbi et al. [119], Brazil	1	20/200	PPV + ERM/ ILM peeling (ERM)	BGG 0.025%	NS	1	NS	fluid	20/40	1	RPE atrophy not involving the fovea	NS	RPE atrophy corresponding to the area of SR BBG
Jain et al. [120], India	1	20/200	PPV + ILM peeling + C_3F_8 (FTMH)	TB 0.06%	NS	2	2 min each	air	CF	24	1 m: peri-hole hypopigmentation; 7 m: subfoveal RPE atrophy	Month 7: RPE atrophy, IS/OS junction defect	Progressive enlargement of atrophic area
Savary and Kodjikian [121], France	1	20/30	PPV + ERM/ ILM peeling	BBG 0.025%	NS	2	NA	BSS	20/25	36	BBG infiltration of the superior and temporal macula, progressively disappeared	Progressive IRL atrophy corresponding to the area of infiltration	BBG infiltration noted during 2nd injection
Jindal et al. [122], Nepal	3	20/400	PPV + ILM peeling + C_3F_8 (FTMH)	BBG 0.025%	NS	1	1 min	BSS (partial FAX)	2/200	2	hyperpigmentation and atrophic changes in the macula	RPE irregular thickening and atrophy, foveal thinning	
		20/60							20/160				
		20/400							20/400				

(continued)

Table 2 (continued)

Authors, country	Eyes (n)	Preop VA	Surgery (baseline diagnosis)	Dye used	Operative time (min)	Staining (n)	Staining time	Eye filling at the time of staining	Final VA	Final FU (months)	Fundus signs	OCT signs	Other
Almeida et al. [123], Brazil	1	20/70	phacoPPV + ERM/ILM peeling (ERM)	BBG 0.05%	NS	1	NS	BSS	20/25	24	Macular staining at day 1, disappeared at day 7	3 m: CME 5 m: worsened CME, resolved after IVT TA	BBG flush during the infusion followed by detection of SR BBG in the macula mfERG reduced amplitude, increased IT at 1 m; residual central amplitude reduction at 2y
Singh and Chhablani [124], India	1	20/125	PPV + ILM peeling (FTMH)	BBG 0.025%	40	1	NS	BSS	CF 1 m	6	3-DD RPE atrophy fovea-involving	RPE atrophy, inner choroidal layers loss, subfoveal choroidal thinning	Initial VA improvement 1 month after sx
Venkatesh et al. [125], India	1	20/80	PPV + ILM peeling + SF_6	BBG 0.05%	90	2	2 min each	air	20/320	3	NA	ORL disruption	FAF: hypo/hyper autofluorescence
Soni et al. [126], USA	3	20/60	PPV + ILM peeling + C_3F_8 (FTMH)	BBG 0.05%	129	2	1 min	BSS/air	CF	1	RPE mottling	ORL and RPE atrophy, foveal thinning, CC loss	
		20/200			131		2 min	NS	CF				
		20/125			116		1 min	BSS/air	HM				

(continued)

Table 2 (continued)

Authors, country	Eyes (n)	Precp VA	Surgery (baseline diagnosis)	Dye used	Operative time (min)	Staining (n)	Staining time	Eye filling at the time of staining	Final VA	Final FU (months)	Fundus signs	OCT signs	Other
		20/50			123		1 min	BSS/air	20/160				
Federico et al. [127], Spain	1	20/40	PPV + ILM peeling + inverted ILM flap	BBG 0.025%	<45	2	6–10 s	N/A	20/400	12	RPE mottling in the macular area and upper mid-periphery, progressing to atrophic changes	Severe ORL disruption, RPE migration and thickening	Progressive RPE atrophy over the FU
Rivera-Valdivia et al. [128], Colombia	1	20/100	PhacoPPV + ILM peeling (FTMH)	None	NS	NS	NS	N/A	HM	24	RPE mottling, atrophic changes in the peeling area	irregular RPE, IS/OS disruption. disorganization of retinal layers	
		20/30	PhacoPPV + ERM/ILM peeling (ERM)	BBG				NS	20/40				CME treated with 1 intravitreal injection of Ozurdex ®

(continued)

Table 2 (continued)

Authors, country	Eyes (n)	Preop VA	Surgery (baseline diagnosis)	Dye used	Operative time (min)	Staining (n)	Staining time	Eye filling at the time of staining	Final VA	Final FU (months)	Fundus signs	OCT signs	Other
Torres-Villaros et al. [129], France	1	20/40	PPV + FTMH ERM peeling (ERM)	BBG 0.025% + TB 0.15% + PEG 4%	111	3	1 min, 30 s, 30 s	BSS	20/20	4	RPE mottling	ORL disruption, irregular RPE thickening with SR deposits	Self-closed iatrogenic extracentral MH Postop VA improved from 20/80 with residual persistent central scotoma
Venkatesh et al. [130], India	1	20/200	PhacoPPV + ILM peeling (FTMH)	BBG 0.05%	87	2	2 min	air	20/630	48	Atrophic areas involving the foveal centre and inferior macula	ORL disruption, absent RPE, choroidal thinning	

CC choriocapillaris, *CME* cystoid macular edema, *CF* counting fingers, *DD* disc diameter, *ERM* epiretinal membrane, *EZ* ellipsoid band, *FAF* fundus autofluorescence, *FAX* fluid-air exchange, *FFA* fundus fluorescein angiography, *FTMH* full-thickness macular hole, *FU* follow-up, *HM* hand movements, *ILM* internal limiting membrane, *IRL* inner retinal layers, *IS/OS* inner segment/outer segment, *IT* implicit time, *IVT* intravitreal, *mfERG* multifocal electroretinography, *MP* microperimetry, *N/A* not applicable, *NS* not specified, *ON* optic nerve, *ORL* outer retinal layers, *Op* operative, *phacoIOL* phacoemulsification and intraocular lens implantation, *PPV* pars plana vitrectomy, *postop* postoperative, *preop* preoperative, *RNFL* retinal nerve fiber layer, *RPE* retinal pigment epithelium, *sx* surgery, *SR* subretinal, *TA* triamcinolone acetonide, *UK* United Kingdom damage through mechanical, thermal, or photochemical mechanisms, depending on light intensity, wavelength, distance, and duration [1, 132]. On the one hand, vital dyes, especially with regard to ICG, can act as photosensitizing substances under specific condition and they can exacerbate this injury increasing the retinal absorbance [1, 133]; on the other hand, the illumination-induced decomposition of dyes results in the formation of free radicals and photoproducts, harmful to the retina [134]. The absorbance of the dye can also be influenced by the solvent [135]. The RPE damage could be enhanced by lights of different wavelengths also in presence of subretinal dyes [136]. Further studies are necessary to better address this topic.

5.5 *How to Recognize Vital Dye-Related Toxicity*

Dye-related retinal toxicity can be associated with significant visual impairment [118, 120, 122, 124–128, 130] and, less frequently, with central scotoma [127, 129]. Functional retinal damage can be also detected as visual field defects [129], decreased sensitivity at microperimetry [118, 123] and decreased amplitude and increased latency on ERG tests [123].

Fundus examination can show RPE changes [119, 126, 127], mottled hyperpigmentated areas [118, 122, 126–128], evolving in atrophic areas, that can become confluent over time [122, 124, 127, 128]; early persistent retinal whitening in the peeling area has also been described [129].

In addition to fundus examination, the following imaging investigations can be performed:

- Optical coherence tomography (OCT): the structural signs more commonly described in association with dye-related retinal toxicity are foveal thinning [120, 122, 124, 126, 130], disruption of the external retinal layers [120, 124, 125, 127–130], photoreceptor loss [127], RPE migration and irregular thickening, appearing as hyperreflective subretinal material [122, 126–129], evolving in RPE atrophy [120, 124, 126–128, 130]. Less common findings may be disruption of the inner retinal layers [128], intraretinal fluid [123, 128], and retinal nerve fiber layer defects progressively evolving in localized atrophic inner retinal areas in case of retinal dye infiltration [121]. Progressive subfoveal choroidal thinning with choriocapillaris loss has also been described [124, 126, 130]. Due to the presence of RPE atrophy and choriocapillaris loss, OCT angiography can show prominent medium choroidal vessels [124].
- Infra-red (IR) imaging: macular speckled hyperreflective dots have been described in the early postoperative period, progressively disappearing, followed by residual atrophic patches [130]. An increased visibility of choroidal vessels of large size may also be noted [124].
- Fundus autofluorescence (FAF): areas of mized hypo- and hyperautofluorescence, more commonly but not always limited to the peeling area, have been described as

sign of outer retinal and RPE damage [125–127]. These areas can evolve in large hypoautofluorescent areas, consistent with RPE atrophy [124, 127, 128, 130].

- Fluorescein angiography (FA): hyperfluorescent window defect, in absence of leakage occasionally surrounded by an area of hypofluorescence, can be detected in the areas of RPE atrophy [118, 119, 123].

Clinical Pearls

- An adequate knowledge of the chemical structure of a given vital dye is crucial to better understand its intraocular behavior.
- Consider binding affinity, selectivity and purity to choose the best dye for a given target tissue.
- Avoid multiple injections of dye, prolonged staining (>1 min) and staining under air.
- Perform a careful removal of residues of intraocular medical devices to avoid iatrogenic interactions.

References

1. Rodrigues EB, Costa EF, Penha FM, Melo GB, Bottós J, Dib E, Furlani B, Lima VC, Maia M, Meyer CH, Höfling-Lima AL, Farah ME. The use of vital dyes in ocular surgery. Surv Ophthalmol. 2009;54:576–617.
2. Rodrigues EB, Meyer CH, Kroll P. Chromovitrectomy: a new field in vitreoretinal surgery. Graefes Arch Clin Exp Ophthalmol. 2005;243:291–3.
3. Schumann RG, Haritoglou C. International chromovitrectomy collaboration. Chromovitrectomy and the vitreoretinal interface. Ophthalmologica. 2013;230(Suppl 2):3–10.
4. Romano MR, Ferrara M, Nepita I, D'Amato Tothova J, Giacometti Schieroni A, Reami D, Mendichi R, Liggieri L, Repetto R. Biocompatibility of intraocular liquid tamponade agents: an update. Eye. 2021;35:2699–713.
5. Peyman GA, Cheema R, Conway MD, Fang T. Triamcinolone acetonide as an aid to visualization of the vitreous and the posterior hyaloid during pars Plana vitrectomy. Retina. 2000;20:554–5.
6. Bakri SJ, Shah A, Faulk NS, Beer PM. Intravitreal preservative-free triamcinolone acetonide for the treatment of macular oedema. Eye. 2005;19:686–8.
7. Lazzara F, Conti F, Ferrara M, Lippera M, Coppola M, Rossi S, Drago F, Bucolo C, Romano MR. Safety profile of lutein-versus triamcinolone acetonide-based vitreous staining. Transl Vis Sci Technol. 2023;12:5.
8. Sasaki M, Ozawa Y, Kurihara T, Noda K, Imamura Y, Kobayashi S, Ishida S, Tsubota K. Neuroprotective effect of an antioxidant, lutein, during retinal inflammation. Invest Ophthalmol Vis Sci. 2009;50:1433–9.
9. Wilson LM, Tharmarajah S, Jia Y, Semba RD, Schaumberg DA, Robinson KA. The effect of lutein/zeaxanthin intake on human macular pigment optical density: a systematic reviewand metaanalysis. Adv Nutr. 2021;12:2244–54.
10. Spadaro A, Rao M, Lorenti M, Romano MR, Augello A, Eandi CM, Platania CBM, Drago F, Bucolo C. New brilliant Blue G derivative as pharmacological tool in retinal surgery. Front Pharmacol. 2020;11:708.
11. Badaro E, Novais EA, Penha FM, et al. Vital dyes in ophthalmology: a chemical perspective. Curr Eye Res. 2014;39:649–58.

12. Wollensak G, Spoerl E, Wirbelauer C, Pham DT. Influence of indocyanine green staining on the biomechanical strength of porcine internal limiting membrane. Ophthalmologica. 2004;218:278–82.
13. Haritoglou C, Mauell S, Benoit M, Schumann RG, Henrich PB, Wolf A, Kampik A. Vital dyes increase the rigidity of the internal limiting membrane. Eye. 2013;27:1308–15.
14. Kenawy N, Wong D, Stappler T, Romano MR, Das RA, Hebbar G, Prime W, Heimann H, Gibran SK, Sheridan CM, Cheung YH, Hiscott PS. Does the presence of an epiretinal membrane alter the cleavage plane during internal limiting membrane peeling? Ophthalmology. 2010;117:320–3.
15. Ho JD, Tsai RJ, Chen SN, Chen HC. Toxic effect of indocyanine green on retinal pigment epithelium related to osmotic effects of the solvent. Am J Ophthalmol. 2003;135:258.
16. Haritoglou C, Gandorfer A, Schaumberger M, Tadayoni R, Gandorfer A, Kampik A. Light-absorbing properties and osmolarity of indocyanine-green depending on concentration and solvent medium. Invest Ophthalmol Vis Sci. 2003;44:2722–9.
17. Melles GRJ, De Waard PWT, Pameyer JH, et al. Trypan blue capsule staining to visualize the capsulorhexis in cataract surgery. J Cataract Refract Surg. 1999;25:7–9.
18. Georgiou CD, Grintzalis K, Zervoudakis G, Papapostolou I. Mechanism of coomassie brilliant blue G-250 binding to proteins: a hydrophobic assay for nanogram quantities of proteins. Anal Bioanal Chem. 2008;250:669–77.
19. Mohr A, Cendoya P, Wilinska J, Apostu M, Apostu E, Janku J, Wilfling T, Ramos G, Al-Joumhawy M, Gabel D. New dual dye for vitreoretinal surgery with increased transparency. BMJ Open Ophthalmol. 2022;7:e001116.
20. Chen TY, Yang CM, Liu KR. Intravitreal triamcinolone staining observation of residual undetached cortical vitreous after posterior vitreous detachment. Eye. 2006;20:423–7.
21. Doi N, Uemura A, Nakao K, Sakamoto T. Vitreomacular adhesion and the defect in posterior vitreous cortex visualized by triamcinolone-assisted vitrectomy. Retina. 2005;25:742–5.
22. Furino C, Micelli Ferrari T, Boscia F, Cardascia N, Recchimurzo N, Sborgia C. Triamcinolone-assisted pars Plana vitrectomy for proliferative vitreoretinopathy. Retina. 2003;23:771–6.
23. Jermak CM, Dellacroce JT, Heffez J, Peyman GA. Triamcinolone acetonide in ocular therapeutics. Surv Ophthalmol. 2007;52:503–22.
24. Fukukita M, Sasoh M, Matsubara H, Furuta M, Okawa C, Ito Y, Wakitani Y, Uji Y. Triamcinolone acetonide remaining on the fovea after successful macular hole closure. Retina. 2007;27:122–3.
25. Payne JF, Bergstrom C, Yan J, Aaberg TM, Srivastava SK. Residual triamcinolone acetonide sequestered in the fovea after macular hole repair. Retina. 2011;31:148–53.
26. Zacharias LC, Lin T, Migon R, Ghosn C, Orilla W, Feldmann B, Ruiz G, Li Y, Burke J, Kuppermann BD. Assessment of the differences in pharmacokinetics and pharmacodynamics pharmacodynamics between four distinct formulations of triamcinolone acetonide. Retina. 2013;33:522–31.
27. Rodrigues EB, Meyer CH. Meta-analysis of chromovitrectomy with indocyanine green in macular hole surgery. Ophthalmologica. 2008;222:123–9.
28. Li SS, Li M, You R, Wang HH, Zhao L, Wang YL, Chen X. Efficacy of different doses of dye-assisted internal limiting membrane peeling in idiopathic macular hole: a systematic review and network meta-analysis. Int Ophthalmol. 2021;41:1129–40.
29. Wakabayashi T, Shiraki N, Tsuboi K, Oshima Y, Abe K, Yamamoto Y, Hisashi F, Baba K, Ishida Y, Otsuka Y, Shiraki A, Suzue M, Hashimoto R, Venkatesh R, Chhablani J, Gomi F, Kamei M, Maeno T, Regillo CD, Yonekawa Y, Ikuno Y, SCHISIS Study Group. Risk factors and outcomes of postoperative macular hole formation after vitrectomy for myopic traction maculopathy: SCHISIS report no. 2. Ophthalmol Retina. 2023;7:779–87.
30. Rodrigues EB, Meyer CH, Farah ME, et al. Intravitreal staining of the internal limiting membrane using indocyanine green in the treatment of macular holes. Ophthalmologica. 2005;219:251–62.
31. Veritti D, Toneatto G, Lanzetta P. Low-concentration infracyanine green-assisted internal limiting membrane peeling in idiopathic macular pucker 25-gauge surgery. Eur J Ophthalmol. 2012;22:626–34.

32. Lanzetta P, Polito A, Del Borrello M, Narayanan R, Shah VA, Frattolillo A, Bandello F. Idiopathic macular hole surgery with low-concentration infracyanine green-assisted peeling of the internal limiting membrane. Am J Ophthalmol. 2006;142:771–6.
33. Balayre S, Boissonnot M, Paquereau J, Dighiero P. Evaluation of trypan blue toxicity in idiopathic epiretinal membrane surgery with macular function test using multifocal electroretinography: seven prospective case studies. J Fr Ophtalmol. 2005;28:169–76.
34. Haritoglou C, Eibl K, Schaumberger M, Mueller AJ, Priglinger S, Alge C, Kampik A. Functional outcome after trypan blue assisted vitrectomy for macular pucker: a prospective, randomized, comparative trial. Am J Ophthalmol. 2004;138:1–5.
35. Haritoglou C, Gandorfer A, Schaumberger M, Priglinger SG, Mueller AJ, Gass CA, Kampik A. Trypan blue in macular pucker surgery: an evaluation of histology and functional outcome. Retina. 2004;24:582–90.
36. Li K, Wong D, Hiscott P, Groenewald C, McGalliard J. Trypan blue staining of internal limiting membrane and epiretinal membrane during vitrectomy: visual results and histopathological findings. Br J Ophthalmol. 2003;87:216–9.
37. Beutel J, Dahmen G, Ziegler A, Hoerauf H. Internal limiting membrane peeling with indocyanine green or trypan blue in macular hole surgery: a randomized trial. Arch Ophthalmol. 2007;125:326–32.
38. Lee KL, Dean S, Guest S. A comparison of outcomes after indocyanine green and trypan blue assisted internal limiting membrane peeling during macular hole surgery. Br J Ophthalmol. 2005;89:420–4.
39. Kwok AK, Lai TYY, Li WWY, Yew DTW, Wong VWY. Trypan blue- and indocyanine green-assisted epiretinal membrane surgery: clinical and histopathological studies. Eye. 2004;18:882–8.
40. Azuma K, Noda Y, Hirasawa K, Ueta T. Brilliant blue G-assisted internal limiting membrane peeling for macular hole: a systematic review of literature and meta-analysis. Retina. 2016;36:851–8.
41. Li SS, You R, Li M, Guo XX, Zhao L, Wang YL, Chen X. Internal limiting membrane peeling with different dyes in the surgery of idiopathic macular hole: a systematic review of literature and network Meta-analysis. Int J Ophthalmol. 2019;12:1917–28.
42. Cervera E, Diaz-Llopis M, Salom D, Udaondo P, Amselem L. Internal limiting membrane staining using intravitreal brilliant blue G: good help for vitreo-retinal surgeon in training. Arch Soc Esp Oftalmol. 2007;82:71–2.
43. Enaida H, Hisatomi T, Hata Y, Ueno A, Goto Y, Yamada T, Kubota T, Ishibashi T. Brilliant blue G selectively stains the internal limiting membrane/brilliant blue G-assisted membrane peeling. Retina. 2006;26:631–6.
44. Machida S, Toba Y, Nishimura T, Ohzeki T, Murai K, Kurosaka D. Comparisons of cone electroretinograms after indocyanine green-, brilliant blue G-, or triamcinolone acetonide-assisted macular hole surgery. Graefes Arch Clin Exp Ophthalmol. 2014;252:1423–33.
45. Mochizuki N, Yamamoto T, Enaida H, Ishibashi T, Yamashita H. Long-term outcomes of 3 surgical adjuvants used for internal limiting membrane peeling in idiopathic macular hole surgery. Jpn J Ophthalmol. 2014;58:455–61.
46. Martins D, Neves P. Epiretinal membrane negative staining and double peeling in a single block with brilliant blue G. Eur J Ophthalmol. 2018;28:112–6.
47. Badaro E, Furlani B, Prazeres J, Maia M, Alves Souza Lima A, Souza-Martins D, Muccioli C, Adami Lucatto LF, Belfort R Jr. Soluble lutein in combination with brilliant blue as a new dye for chromovitrectomy. Graefes Arch Clin Exp Ophthalmol. 2014;252:1071–8.
48. Maia M, Furlani BA, Souza-Lima AA, Martins DS, Navarro RM, Belfort R Jr. Lutein: a new dye for chromovitrectomy. Retina. 2014;34:262–72.
49. Romano MR, Ilardi G, Ferrara M, Cennamo G, Parolini B, Mariotti C, Staibano S, Cennamo G. Macular peeling-induced retinal damage: clinical and histopathological evaluation after using different dyes. Graefes Arch Clin Exp Ophthalmol. 2018;256:1573–80.
50. Röhrig S, Farecki ML, Boden KT, Haus A, Gutfleisch M, Jung S, Lommatzsch A, Szurman P, Januschowski K. Negative effects of vital dyes after uneventful vitreomacular surgery. Retina. 2019;39:1772–8.

51. Soiberman U, Shai D, Loewenstein A, Barak A. Macular hole surgery with internal limiting membrane peeling facilitated by Membrane-Blue® versus Membrane-Blue-Dual®: a retrospective comparative study. J Ophthalmol. 2016;2016:1292735.
52. Tognetto D, De Giacinto C, D'Aloisio R, Papagno C, Pastore M, Zweyer M. The combination of Trypan Blue and Brilliant Blue G-assisted vitrectomy for macular pucker: histopathological findings. Ophthalmologica. 2018;239:167–75.
53. Veckeneer M, Mohr A, Alharthi E, Azad R, Bashshur ZF, Bertelli E, Bejjani RA, Bouassida B, Bourla D, Crespo IC, Fahed C, Fayyad F, Mura M, Nawrocki J, Rivett K, Scharioth GB, Shkvorchenko DO, Szurman P, Van Wijck H, Wong IY, Wong DS, Frank J, Oellerich S, Bruinsma M, Melles GR. Novel 'heavy' dyes for retinal membrane staining during macular surgery: multicenter clinical assessment. Acta Ophthalmol. 2014;92:339–44.
54. Iuliano L, Kacerik E, Corbelli E, Bandello F, Codenotti M. Intraoperative efficacy and clinical outcomes of two commercial staining solutions used in idiopathic epiretinal membrane surgery. Int Ophthalmol. 2021;41:1033–41.
55. Romano MR, Gatto C, Giurgola L, Ragazzi E, D'Amato TJ. Toxicity threshold of perfluorocarbon liquids for intraocular use: dose-response assessment of in vitro cytotoxicity of possible contaminants. Transl Vis Sci Technol. 2021;10:24.
56. International Organization for Standardization. ISO 10993-5:2009. Biological evaluation of medical devices—part 5: tests for in vitro cytotoxicity. https://www.iso.org/standard/36406.html
57. Gatto C, Romano MR, Giurgola L, Ferrara M, Ragazzi E, D'Amato TJ. Ex vivo evaluation of retinal cytotoxicity after the use of multiple medical devices in pars Plana vitrectomy in porcine eyes. Exp Eye Res. 2021;213:108837.
58. Spitzer MS, Mlynczak T, Schultheiss M, Rinker K, Yoeruek E, Petermeier K, Januschowski K, Szurman P. Preservative-free triamcinolone acetonide injectable suspension versus "traditional" triamcinolone preparations: impact of aggregate size on retinal biocompatibility. Retina. 2011;31:2050–7.
59. Yeung CK, Chan KP, Chiang SWY, Pang CP, Lam DSC. The toxic and stress responses of cultured human retinal pigment epithelium (ARPE19) and human glial cells (SVG) in the presence of triamcinolone. Invest Ophthalmol Vis Sci. 2003;44:5293–300.
60. Yeung CK, Chan KP, Chan CKM, Pang CP, Lam DSC. Cytotoxicity of triamcinolone on cultured human retinal pigment epithelial cells: comparison with dexamethasone and hydrocortisone. Jpn J Ophthalmol. 2004;48:236–42.
61. Szurman P, Kaczmarek R, Spitzer MS, Jaissle GB, Decker P, Grisanti S, Henke-Fahle S, Aisenbrey S, Bartz-Schmidt KU. Differential toxic effect of dissolved triamcinolone and its crystalline deposits on cultured human retinal pigment epithelium (ARPE19) cells. Exp Eye Res. 2006;83:584–92.
62. Chang YS, Wu CL, Tseng SH, Kuo PY, Tseng SY. In vitro benzyl alcohol cytotoxicity: implications for intravitreal use of triamcinolone acetonide. Exp Eye Res. 2008;86:942–50.
63. Chang YS, Lin CF, Wu CL, Kuo PY, Wu FS, Shieh CC, Gean PW, Chen ST, Chen MS, Wu WC, Tai MH, Tseng SH. Mechanisms underlying benzyl alcohol cytotoxicity (triamcinolone acetonide preservative) in human retinal pigment epithelial cells. Invest Ophthalmol Vis Sci. 2011;52:4214–22.
64. Shaikh S, Ho S, Engelmann LA, Klemann SW. Cell viability effects of triamcinolone acetonide and preservative vehicle formulations. Br J Ophthalmol. 2006;90:233–6.
65. Li Y, Chen H, Hou J, Zhang Y, Li G, Gu X, Luo L, Shen H, Qu J, Cheng L. Further characterization of ocular safety profile of commercially available preserved and preservative-free triamcinolone acetonide. Retina. 2012;32:364–74.
66. Moshfeghi AA, Nugent AK, Nomoto H, Sanislo SR, Kitchens JW, Moshfeghi DM. Triamcinolone acetonide preparations: impact of crystal size on in vitro behavior. Retina. 2009;29:689–98.
67. Kodjikian L, Richter T, Halberstadt M, Beby F, Flueckiger F, Boehnke M, Garweg JG. Toxic effects of indocyanine green, infracyanine green, and trypan blue on the human retinal pigmented epithelium. Graefes Arch Clin Exp Ophthalmol. 2005;243:917–25.

68. Iriyama A, Uchida S, Yanagi Y, Tamaki Y, Inoue Y, Matsuura K, Kadonosono K, Araie M. Effects of indocyanine green on retinal ganglion cells. Invest Ophthalmol Vis Sci. 2004;45:943–7.
69. Matsui H, Karasawa Y, Sato T, Kanno S, Nishikawa S, Okisaka S. Toxicity of indocyanine green dye on Muller cells. Nippon Ganka Gakkai Zasshi. 2007;111:587–93.
70. Enaida H, Sakamoto T, Hisatomi T, Goto Y, Ishibashi T. Morphological and functional damage of the retina caused by intravitreous indocyanine green in rat eyes. Graefes Arch Clin Exp Ophthalmol. 2002;240:209–13.
71. Goldstein M, Zemel E, Loewenstein A, Perlman I. Retinal toxicity of indocyanine green in albino rabbits. Invest Ophthalmol Vis Sci. 2006;47:2100–7.
72. Maia M, Kellner L, de Juan E Jr, Smith R, Farah ME, Margalit E, Lakhanpal RR, Grebe L, Eong KGA, Humayun MS. Effects of indocyanine green injection on the retinal surface and into the subretinal space in rabbits. Retina. 2004;24:80–91.
73. Maia M, Margalit E, Lakhanpal R, Tso MO, Grebe R, Torres G, Au Eong KG, Farah ME, Fujii GY, Weiland J, de Juan E Jr, D'Anna SA, Humayun MS. Effects of intravitreal indocyanine green injection in rabbits. Retina. 2004;24:69–79.
74. Kwok AK, Lai TY, Yeung CK, Yeung YS, Li WW, Chiang SW. The effects of indocyanine green and endoillumination on rabbit retina: an electroretinographic and histological study. Br J Ophthalmol. 2005;89:897–900.
75. Rodrigues EB, Meyer CH, Mennel S, Farah ME. Mechanisms of intravitreal toxicity of indocyanine green dye: implications for chromovitrectomy. Retina. 2007;27:958–70.
76. Penha FM, Pons M, Costa EF, Rodrigues EB, Maia M, Marin-Castaño ME, Farah ME, International Chromovitrectomy Collaboration. Effect of vital dyes on retinal pigmented epithelial cell viability and apoptosis: implications for chromovitrectomy. Ophthalmologica 2013;230:41–50
77. Penha FM, Pons M, Costa EF, Barros NM, Rodrigues EB, Cardoso EB, Dib E, Maia M, Marin-Castaño ME, Farah ME. Retinal pigmented epithelial cells cytotoxicity and apoptosis through activation of the mitochondrial intrinsic pathway: role of indocyanine green, brilliant blue and implications for chromovitrectomy. PLoS ONE 2013;10(8):e64094
78. Haritoglou C, Freyer W, Priglinger SG, Kampik A. Light absorbing properties of indocyanine green (ICG) in solution and after adsorption to the retinal surface: an ex-vivo approach. Graefes Arch Clin Exp Ophthalmol. 2006;244:1196–202.
79. Haritoglou C, Priglinger S, Gandorfer A, Welge-Lussen U, Kampik A. Histology of the vitreoretinal interface after indocyanine green staining of the ILM, with illumination using a halogen and xenon light source. Invest Ophthalmol Vis Sci. 2005;46:1468–72.
80. Gandorfer A, Haritoglou C, Gandorfer A, Kampik A. Retinal damage from indocyanine green in experimental macular surgery. Invest Ophthalmol Vis Sci. 2003;44:316–23.
81. Ho JD, Tsai RJ, Chen SN, Chen HC. Removal of sodium from the solvent reduces retinal pigment epithelium toxicity caused by indocyanine green: implications for macular hole surgery. Br J Ophthalmol. 2004;88:556–9.
82. Marmor MF. Retinal detachment from hyperosmotic intravitreal injection. Invest Ophthalmol Vis Sci. 1979;18:1237–44.
83. Stalmans P, Van Aken EH, Veckeneer M, Feron EJ, Stalmans I. Toxic effect of indocyanine green on retinal pigment epithelium related to osmotic effects of the solvent. Am J Ophthalmol. 2002;134:282–5.
84. Haritoglou C, Gandorfer A, Gass CA, Schaumberger M, Ulbig MW, Kampik A. The effect of indocyanine-green on functional outcome of macular pucker surgery. Am J Ophthalmol. 2003;135:328–37.
85. Engel E, Schraml R, Maisch T, Kobuch K, König B, Szeimies RM, Hillenkamp J, Bäumler W, Vasold R. Light-induced decomposition of indocyanine green. Invest Ophthalmol Vis Sci. 2008;49:1777–83.
86. Wollensak G. Biomechanical changes of the internal limiting membrane after indocyanine green staining. Dev Ophthalmol. 2008;42:82–90.

87. Sousa-Martins D, Caseli L, Figueiredo MC, Sa E, Cunha C, Mota-Filipe H, Souza-Lima A, Belfort R Jr, Rodrigues E, Maia M. Comparing the mode of action of intraocular lutein-based dyes with synthetic dyes. Invest Ophthalmol Vis Sci. 2015;19:1993–2000.
88. Jin Y, Uchida S, Yanagi Y, Aihara M, Araie M. Neurotoxic effects of trypan blue on rat retinal ganglion cells. Exp Eye Res. 2005;81:395–400.
89. Awad D, Schrader I, Bartok M, Mohr A, Gabel D. Comparative toxicology of trypan blue, brilliant blue G, and their combination together with polyethylene glycol on human pigment epithelial cells. Invest Ophthalmol Vis Sci. 2011;52:4085–90.
90. Lüke M, Grisanti S, Lüke J, International Chromovitrectomy Collaboration. The retinal biocompatibility of dyes in the ex vivo model of the isolated superfused vertebrate retina. Ophthalmologica. 2013;230(Suppl 2):21–6.
91. Grisanti S, Szurman P, Tatar O, Gelisken F, Aisenbrey S, Oficjalska-Mlynczak J, Kaczmarek R, Bartz-Schmidt KU. Histopathological analysis in experimental macular surgery with trypan blue. Br J Ophthalmol. 2004;88:1206–8.
92. Veckeneer M, van Overdam K, Monzer J, Kobuch K, van Marle W, Spekreijse H, van Meurs J. Ocular toxicity study of trypan blue injected into the vitreous cavity of rabbit eyes. Graefes Arch Clin Exp Ophthalmol. 2001;239:698–704.
93. Penha FM, Maia M, Farah ME, Príncipe AH, Freymüller EH, Maia A, Magalhães O Jr, Smith RL. Effects of subretinal injections of indocyanine green, trypan blue, and glucose in rabbit eyes. Ophthalmology. 2007;114:899–908.
94. Balaiya S, Brar VS, Murthy RK, Chalam KV. Comparative in vitro safety analysis of dyes for chromovitrectomy: indocyanine green, brilliant blue green, bromophenol blue, and infracyanine green. Retina. 2011;31:1128–36.
95. Gerding H. A short review on the safety of bromphenol blue for dye-assisted vitreoretinal interventions. Klin Monbl Augenheilkd. 2020;237:441–5.
96. Awad D, Wilińska J, Gousia D, Shi X, Eddous J, Müller A, Wagner V, Hillner C, Brannath W, Mohr A, Gabel D. Toxicity and phototoxicity in human ARPE-19 retinal pigment epithelium cells of dyes commonly used in retinal surgery. Eur J Ophthalmol. 2018;28:433–40.
97. Morales MC, Freire V, Asumendi A, Araiz J, Herrera I, Castiella G, Corcóstegui I, Corcóstegui G. Comparative effects of six intraocular vital dyes on retinal pigment epithelial cells. Invest Ophthalmol Vis Sci. 2010;51:6018–29.
98. Creuzot-Garcher C, Acar N, Passemard M, Bidot S, Bron A, Bretillon L. Functional and structural effect of intravitreal indocyanine green, triamcinolone acetonide, trypan blue, and brilliant blue g on rat retina. Retina. 2010;30:1294–301.
99. Yuen D, Gonder J, Proulx A, Liu H, Hutnik C. Comparison of the in vitro safety of intraocular dyes using two retinal cell lines: a focus on brilliant blue G and indocyanine green. Am J Ophthalmol. 2009;147:251–9.
100. Notomi S, Hisatomi T, Kanemaru T, Takeda A, Ikeda Y, Enaida H, Kroemer G, Ishibashi T. Critical involvement of extracellular ATP acting on P2RX7 purinergic receptors in photoreceptor cell death. Am J Pathol. 2011;179:2798–809.
101. Enaida H, Hisatomi T, Goto Y, Hata Y, Ueno A, Miura M, Kubota T, Ishibashi T. Preclinical investigation of internal limiting membrane staining and peeling using intravitreal brilliant blue G. Retina. 2006;26:623–30.
102. Sheu S-J, Chen J-L, Bee Y-S, Chen Y-A, Lin S-H, Shu C-W. Differential autophagic effects of vital dyes in retinal pigment epithelial ARPE-19 and photoreceptor 661W cells. PLoS ONE. 2017;12:e0174736.
103. Furlani BA, Barroso L, Sousa-Martins D, Maia M, Moraes-Filho MN, Badaro E, Portella R, Lima-Filho AA, Rodrigues EB, Belfort R Jr. Lutein and zeaxanthin toxicity with and without brilliant blue in rabbits. J Ocul Pharmacol Ther. 2014;30:559–66.
104. Januschowski K, Sebastian M, Spitzer MS, Hoffmann J, Schramm C, Schultheiss M, Bartz-Schmidt K, Szurman P. Investigating the biocompatibility of two new heavy intraocular dyes for vitreoretinal surgery with an isolated perfused vertebrate retina organ culture model and a retinal ganglion cell line. Graefes Arch Clin Exp Ophthalmol. 2012;250:533–45.

105. Lueke C, Lueke M, Dietlein TS, Hueber A, Jordan J, Sickel W, Kirchof B. Retinal tolerance to dyes. Br J Ophthalmol. 2005;89:1188–91.
106. Grossini E, Venkatesan S, Alkabes M, Toma C, de Cillà S. Membrane blue dual protects retinal pigment epithelium cells/ganglion cells-like through modulation of mitochondria function. Biomedicines. 2022;10:2854.
107. Kampougeris G, Cheema R, McPherson R, Gorman C. Safety of triamcinolone acetonide (TA)-assisted pars plana vitrectomy in macular hole surgery. Eye. 2007;21:591–4.
108. Koto T, Inoue M, Shinoda K, Ishida S, Tsubota K. Residual crystals of triamcinolone acetonide in macular hole may prevent complete closure. Acta Ophthalmol Scand. 2007;85:913–4.
109. Maia M, Farah ME, Belfort RN, Penha FM, Lima Filho AA, Aggio FB, Belfort R Jr. Effects of intravitreal triamcinolone acetonide injection with and without preservative. Br J Ophthalmol. 2007;91:1122–4.
110. Roth DB, Chieh J, Spirn MJ, Green SN, Yarian DL, Chaudhry NA. Noninfectious endophthalmitis associated with intravitreal triamcinolone injection. Arch Ophthalmol. 2003;121:1279–82.
111. Tadayoni R, Paques M, Girmens JF, Massin P, Gaudric A. Persistence of fundus fluorescence after use of indocyanine green for macular surgery. Ophthalmology. 2003;110:604–8.
112. Mavrofrides E, Smiddy WE, Kitchens JW, Salicone A, Feuer W. Indocyanine green–assisted internal limiting membrane peeling for macular holes: toxicity? Retina. 2006;26:637–44.
113. Hirata A, Inomata Y, Kawaji T, Tanihara H. Persistent subretinal indocyanine green induces retinal pigment epithelium atrophy. Am J Ophthalmol. 2003;136:353–5.
114. Uemoto R, Yamamoto S, Takeuchi S. Changes in retinal pigment epithelium after indocyanine green-assisted internal limiting lamina peeling during macular hole surgery. Am J Ophthalmol. 2005;140:752–5.
115. Maia M, Haller JA, Pieramici DJ, Margalit E, de Juan E Jr, Farah ME, Lakhanpal RR, Eong K-GA, Guven D, Humayun MS. Retinal pigment epithelial abnormalities after internal limiting membrane peeling guided by indocyanine green staining. Retina. 2004;24:157–60
116. Spaide RF. Persistent intraocular indocyanine green staining after macular hole surgery. Retina. 2002;22:637–9.
117. Weinberger AW, Kirchhof B, Mazinani BE, Schrage NF. Persistent indocyanine green (ICG) fluorescence 6 weeks after intraocular ICG administration for macular hole surgery. Graefes Arch Clin Exp Ophthalmol. 2001;239:388–90.
118. Saeed MU, Heimann H. Atrophy of the retinal pigment epithelium following vitrectomy with trypan blue. Int Ophthalmol. 2009;29:239–41.
119. Malerbi FK, Maia M, Farah ME, Rodrigues EB. Subretinal brilliant blue G migration during internal limiting membrane peeling. Br J Ophthalmol. 2009;93:1687.
120. Jain S, Kishore K, Sharma YR. Progressive atrophy of retinal pigment epithelium after trypan-blue-assisted ILM peeling for macular hole surgery. Indian J Ophthalmol. 2013;61:235–7.
121. Savary P, Kodjikian L. Intraretinal brilliant blue G infiltration during internal limiting membrane peeling. Graefes Arch Clin Exp Ophthalmol. 2014;252:1017–9.
122. Jindal A, Pathengay A, Mithal K, Chhablani J, Pappuru RR, Flynn HW. Macular toxicity following brilliant blue G-assisted macular hole surgery—a report of three cases. Nepal J Ophthalmol. 2014;6:98–101.
123. Almeida FPP, De Lucca AC, Scott IU, Jorge R, Messias A. Accidental subretinal brilliant blue G migration during internal limiting membrane peeling surgery. JAMA Ophthalmol. 2015;133:85–8.
124. Singh SR, Chhablani J. Geographic atrophy with choroidal thinning following brilliant blue staining. BMJ Case Rep. 2019;12:e230242.
125. Venkatesh R, Aseem A, Jain K, Yadav NK. Combined brilliant blue G and xenon light induced outer retinal layer damage following macular hole surgery. Indian J Ophthalmol. 2020;68:247–9.
126. Soni A, Parameswarappa DC, Tyagi M, Sahoo NK, Dogra A, Pappuru RR, Chhablani J. Brilliant Blue G toxicity in macular hole surgeries: a report on combined phototoxicity and dye-induced macular damage. Semin Ophthalmol. 2022;37:117–22.

127. Federico O, Anniken BJ, Carlos M. Diffuse retinal pigment epithelium atrophy following pars plana vitrectomy for high myopic macular hole assisted by brilliant blue G: a case report. Am J Ophthalmol Case Rep. 2021;23:101148.
128. Rivera-Valdivia N, Maeda-Yasunaga H, Cabal-López P, Salgado-Cerrate C, Abdala-Caballero C. Retinal pigment epithelium atrophy after epiretinal membrane and internal limiting membrane peeling: case reports. Rom J Ophthalmol. 2022;66:79–83.
129. Torres-Villaros H, Louis-Philippe S, Amari F, Giocanti-Aurégan A, Janicot L. Macular toxicity of vital dye after pars plana vitrectomy for idiopathic epiretinal membrane: a case report. Am J Ophthalmol Case Rep. 2022;27:101588.
130. Venkatesh R, Mangla R, Sharief S, Chhablani J. Long-term effects of combined brilliant blue G and xenon light induced retinal toxicity following macular hole repair surgery. BMC Ophthalmol. 2023;23:57.
131. Czajka MP, McCuen BW 2nd, Cummings TJ, Nguyen H, Stinnett S, Wong F. Effects of indocyanine green on the retina and retinal pigment epithelium in a porcine model of retinal hole. Retina. 2004;24:275–82.
132. Fominykh OD, Balakina MY, Burganov TI, Katsyuba SA. The effect of stacking arrangement on the conjugation in azochromophores revealed by combination of Raman spectroscopy and DFT calculations. Chem Phys Lett. 2016;659:242–6.
133. Chalam KV, Li W, Koushan K. Effect of distance and duration of illumination on retinal ganglion cells exposed to varying concentrations of brilliant blue green. J Clin Med Res. 2015;7:517–24.
134. Al-Halafi AM. Chromovitrectomy: update. Saudi J Ophthalmol. 2013;27:271–6.
135. Costa EF, Rodrigues EB, Farah ME, Dib E, Penha F, Magalhães O Jr, Furlani BA, Filho AASL, de Miranda A, Maia M. Vital dyes and light sources for chromovitrectomy: comparative assessment of osmolarity, pH, and spectrophotometry. Invest Ophthalmol Vis Sci. 2009;50:385–91.
136. Yanagi Y, Inoue Y, Jang WD, Kadonosono K. A2e mediated phototoxic effects of enlluminators. Br J Ophthalmol. 2006;90:229–32.

Use of Intraoperative Optical Coherence Tomography in Retinal Surgery

S. Tammy Hsu, Vahid Ownagh, and Lejla Vajzovic

Abstract Optical coherence tomography (OCT) has revolutionized the field of ophthalmology, providing noninvasive, high-resolution imaging of the retinal layers. In recent years, use of OCT in the operating room, or intraoperative OCT (iOCT), has emerged as a valuable tool in retinal surgery, enabling real-time visualization and guidance during surgical procedures. This chapter explores the principles, applications, and benefits of iOCT in various retinal surgeries. Different cases are used as examples to discuss the impact of iOCT on intraoperative visualization and surgical decision-making. Additionally, the chapter addresses the current challenges and future directions for the integration of iOCT into routine retinal surgical practice.

Keywords Optical coherence tomography · Intraoperative OCT · Retina · Vitreoretinal surgery · Ophthalmic imaging

1 Introduction

Retinal surgery involves a range of procedures aimed at addressing various retinal pathologies, including vitreoretinal interface disorders, retinal detachments, macular diseases, and optic disc abnormalities. These surgeries require meticulous planning, precise execution, and real-time assessment to achieve optimal outcomes. Technological advancements such as optical coherence tomography (OCT) has allowed for improved methods of visualizing the retina by providing high-resolution cross-sectional imaging of the retina. Intraoperative OCT (iOCT) involves the integration of OCT technology into the operating room, allowing surgeons to obtain real-time,

S. T. Hsu · V. Ownagh · L. Vajzovic (✉)
Department of Ophthalmology, Duke Eye Center, Durham, NC 27705, USA
e-mail: Lejla.vajzovic@duke.edu

S. T. Hsu
e-mail: s.tammyhsu@duke.edu

V. Ownagh
e-mail: vahid.ownagh@duke.edu

F. Patelli et al. (eds.), *Macular Surgery*, https://doi.org/10.1007/978-3-031-63508-3_4

high-resolution images during surgery. By providing intraoperative imaging guidance, iOCT has the potential to enhance surgical precision, decision-making, and overall outcomes in retinal surgery.

2 Optical Coherence Tomography Basics

OCT is a noninvasive imaging modality that produces detailed, cross-sectional images of biological tissue micron-level structures. It uses low-coherence interferometry, in which a beam of near-infrared light is emitted and split into two arms that recombine to generate an image: the sample arm is emitted onto the tissue of interest and the reference arm is directed towards a mirror. When the reference arm and the sample arm recombine, they create interference patterns that are detected by a photodetector. Tissue structures have different levels of reflectivity that create different interference patterns, which then can be used to generate a depth-resolved image. By scanning the light beam across the tissue and acquiring multiple A-scans, a two-dimensional image (B-scan) or a three-dimensional volume can be reconstructed, allowing for the visualization of tissue morphology and pathology in detail [1–3].

OCT has been used in a variety of medical specialties, including ophthalmology, dermatology, cardiology, and oncology [4–8]. Within ophthalmology, OCT is used across multiple subspecialities, including cornea, glaucoma, neuro-ophthalmology, and retina. This chapter focuses on the use of OCT in retinal surgery.

3 Adaptation for Intraoperative Use

OCT was first available in the clinic setting and often used for preoperative and postoperative assessment.

The adaptation of OCT technology for intraoperative use involved addressing several challenges, such as instrument design, sterilization requirements, and integration with surgical microscopes or heads-up displays. Several modifications were required to make OCT systems suitable for use in the operating room and during surgery.

Firstly, intraoperative procedures require real-time imaging feedback to guide surgical decision-making. Therefore, advancements were made to improve the speed and efficiency of OCT imaging systems. High-speed imaging technologies, such as spectral-domain OCT (SD-OCT) or swept-source OCT (SS-OCT), were developed to capture and process images rapidly, providing immediate visualization of tissue structures during the surgical procedure [2, 9–11].

Secondly, traditional OCT systems were bulky and needed to be optimized for the operating room setting. Efforts were made to develop compact, handheld probes or specialized surgical microscope-mounted OCT systems. These compact designs allowed for easy integration into the surgical workflow and improved maneuverability by the surgical team [2, 9, 12–14].

Lastly, an ergonomic and practical method to allow the surgeon to efficiently and seamlessly view the OCT images during surgery was necessary. In order to integrate OCT into the surgical workflow, compatibility with existing visualization systems, such as surgical microscopes or heads-up displays, was essential. Adapters or interfaces were developed to allow for the integration of OCT imaging with these existing visualization platforms, enabling surgeons to visualize OCT images alongside the surgical field without needing to pause the surgery or turn attention away from the operative site [2, 9, 15, 16].

Intraoperative OCT (iOCT) imaging was first introduced using early hand-held OCT (HH-OCT) devices (Fig. 1). Envisu (Leica microsystems) spectral domain HH-OCT was the first HH-OCT device to receive clearance from Food and Drug Administration [17]. A new generation of investigational swept source HH-OCT system developed at Duke University is capable of high speed 400 kHz 750 B-scan/volume imaging [18]. HH-OCT imaging generally requires pause in during the surgery, limiting its application in operating theater and it is incapable of imaging dynamic surgical maneuvers. These limitations led to development of microscope integrated OCT (MIOCT) imaging. Currently there are commercially available spectral domain MIOCT systems as well as an investigational swept source MIOCT (SS-MIOCT) prototype developed at Duke University [19]. The advantage of SS-MIOCT is increased depth of imaging to provide clear images of deeper structures including large subretinal blebs [14].

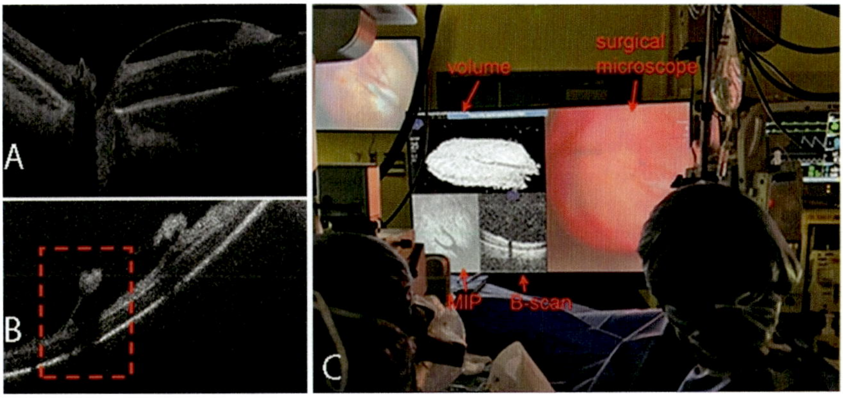

Fig. 1 iOCT evolution. HH-OCT is capable of static intraoperative imaging. Envisu HH-OCT displaying subhyaloid hemorrhage in a child with abusive head trauma (**A**). Duke investigational swept source HH-OCT is capable of peripheral OCT imaging, demonstrating vascular tufts in a baby with retinopathy of prematurity (red dashed line, **B**). Duke investigational SS-MIOCT integrated with heads up display, provides real time dynamic imaging of instrument-retina interactions (**C**)

4 Applications of Intraoperative Optical Coherence Tomography in Retinal Surgery

iOCT offers real-time visualization of surgical maneuvers and tissue changes, enhancing surgical precision and offering more information for surgical decision-making [7, 8]. The availability of real-time iOCT imaging during surgery enables surgeons to make informed decisions regarding tissue manipulation, tissue removal, and the need for additional procedures. This section describes cases in which iOCT was used to guide surgeries by improving visualization of critical structures and more accurate tissue manipulation.

5 Clinical Applications

Application of iOCT has shown promise in numerous vitreoretinal disorders such as macular hole[20], epiretinal membrane[21], vitreomacular traction [22], retinal detachments[23], optic pit maculopathy[24], subretinal drug delivery and gene therapy [25]. iOCT enables real time visualization of subtle retinal structural details such as partially peeled membranes to assist with intraoperative decision-making. iOCT has been shown to be valuable for intraoperative validation of vitreomacular traction release and identification of occult residual membranes [26, 27]. In DISCOVER study, data provided by iOCT altered surgical decision making in 12% of vitrectomy surgeries for macular hole repair [28].

In one of the largest prospective studies of iOCT feasibility and utility (PIONEER), intraoperative OCT altered surgeon understanding of underlying tissue configurations in 43% (63 from 146) of membrane peeling procedures. The most common reported impact of the intraoperative OCT was helping to assess completeness of the membrane peeling [29].

iOCT can provide information on anatomical dynamics of macular hole closure and provide insights to pathophysiology of macular interface disorders. Intraoperative structural study of macular holes using handheld OCT revealed shorter macular hole base diameter after fluid air exchange in comparison with after ILM peeling measurements [30]. Some structural characteristics provided by iOCT such as post-ILM peel expansion of ellipsoid zone-retinal pigment epithelium (EZ-RPE) or change in macular hole volume and width, have been shown to be useful predictors of closure speed after macular hole repair surgery [31].

Intraoperative OCT can also detect the residual tissue fragments at the edge of the MH and may be an indicator of hyperreflective inner tissue observed postoperatively in closed macular holes. The presence of these residual fragments is reported to be associated with limited postoperative recovery of visual acuity [32].

In vitreoretinal procedures requiring ILM peeling, utilizing iOCT may increase successful membrane peeling without re-staining with dye. In the study of 70 eyes by

Falkner et al., MIOCT allowed performing membrane peeling without using retinal dyes in 40% of cases.

Interestingly, iOCT contribution to macular hole surgery goes beyond intraoperative management. Lorusso et al. advocated shorter (12–24 h) instead of conventional (3–5 days) face down positioning after macular hole repair surgery if iOCT confirms closure of the hole at the end of surgery [33].

Although iOCT has been shown to provide better visualization and may alter surgical planning, there is very limited data on whether this may translate to better visual and anatomic outcomes for patients. iOCT-guided ERM removal provided comparable visual and anatomic results to conventional ILM peeling [34]. Future randomized prospective studies should address the role of iOCT in improving real world functional and structural outcomes.

6 Clinical Cases

Case 1: A 12-year-old patient presented with a history of optic nerve coloboma/pit and persistent serous retinal detachment in left eye. Despite previous pars plana vitrectomy and endolaser, she still had persistent serous retinal detachment with decreasing vision. The surgeon proceeded with ILM peeling, amniotic membrane graft and long acting gas tamponade. iOCT was used to delineate the communication site between perineural and subretinal/intraretinal spaces (Fig. 2A) and to confirm that amniotic membrane graft covered the area of optic pit (Fig. 2B).

Case 2: A 68-year-old patient was evaluated for vitreomacular traction and epiretinal membrane causing significant metamorphopsia. iOCT helped to intraoperative visualization of the epiretinal membrane and macular traction (Fig. 3A), as well as validating successful membrane peeling and release of macular traction (Fig. 3B). At the post-op month three visit, the patient's visual acuity improved from baseline 20/100 to 20/32.

Case 3: A 69-year-old patient with retinitis pigmentosa and degenerative myopia exhibited a lamellar macular hole and epiretinal membrane (ERM). The ERM with lamellar hole was evident on the iOCT volumetric images with demonstration of the interaction between surgical instruments such as the Flex loop and the retinal surface. iOCT showed successful peeling of the dense ERM (Fig. 4).

Case 4: A 74-year-old patient with history of neovascular AMD and multiple anti-VEGF injections presented with subretinal hemorrhage and exudative macular detachment (Fig. 5A). The patient underwent subretinal injection of tissue plasminogen activator (t-PA) with iOCT guidance.

In subretinal injections of t-PA, iOCT may play a crucial role by providing real time data on the exact location of drug delivery. Verification of subretinal rather than sub-RPE injection and visualizing subsequent propagation of the drug towards the fovea

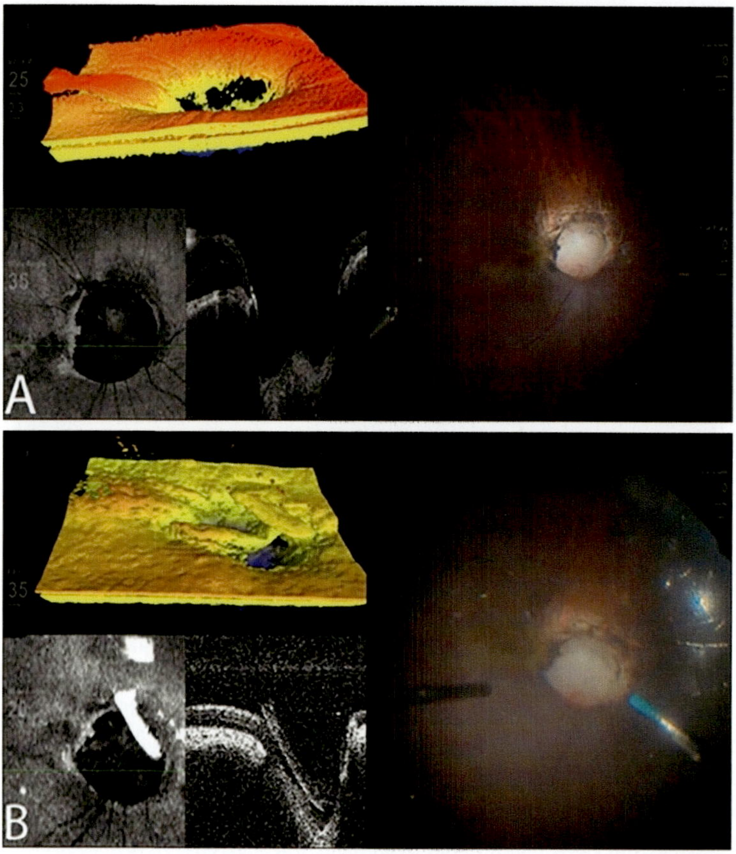

Fig. 2 iOCT demonstrated the suspected communication between perineural and subretinal spaces, and showed the exudative retinal detachment and retinoschisis cavities (**A**). A 4.0 mm amniotic membrane graft was introduced through a 23-gauge cannula and placed into the cup of the optic nerve in order to tamponade the temporal edge at the location of the suspected optic nerve pit. At the completion of the surgery, iOCT confirmed the appropriate position of amniotic membrane to provide adequate coverage of the optic pit and intercalary membrane (**B**)

is difficult to achieve without employing iOCT (Fig. 5B). Total amount of 0.14 mL of Alteplase was delivered subretinally. No iatrogenic macular hole was visualized on iOCT.

Case 5: A 76-year-old patient with neovascular AMD underwent subretinal injection of gene therapy vectors. iOCT was used to confirm successful subretinal delivery of the agent (Fig. 6). Care was taken to avoid the prior noted areas of chorioretinal scarring.

Case 6: A 77-year-old patient with macular hole of right eye was scheduled for a macular hole repair surgery. After ILM peeling, subretinal perifoveal injection of

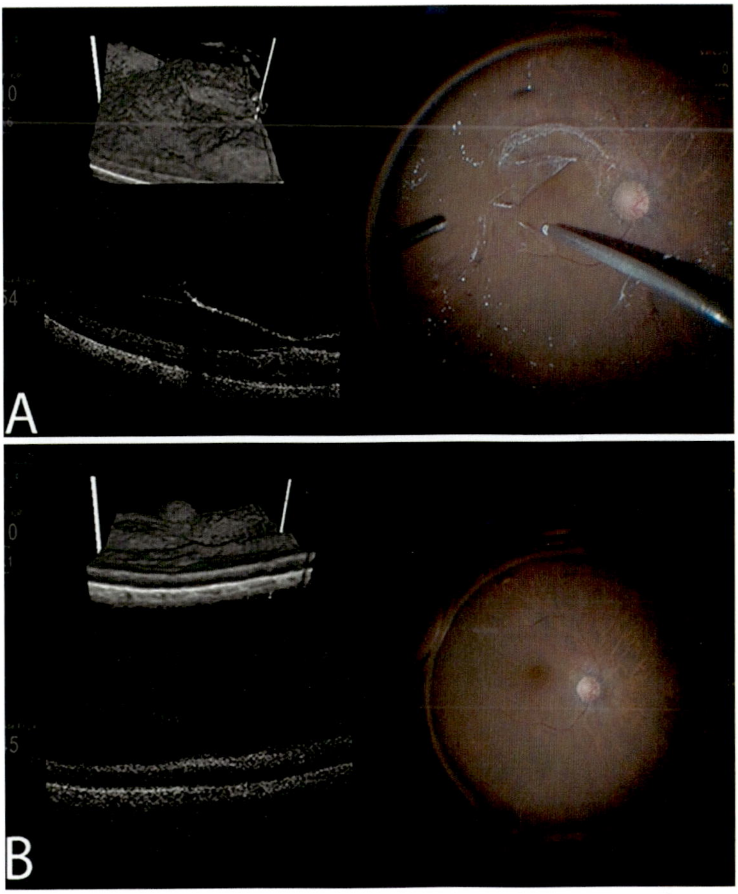

Fig. 3 SS-MIOCT system demonstrated vitreomacular traction, epiretinal membrane, and macular schisis (**A**). iOCT was used throughout the surgery to confirm adequate removal of the posterior hyaloid and epiretinal membrane without the creation of a macular hole (**B**)

fluid was performed to further mobilize the retina and promote macular hole closure (Fig. 7).

iOCT is an invaluable tool to validate safe perifoveal subretinal injection of fluid. Subretinal injections of BSS has been previously introduced for surgical repair of refractory large macular holes. Creating subretinal blebs may facilitate release of subretinal adhesions, mobilization of overlying retina and subsequent anatomic hole closure [35].

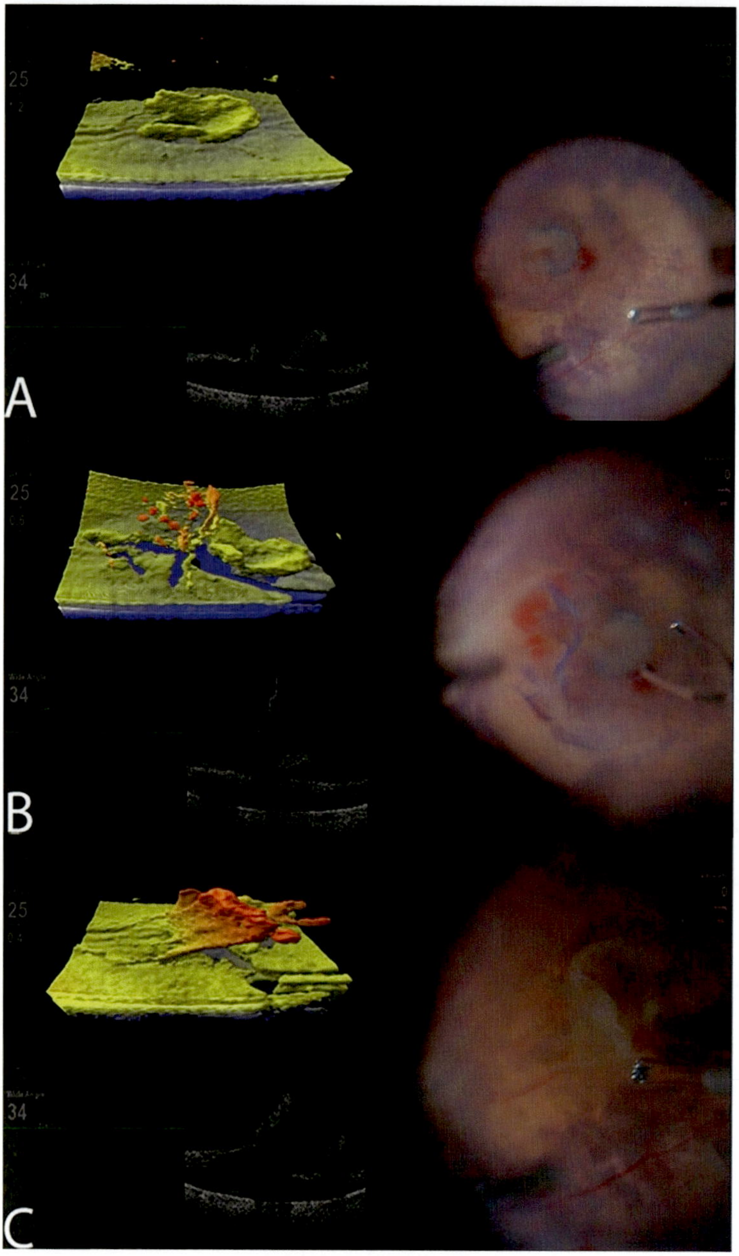

Fig. 4 Pars plana vitrectomy for dense ERM and lamellar macular hole. ILM and existing epiretinal membrane were peeled using an ILM forceps. After removing membranes, iOCT showed residual dense perifoveal epiretinal membrane (**A**). iOCT demonstrated partially peeled ILM (**B**). iOCT showed real time peeling of the ERM from retinal surface and creation of correct dissection plane (**C**)

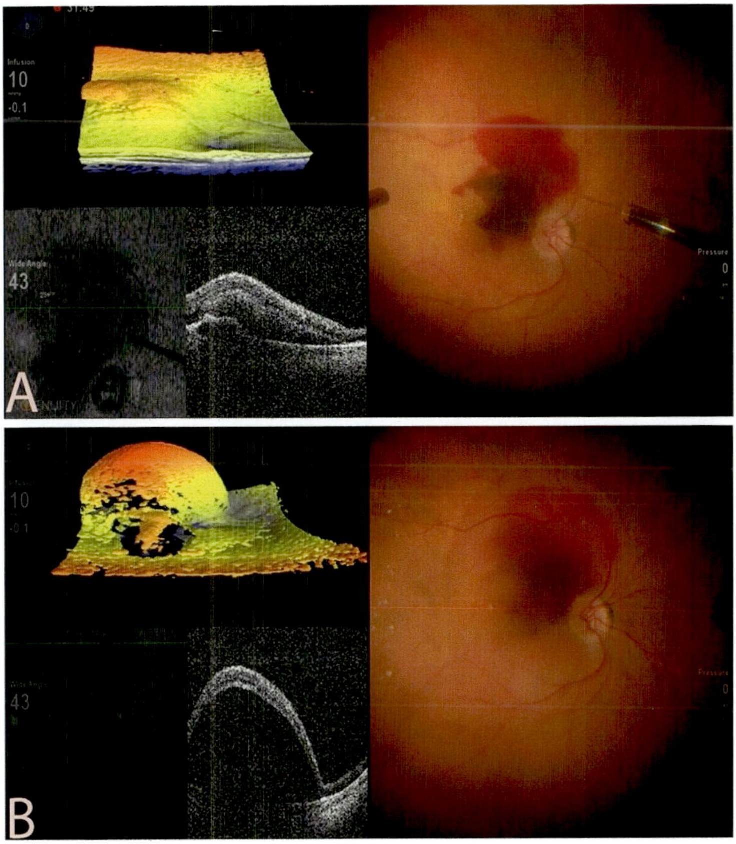

Fig. 5 A pars plana vitrectomy for subretinal injection of t-PA was performed for a subretinal hemorrhage. iOCT displayed subretinal hemorrhage superimposed on a previous hemorrhagic pigment epithelium detachment (**A**). Proper subretinal injection of alteplase and the formation of well distributed subretinal bleb were validated by iOCT (**B**)

7 Challenges

The integration of iOCT into the surgical workflow poses some challenges including set up, training, surgeon ergonomics, and cost.

As with all new technology, there is a learning curve associated with iOCT. The adoption of iOCT requires the operating room staff to develop proficiency in setting up the machine and assisting with acquiring iOCT images. Then, once the data has been acquired, the images need to be displayed to the surgeon as ergonomically as possible, such as through a microscope-integrated heads-up display viewing system or 3D heads-up Ngenuity visualization system [14, 16, 36–38]. Optimal display options are still being explored.

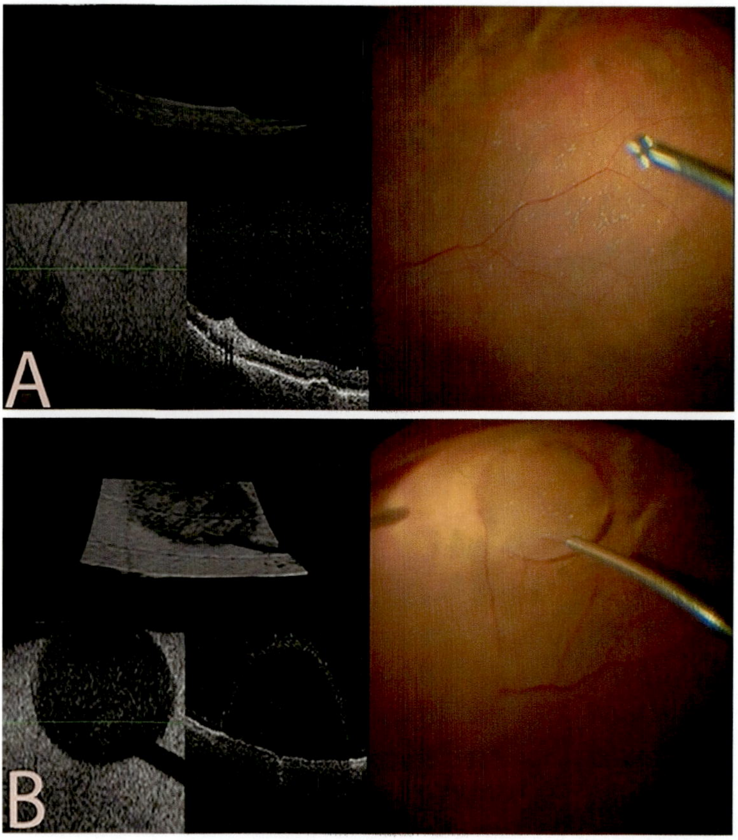

Fig. 6 A 23-gauge pars plana vitrectomy was performed to deliver gene therapy vectors in a patient with neovascular AMD. AMD associated retinal changes such as drusenoid pigment epithelium detachment were evident on iOCT (**A**). Successful subretinal delivery of the agent was confirmed by iOCT imaging (**B**)

Upon viewing the images, surgeons need to be able to interpret the iOCT images in real time while operating in order to guide surgical decision making. The surgeons need to be able to interpret artifacts as well as they still unfortunately exist on imaging.

Furthermore, the cost of iOCT systems can also be a significant barrier to widespread adoption. While the benefits of intraoperative OCT are appreciated, the reimbursement for the technology may not be enough to outweigh the costs.

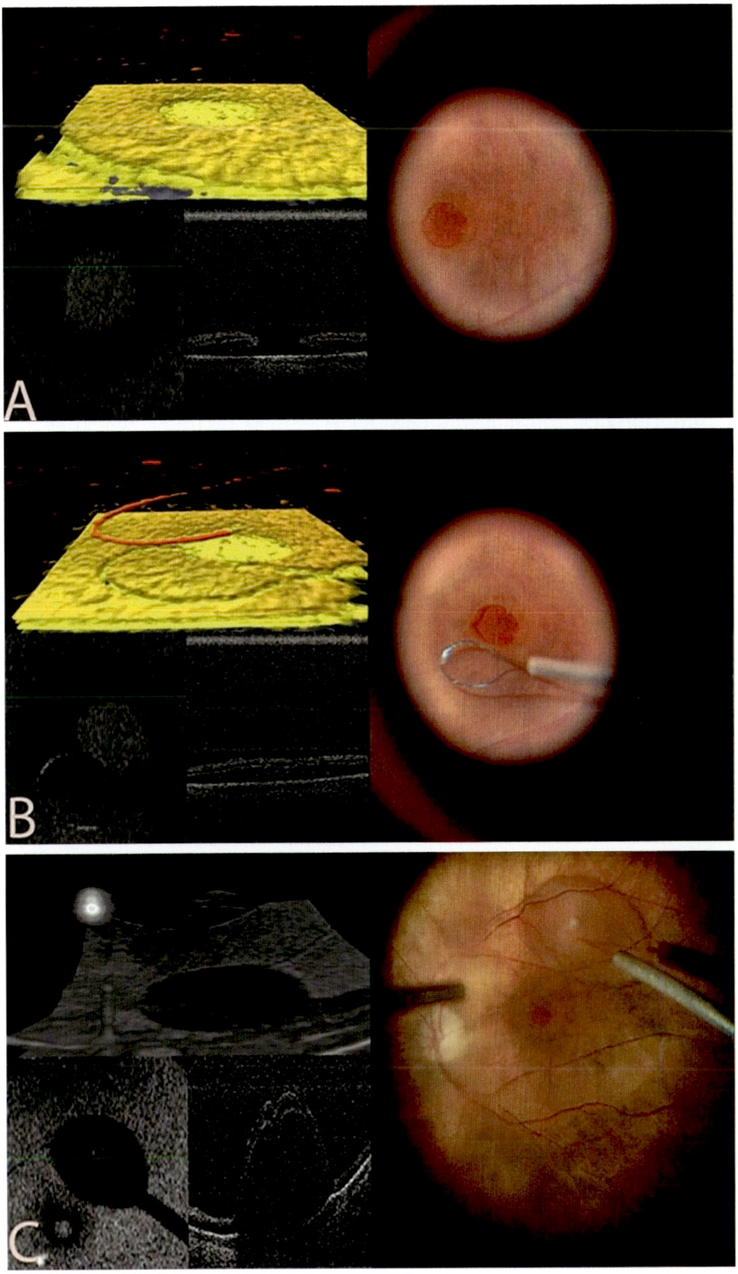

Fig. 7 A 25-gauge pars plana vitrectomy with subretinal BSS injection was carried out to repair a large macular hole. A full thickness macular hole was evident in volumetric and B-scan images of iOCT (**A**). A Flex loop was introduced to stretch and mobilize the retina surrounding the macular hole. iOCT illustrating tool-tissue interaction (**B**). iOCT was used to verify subretinal delivery of fluid for perifoveal retinal expansion (**C**)

8 Future Directions

Ongoing advancements in iOCT technology aim to further enhance image quality, speed, and ease of use to seamlessly integrate visualization with surgeon response and feedback. To improve image capture and visualization of surgical instruments and tissue planes, OCT-compatible instruments are being developed [37, 39, 40].

Applications of iOCT is beyond diagnostic intraoperative imaging and it is capable of potentially guiding intraocular robotic surgery. Chen et al. has applied a semi-automated OCT guided robotic surgery system to perform cataract surgery on porcine lenses [41]. Mach et al. have introduced a deep learning based OCT guided robotic needle for subretinal injections [42].

Research is also being conducted on using artificial intelligence and machine learning algorithms to automate image analysis and facilitate real-time decision support during iOCT-guided surgeries.

Clinical Pearls

- Intraoperative OCT can be used to guide retinal cases by improving visualization of tissue planes and providing information for real-time intraoperative surgical decision making
- The successful adoption of iOCT requires surgeons and operating room staff to develop proficiency in acquiring and interpreting iOCT images which can be subject to artifacts

References

1. Huang D, Swanson EA, Lin CP, et al. Optical coherence tomography. Science. 1991;254(5035):1178–81.
2. Carrasco-Zevallos OM, Viehland C, Keller B, et al. Review of intraoperative optical coherence tomography: technology and applications [Invited]. Biomed Opt Exp. 2017;8(3):1607–37. https://doi.org/10.1364/BOE.8.001607.
3. Saad A, Guilbert E, Grise-Dulac A, Sabatier P, Gatinel D. Intraoperative OCT-assisted DMEK: 14 consecutive cases. Cornea. 2015;34(7):802–7. https://doi.org/10.1097/ico.0000000000000462.
4. Bezerra HG, Costa MA, Guagliumi G, Rollins AM, Simon DI. Intracoronary optical coherence tomography: a comprehensive review. JACC Cardiovasc Interv. 2009;2(11):1035–46. https://doi.org/10.1016/j.jcin.2009.06.019.
5. Sattler E, Kästle R, Welzel J. Optical coherence tomography in dermatology. J Biomed Opt. 2013;18(6): 061224.
6. Wang J, Xu Y, Boppart S. Review of optical coherence tomography in oncology. J Biomed Opt. 2017;22(12): 121711.
7. Cai S, Therattil A, Vajzovic L. Pediatric Vitreoretinal surgery and integrated intraoperative optical coherence tomography. In: Nischal KK, Nischal KK, editors. Integrated Intraoperative Ocular Coherence Tomography for Pediatric Ocular Surgery. S. Karger AG (2021)
8. Finn AP, Grewal DS, Vajzovic L. Argus II retinal prosthesis system: a review of patient selection criteria, surgical considerations, and post-operative outcomes. Clin Ophthalmol. 2018;12:1089–97. https://doi.org/10.2147/OPTH.S137525.

9. Ehlers JP. Intraoperative optical coherence tomography: past, present, and future. Eye. 2016;30(2):193–201. https://doi.org/10.1038/eye.2015.255.
10. Chen TC, Cense B, Pierce MC, et al. Spectral domain optical coherence tomography: ultra-high speed. Ultra-high resolution ophthalmic imaging. Arch Ophthalmol. 2005;123(12):1715–20. https://doi.org/10.1001/archopht.123.12.1715.
11. YasinAlibhai A, Or C, Witkin AJ. Swept source optical coherence tomography: a review. Curr Ophthalmol Rep. 2018;6(1):7–16. https://doi.org/10.1007/s40135-018-0158-3.
12. Viehland C, Chen X, Tran-Viet D, et al. Ergonomic handheld OCT angiography probe optimized for pediatric and supine imaging. Biomed Opt Exp. 2019;10(5):2623–38. https://doi.org/10.1364/BOE.10.002623.
13. Carrasco-Zevallos OM, Keller B, Viehland C, et al. Optical coherence tomography for retinal surgery: perioperative analysis to real-time four-dimensional image-guided surgery. Invest Ophthalmol Vis Sci. 2016;57(9):37–50. https://doi.org/10.1167/iovs.16-19277.
14. Carrasco-Zevallos OM, Keller B, Viehland C, et al. Live volumetric (4D) visualization and guidance of in vivo human ophthalmic surgery with intraoperative optical coherence tomography. Sci Rep. 2016;6:31689. https://doi.org/10.1038/srep31689.
15. Ehlers JP, Uchida A, Srivastava SK. The integrative surgical theater: combining intraoperative optical coherence tomography and 3D digital visualization for vitreoretinal surgery in the DISCOVER study. Retina. 2018;38:S88–96.
16. Tao YK, Srivastava SK, Ehlers JP. Microscope-integrated intraoperative OCT with electrically tunable focus and heads-up display for imaging of ophthalmic surgical maneuvers. Biomed Opt Express. 2014;5(6):1877–85. https://doi.org/10.1364/BOE.5.001877.
17. Chopra R, Wagner SK, Keane PA. Optical coherence tomography in the 2020s-outside the eye clinic. Eye (Lond). 2021;35(1):236–43. https://doi.org/10.1038/s41433-020-01263-6.
18. Viehland C, Chen X, Tran-viet D, et al. 400 kHz handheld OCTA system for bedside imaging of infant. Investig Ophthalmol Visual Sci. 2022;63(7):2906.
19. Hsu ST, Gabr H, Viehland C, et al. Volumetric measurement of subretinal blebs using microscope-integrated optical coherence tomography. Transl Vis Sci Technol. 2018;7(2):19. https://doi.org/10.1167/tvst.7.2.19.
20. Confalonieri F, Haave H, Bragadottir R, et al. Intraoperative optical coherence tomography in the management of macular holes: state of the art and future perspectives. Biomedicines. 2022;10(11):2873.
21. Carrasco-Zevallos OM, Viehland C, Keller B, et al. Review of intraoperative optical coherence tomography: technology and applications. Biomed Opt Express. 2017;8(3):1607–37.
22. Huang HJ, Sevgi DD, Srivastava SK, Reese J, Ehlers JP. Image-guided surgical intervention in vitreomacular traction from the DISCOVER study: intraoperative OCT utility, ellipsoid zone dynamics, and anatomic/functional outcomes. Invest Ophthalmol Vis Sci. 2020;61(7):4381–4381.
23. Toygar O, Riemann C. Intraoperative optical coherence tomography in macula involving rhegmatogenous retinal detachment repair with pars plana vitrectomy and perfluoron. Eye. 2016;30(1):23–30.
24. Ehlers JP, Kernstine K, Farsiu S, Sarin N, Maldonado R, Toth CA. Analysis of pars plana vitrectomy for optic pit–related maculopathy with intraoperative optical coherence tomography: a possible connection with the vitreous cavity. Arch Ophthalmol. 2011;129(11):1483–6.
25. Vasconcelos HM, Lujan BJ, Pennesi ME, Yang P, Lauer AK. Intraoperative optical coherence tomographic findings in patients undergoing subretinal gene therapy surgery. Int J Retina Vitreous. 2020;6(1):1–10.
26. Khan M, Ehlers JP. Clinical utility of intraoperative optical coherence tomography. Curr Opin Ophthalmol. 2016;27(3):201.
27. Falkner-Radler CI, Glittenberg C, Gabriel M, Binder S. Intrasurgical microscope-integrated spectral domain optical coherence tomography–assisted membrane peeling. Retina. 2015;35(10):2100–6.
28. Yee P, Sevgi DD, Abraham J, et al. IOCT-assisted macular hole surgery: outcomes and utility from the DISCOVER study. Br J Ophthalmol. 2021;105(3):403–9.

29. Ehlers JP, Dupps WJ, Kaiser PK, et al. The prospective intraoperative and perioperative ophthalmic imaging with optical coherence tomography (PIONEER) study: 2-year results. Am J Ophthalmol. 2014;158(5):999-1007.e1.
30. Hayashi A, Yagou T, Nakamura T, Fujita K, Oka M, Fuchizawa C. Intraoperative changes in idiopathic macular holes by spectral-domain optical coherence tomography. Case Report Ophthalmol. 2011;2(2):149–54.
31. Ehlers JP, Uchida A, Srivastava SK, Hu M. Predictive model for macular hole closure speed: insights from intraoperative optical coherence tomography. Transl Vis Sci Technol. 2019;8(1):18–18.
32. Inoue M, Itoh Y, Koto T, Kurimori HY, Hirakata A. Intraoperative OCT findings may predict postoperative visual outcome in eyes with idiopathic macular hole. Ophthalmol Retina. 2019;3(11):962–70.
33. Lorusso M, Micelli Ferrari L, Cicinelli MV, et al. Feasibility and safety of intraoperative optical coherence tomography-guided short-term posturing prescription after macular hole surgery. Ophthalmic Res. 2020;63(1):18–24.
34. Tuifua TS, Sood AB, Abraham JR, et al. Epiretinal membrane surgery using Intraoperative OCT-guided membrane removal in the DISCOVER study versus conventional membrane removal. Ophthalmol Retina. 2021;5(12):1254–62.
35. Meyer CH, Borny R, Horchi N. Subretinal fluid application to close a refractory full thickness macular hole. Int J Retina Vitreous. 2017;3(1):1–4.
36. Kantor P, Matonti F, Varenne F, et al. Use of the heads-up NGENUITY 3D Visualization System for vitreoretinal surgery: a retrospective evaluation of outcomes in a French tertiary center. Sci Rep. 2021;11(1):10031. https://doi.org/10.1038/s41598-021-88993-z.
37. Ehlers JP, Srivastava SK, Feiler D, Noonan AI, Rollins AM, Tao YK. Integrative advances for OCT-guided ophthalmic surgery and intraoperative OCT: microscope integration, surgical instrumentation, and heads-up display surgeon feedback. PLoS One. 2014;9(8): e105224.
38. Gabr H, Zhang W, Viehland C, et al. Heads-up ocular microsurgery with integrated live volumetric intraoperative optical coherence tomography. Invest Ophthalmol Vis Sci. 2021;62(8):2292.
39. Ehlers JP, Uchida A, Srivastava SK. Intraoperative optical coherence tomography-compatible surgical instruments for real-time image-guided ophthalmic surgery. Br J Ophthalmol. 2017;101(10):1306–8.
40. El-Haddad MT, Tao YK. Advances in intraoperative optical coherence tomography for surgical guidance. Curr Opin Biomed Eng. 2017;3:37–48.
41. Chen CW, Francone AA, Gerber MJ, et al. Semiautomated optical coherence tomography-guided robotic surgery for porcine lens removal. J Cataract Refract Surg. 2019;45(11):1665–9. https://doi.org/10.1016/j.jcrs.2019.06.020.
42. Mach K, Wei S, Kim JW, et al. OCT-guided robotic subretinal needle injections: a deep learning-based registration approach. Proc IEEE Int Conf Bioinform Biomed. 2022;2022:781–6. https://doi.org/10.1109/bibm55620.2022.9995143.

Macular Pucker Staging System and Surgery

Andrea Govetto and Paolo Radice

Abstract Over the last decade, tremendous advances has been made in the evaluation and surgical management of macular pucker. Macular pucker can be staged according to a 4-stages OCT staging system based on the presence of the ectopic inner foveal layers (EIFL), a continuous layer of inner retinal tissue covering the whole foveal roof, sign of chronic tangential traction. Centripetal traction in macular pucker lead to the formation of EIFL, whether centrifugal traction causes the formation of epiretinal membrane-foveoschisis, an entity previously included in the lamellar macular hole spectrum (tractional subtype). Axial traction in macular pucker may cause the abnormalities of the central cone bouquet, an important anatomical landmark particularly susceptible to mechanical stress. The cotton ball sign, the foveolar detachment and the pseudovitelliform lesion are part of the same clinical spectrum and represent different stages of cone bouquet tractional alterations. Macular pucker may cause both exudative and tractional macular edema, the first with petaloid appearance as seen with OCT, the second with a spoke-wheel morphology. Surgery in macular pucker should be tailored to the patient's characteristics and expectations, but earlier intervention is recommended to avoid the development of irreversible damage. Centripetal peeling may better preserve the integrity of the central fovea.

Keywords Macular pucker · Epiretinal membrane · Macular edema · Cone bouquet · Central fovea · Müller cell

Contractile epiretinal membrane (ERM), is a premacular proliferation of glial cells which may result in *Macular Pucker (*from the word "*puckering*", i.e. a fold or

Supplementary Information The online version contains supplementary material available at https://doi.org/10.1007/978-3-031-63508-3_5.

A. Govetto (✉)
Department of Biomedical Sciences, Humanitas University, Milan, Italy
e-mail: a.govetto@gmail.com

P. Radice
Circolo and Macchi Foundation Hospital, Varese, Italy

F. Patelli et al. (eds.), *Macular Surgery*, https://doi.org/10.1007/978-3-031-63508-3_5

pinched bunch of fabric caused by the shrinkage of one layer among many), a vitreo-maculopathy causing macular wrinkling and retinal displacement, resulting in vision loss and metamorphopsia [1].

Since the first report of macular pucker by Iwanoff in 1865, tremendous advances have been made in the understanding of the pathophysiology, classification, and evolution of macular pucker, with a significant impact on current clinical practice, including surgical recommendations.

In particular, the ability to understand the microanatomical retinal changes caused by macular pucker dramatically increased with the advent of high-resolution, high-speed optical coherence tomography (OCT) machines, which represented a transformative shift in macular pucker assessment, and are currently the *gold standard* diagnostic tool in these patients [2]. Further, improvements in surgical techniques, vitrectomy platforms, dyes and instrumentations, allow surgeons to face macular pucker surgery in a safer and more effective way if compared to the past [3].

Before focusing on the purpose of this chapter, i.e. current clinical classification and surgical indications of macular pucker, there is the need to clarify the terminology referred to this specific macular condition, as there is no universal consensus on this issue. Just listing some of the terms used for macular pucker highlights the problem: epiretinal membrane (ERM), epimacular membrane, preretinal membrane, cellophane maculopathy, and retinal wrinkle. Some authors believe that the term ERM lacks specificity as it may refer to membranes developing in any region of the retina, whether premacular membrane may be more specific as it relates exclusively to those membranes developing over the inner side of the internal limiting membrane in the macular region [1]. This chapter will use the term Macular pucker referring to the *effects* of contractile membranes over the macula.

The issue of classifying macular puckers is critical, as is it is intimately connected to surgical indications which, in recent years, have switched from a conservative and observational attitude to a more interventional and aggressive approach.

To understand and classify macular pucker, it is critical to focus on the profound retinal alterations that such disease may cause, which can be roughly classified in mechanical (i.e. retinal displacement, which may be either axial or tangential) and biological (i.e. intraretinal gliosis, disruption of the blood-retinal barrier).

1 Tangential Centripetal Traction and the Development of the Ectopic Inner Foveal Layers

Although clinicians have been classically focused on outer retinal alterations in macular puckers (i.e. ellipsoid zone and external limiting membrane defects) [4–7], the description of the ectopic inner foveal layers (EIFL) in 2017 represented a change in such trend, focusing more on inner retinal changes [2]. This seems logical, as the inner retina is directly exposed to the mechanical stress exerted by contractile ERMs.

The EIFL are defined as a continuous layer of inner retinal tissue covering the whole foveal area, with similar reflectivity to the inner nuclear layer and inner plexiform layer (Video 1) [2]. This entity was discovered by observing that in many eyes with macular pucker, there was inner retina over the foveal region, a finding normally exclusive of congenital conditions such as albinism or fovea plana.

The EIFL are pathological, as in normal foveal development the inner retina is shifted outwards while the cone mosaic is packed inwards (i.e. the foveation phenomenon as described by Spaide) [8]. This configuration is similar to other predatory animals (i.e. birds of prey) and it is supposed to guarantee the highest visual acuity as the impending light may directly reach the central cone mosaic. What happens in advanced puckers is that, due to the centripetal contraction of the contractile ERMs, the inner retina is dragged toward the fovea up to its complete cover. This ectopic tissue may then degrade or obstruct the impending light causing a decrease in visual acuity [2].

It is still matter of speculation whether the EIFL may be just the result of mechanical forces or if they may be caused by biological mechanisms as well (i.e. Müller cell proliferation). Since at this time there is no histology analysis of EIFL, such issue will only be resolved by future research.

The identification of EIFL served as the centrepiece of the current structural OCT staging system of macular pucker, which divides such lesions in four stages (Fig. 1):

Stage 1: early macular pucker with a well-preserved foveal microanatomy, presence of the foveal depression, absence of EIFL
Stage 2: intermediate macular pucker with loss of the foveal depression, but well-preserved retinal layers and absence of EIFL
Stage 3: advanced macular pucker with loss of the foveal depression, well-preserved retinal layers and presence of EIFL covering the foveal roof.
Stage 4: ends-stage macular pucker with loss of the foveal depression, presence of EIFL and generalized disruption of retinal layers.

Since its publication, the EIFL staging system has been validated by many independent reports, and it is clinically relevant as well, as macular pucker stages and severity correlates well with visual acuity, providing a nice correspondence between OCT findings and visual function.

There is a broad agreement on the negative correlation of EIFL with visual acuity (i.e. worse visual acuity in eyes with EIFL) both preoperatively and postoperatively, suggesting that eyes with EIFL may not fully recover after surgery [9–12]. This is important, as the evidence suggests that to obtain the best possible functional results, surgery needs to be performed prior to the development of EIFL (i.e. Stage 1 or 2) [3].

The development of EIFL has been found to significantly relate with metamorphopsia (i.e. distorted images) [13].

Once the EIFL are established, the foveal microanatomy rarely returns to its original morphology [3]. However, the EIFL do show some form of regression and

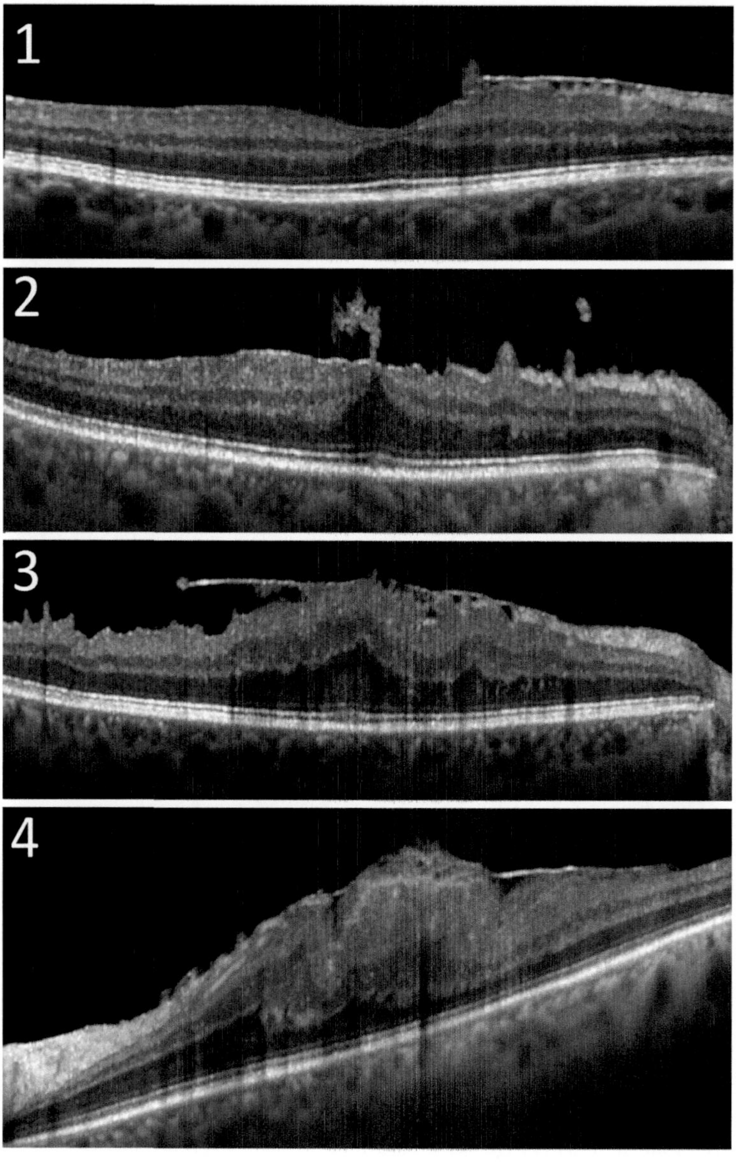

Fig. 1 Ectopic inner foveal layers OCT classification of macular pucker: 1. **Stage 1 macular pucker**: very mild epiretinal membrane with preserved foveal depression and well-defined retinal layers. 2. **Stage 2 macular pucker**: more advanced macular pucker with loss of the foveal depression, but well-preserved retinal layers. 3. **Stage 3 macular pucker**: advanced macular pucker with loss of the foveal depression, well preserved retinal layers, and appearance of continuous ectopic inner foveal layers covering the central fovea. 4. **Stage 4 macular pucker**: Very advanced membrane, with loss of foveal depression, thick ectopic inner foveal layers and complete disruption of all retinal layers

thinning in the postoperative period, suggesting that the main driving force in their development is indeed mechanical traction.

2 Tangential Centrifugal Traction, the Development of ERM Foveoschisis and the Concept of Tractional Macular edema

Oppose to centripetal traction leading to the formation of EIFL, centrifugal traction may cause the membrane to generate an outer retinal schisis (i.e. within the Henle Fiber Layer), effectively becoming an entity known as ERM-foveoschisis, as proposed by a recent consensus (Fig. 2) [14].

This entity was previously considered as a lamellar macular hole, and later redefined tractional lamellar macular hole due to its evident mechanical pathophysiology [15]. However, it was recently included in the ERM-macular pucker spectrum, therefore it seems appropriate to include ERM-foveoschisis in this chapter.

The clinical diagnosis of ERM-foveoshisis is based upon 2 major and 3 minor diagnostic criteria, as summarized below [14]. The diagnosis of ERM foveoschisis requires fulfilment of all major criteria.

- The major criteria for the diagnosis of ERM foveoschisis were the presence of: 1. contractile ERM; 2. foveoschisis at the level of Henle's fiber layer.
- The minor criteria were the presence of: 1. microcystoid spaces in the INL; 2. retinal thickening; 3. retinal wrinkling.

The terminology "*epiretinal membrane foveoschisis*" differentiates this condition from myopic foveoschisis or stellate non-hereditary idiopathic foveomacular retinoschisis, in which a tractional ERM may not be present. Further, the term underscores a causative association between the presence of a tractional ERM and the development of foveoschisis.

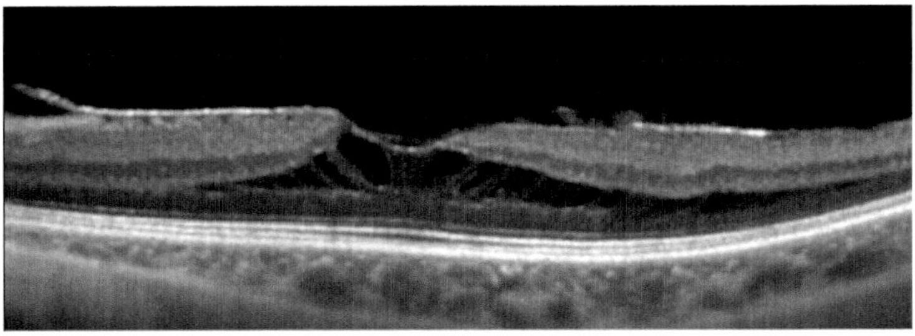

Fig. 2 Epiretinal membrane foveoschisis: in this case of ERM foveoschisis, all major criteria are fulfilled: contractile ERM and foveoschisis at the level of Henle's fiber layer. Fulfilled minor criteria are: retinal thickening, retinal wrinkling. There are no microcystoid spaces in the inner nuclear layer

Normally, such lesions tend to be stable, with a very low risk of developing full thickness macular holes [15]. Despite the profound alterations as seen with OCT, these patients normally present with good visual acuity and low metamorphopsia scores [15].

The peculiar morphology of ERM-foveoschisis has an intimate relationship with the specific disposition of Müller cell in the parafoveal area which, differently from straight Müller cell cone cells within the very central fovea, display a Z-shape [16].

Traditionally considered as a weak part of the retina, the Henle fiber layer has been greatly reconsidered in recent years. Theorical biomechanical physical models have shown that with traction, the *Z-shaped* Müller cells tend to assume a bevelled disposition, which act as a "*damping mechanism*" protecting the outer retina and the underlying photoreceptors from mechanical stress (Video 2) [16]. The hypothesis of the '*damping*' role of the parafoveal HFL is supported by previous laboratory studies. It has been shown that glial fibrillar acidic protein (GFAP) may contribute to the biomechanical properties of Müller cells by upregulation of intermediate filaments after mechanical stimulation [17]. As proposed by Bringmann et al., GFAP expression in Müller cells is a very sensitive indicator of stress, and this molecule is constitutively expressed in the OPL and HFL [18]. This may signify the presence of ongoing mechanical stress in these layers. Therefore, some authors hypothesised that GFAP distribution may support the assumption that Müller cell processes in the Henle fibres underlie the structural stability of the parafovea [19].

The hyporeflective spaces as seen with structural OCT in ERM-foveoschisis call for investigation on their origin and pathophysiology, as they may be confused with exudative cystoid macular edema, which is a condition normally not related to traction but rather to the disruption of the blood-retinal barrier (i.e. of vascular aetiology). In exudative macular edema, leaking fluid from pathologic vessels accumulates within the retinal parenchyma, displacing tissue and creating cystoid spaces, normally seen as petaloid with en-face OCT (Fig. 3a). Differently, in tractional disorders the retinal plexuses are normally intact, and the fluid accumulates within clusters of cells displaced by traction, with a spoke-wheel morphology (Fig. 3b) [20].

Retinal capillaries are normally impermeable to proteins, electrolytes, and water-soluble non-electrolytes. However, when there is a breakdown of the BRB, retinal edema follow the principles of Starling's law).

Compromise of the BRB would present dye leakage or pooling with FA and by the presence of cystoid spaces in both the INL and HFL, contiguous with the deep retinal capillary plexus. Intraretinal cystoid spaces may also be observed in tractional macular disorders [20]. However, in such cases there is no disruption of the blood-retinal barriers, as mechanical forces may physically separate and displace Müller cell processes in the HFL. As stated above, interstitial fluid may flow freely within such anatomic "spaces," created and maintained by traction and independent from Starling's equation. Such cystoid spaces may not resolve unless such mechanical forces are released.

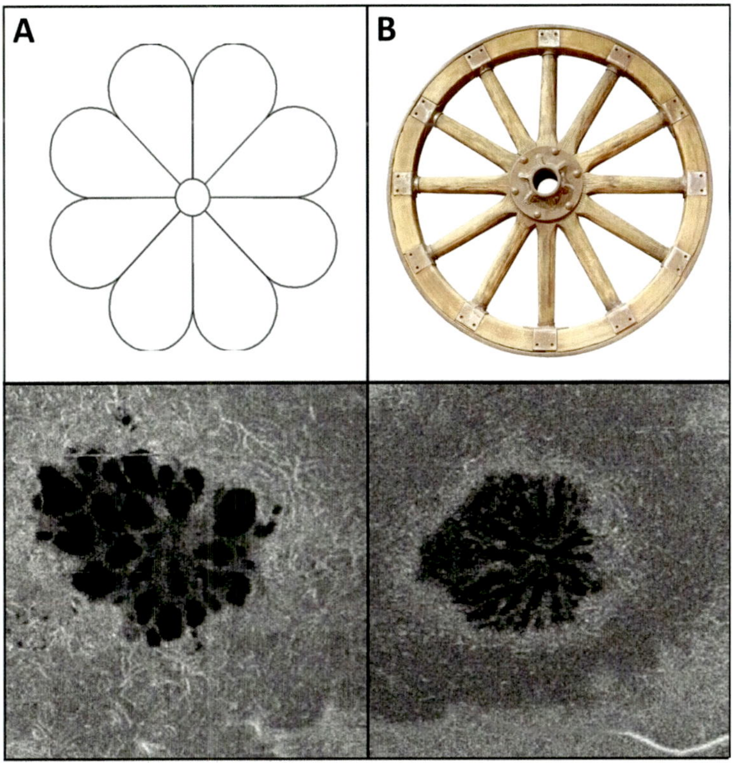

Fig. 3 En face distinctive patterns in tractional and exudative intraretinal cystoid spaces. **a** Exudative intraretinal cystoid spaces. Petaloid pattern. Multiple hyporeflective cystoid spaces display a petaloid pattern. **b** Tractional intraretinal cystoid spaces. Spoke-wheel pattern. Multiple hyporeflective cystoid spaces radiating from the foveal center

3 Anteroposterior Traction and the Abnormalities of the Central Cone Bouquet

Differently from parafoveal photoreceptors which are protected by the HFL from tangential and axial mechanical forces, central photoreceptors are particularly susceptible to traction as there is no damping mechanism to protect them. At the very center of the fovea lies the bouquet of cone of Rochon Duvigneaud's, defined as a small circular island, less than 100 mm in diameter, composed of approximately 2000 of the thinnest cone photoreceptors [21].

The precise anatomical composition of this specific central area has always puzzled clinician and investigators, especially regarding its glial architecture. Based on an electron microscopic study by Yamada [22], Gass proposed the existence of a peculiar formation of Müller cells, referred to as the Müller cell cone, a plug of tissue located in the center of the foveal floor, which was not displayed in the original illustration by Rochon-Duvigneaud [23]. Further, recent evidence suggests that Müller cells may be numerous, equal or higher in number to cone photoreceptors, at 200 mm from the foveal center in nonhuman primates [24].

The glial architecture of the central fovea is of utmost importance for surgical macular pathology. An indirect proof of the existence of the Müller cell cone was provided by the observation of specific outer retinal abnormalities, named cotton ball sign, foveolar detachment, and pseudovitelliform lesion, which represent a continuum in the same clinical spectrum of tractional abnormalities of the central cone bouquet in macular pucker [25].

The idea is that straight Müller cell cone may efficiently transmit mechanical forces to the underlying photoreceptors, with which they are intimately connected through their outer processes. With OCT, the EZ and ELM appears as exquisitely straight and parallel hyperreflective line due to a precise disposition and alignment of cells. When the photoreceptors are lifted vertically, such alignment is lost and a small area of hyperreflectivity is seen within the EZ and the ELM, and it was called "cotton ball" sign by Tsunoda [26]. This condition is fully reversible once the traction has been released and it does not cause irreversible damage to the photoreceptors.

If the tractional force is strong enough to detach the central cones from the retinal pigment epithelium, a small foveolar detachment with accumulation of a pocket of subretinal fluid will develop. Like cotton ball sign, foveolar detachment will resolve once the mechanical traction is released. It is unclear whether in these cases photoreceptors may experience irreversible damage.

When axial traction persists chronically, the subretinal fluid is slowly replaced by vitelliform material, as the normal metabolism of the photoreceptors outer segment is disrupted, and the RPE ability to clear up the photoreceptor waste material is reduced. In this case, the damage to the photoreceptor may be irreversible, and there is a risk to create a collapse of the lesion and subsequent foveal atrophy after surgery. If the ELM is compromised, the vitelliform material may migrate toward the outer nuclear layer, causing the resolution of the vitelliform lesion, often resulting in photoreceptor atrophy [25].

4 Macular Pucker Surgery

The surgical indication for macular pucker has dramatically changed over the last decade. The tendency, differently from the past, is to operate earlier to avoid the development of potentially irreversible retinal damage, i.e. the ectopic inner foveal layers. Evolutions in surgical techniques, instrumentation and vitrectomy platform allow safer interventions, improve patient comfort, and decrease intraoperative complications. However, accurate postoperative prediction of functional and anatomical result may still be elusive.

That said, the surgical indication must be tailored to the patient's characteristics and expectations. What may be unbearable symptoms for a patient may be perfectly tolerable for others, and as a rule it is not advisable to operate on macular pucker patients who are happy with their vision.

Many anatomical and functional parameters have been analysed to provide reliable predictors of postoperative results. A recent study in which a new artificial intelligence analysis was employed, found preoperative factors correlated with lower postoperative anatomical recovery: foveal detachment, EZ interruption, central macular thickness, and EIFL [27]. Ideally, one should operate on macular pucker before the development of such abnormalities.

Once the EIFL are established, they rarely disappear after surgery, although a reduction in their thickness has been shown in published reports [3]. However, EIFL thinning has not been shown to relate with postoperative visual acuity [3].

It is important to remark that all macular puckers, regardless of stage, may benefit form surgery. In example, stage 4 membranes were the ones with the biggest postoperative improvement in terms of visual acuity, despite achieving lower postoperative vision if compared to earlier lesions [3].

An active debate is still ongoing about whether to peel or not the internal limiting membrane together with macular pucker, with a recent systematic review suggesting that removing the ILM may result in less macular pucker recurrence and reoperations [28].

Special consideration may be given to macular puckers with microcystoid macular edema (MME), a specific subtype of macular edema characterized by multiple, numerous cystoid spaced disposed in the parafoveal area, localized exclusively within the inner nuclear layer [29]. Although it has been speculated that their origin may be retrograde transsynaptic maculopathy, their pathophysiology is still controversial. Microcystoid macular edema normally develops preoperatively in advanced macular puckers, but it may appear *de-novo* in the postoperative period [29]. Preoperative microcystoid macular edema has been related to worse postoperative visual acuty, whether the effect of postoperative microcystoid macular edema on vision has not been robustly established [29].

In eyes with MME, the ILM should be spared, as its removal may cause the worsening of the MME, possibly due to increased Müller cell damage. However, t must be noted that it is not always possible to selectively remove macular pucker, leaving and intact ILM below. In many cases, the ILM and Macular pucker will come *en-block*, as they may be tightly adherent one with the other.

Regarding the surgical technique, we prefer to remove macular pucker with centripetal movements, similar to what it is done in the creation of an inverted flap in macular hole surgery (Video 3, Fig. 4). The membrane is slowly peeled from the outside to the center avoiding any axial traction, up to the creation of a small "*ERM flake*" attached to the foveal center. At that point, with slow movements, the macular pucker is detached en-block. When the ILM must be removed as well, the procedure is repeated. In such cases, before the detachment of the macular pucker from the foveal center, another "*flake*" of ILM is created, always with the centripetal peeling technique. At the end, both ILM and ERM are peeled off en-block, avoiding any mechanical stress over the foveal region, as seen in Video 1. Before peeling the ILM,

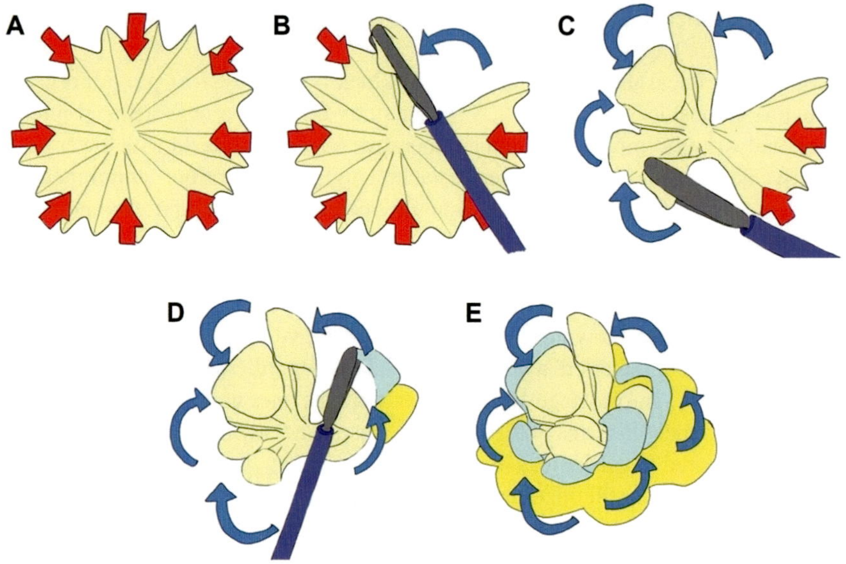

Fig. 4 Centripetal peeling technique in macular pucker. **a** Foveal macular pucker with central contraction center. **b** First the macular pucker is peeled with centripetal movements (**b**), from the outside to the inside, up to the formation of a pucker "*flake*" (**c**). Then, the internal limiting membrane is peeled off as well (**d**), with the same movements performed for the macular pucker, up to the formation of a "flake" of internal limiting membrane (**d**). At the end, with slow manoeuvres, both flakes are removed *en-block*, with minimum mechanical stress over the central fovea

a second stain is advised as in many cases the ILM stains partially when the dye is injected prior to the removal of the macular pucker.

A correct visualization is important, and we feel that narrow-field, flat lenses for macular surgery are superior to wide-field indirect systems, as they provide a very detailed view of the macula, allowing precise grasping.

The use of dyes is also important, compounds containing both trypan blue and brilliant blue-G (i.e. Membrane Blue Dual, DORC, Netherlands) are excellent as they efficiently stain both macular pucker and the ILM. Newer compounds containing lutein are thought to better preserve Müller cell integrity.

The surgical planning is essential, and recent OCT imaging imperative prior do proceed with surgery. Apart from standard B-scan imaging, en-face reconstruction may be useful to identify contraction centers and wrinkling areas. In wrinkled areas, it may be easier to grasp macular pucker due to loose membrane-retina adherences.

The decision whether to perform of not simultaneous cataract surgery depends on the ability of the surgeons to perform both anterior and posterior segment surgery, and on other factors as well. Inflammation may be higher in combined surgeries, and posterior synechiae are not a rare finding in the postoperative period. Further, intraoperative corneal opacification, excessive corneal incision hydration, as well as intracamerular bubbles, are all factors which may complicate macular pucker peeling.

In addition, the incidence of postoperative CME (i.e. Irvine-Gass syndrome) is higher in phacovitrectomies if compared to vitrectomies alone [30].

In cases of very mild macular puckers and significant cataract surgery, it seems wise to operate the cataract first, then decide whether it is appropriate to remove the pucker as well. In many cases, mild membranes are completely asymptomatic and non-surgical.

5 Conclusion

Over the last decade, tremendous advanced in understanding macular pucker evolution has been made. The 4-stage OCT staging system based on the ectopic inner foveal layers is widely used to classify macular puckers and provides useful preoperative and postoperative predictors of functional and anatomical recovery. ERM-foveoschisis is no longer considered as part of the lamellar macular hole pathology, but rather part of the ERM spectrum. Centripetal ERM traction may cause the development of EIFL, whether centrifugal traction will lead to the development of schisis. Axial traction over the fovea causes the abnormalities of the central cone bouquet. Axial traction over the parafovea normally has no effect on the parafoveal photoreceptors. Surgical indications have changed compared to the recent past, and it is common practice to intervene earlier to avoid potentially irreversible retinal changes which would negatively affect postoperative results.

References

1. Sebag J, Gupta P, Rosen RR, Garcia P, Sadun AA. Macular holes and macular pucker: the role of vitreoschisis as imaged by optical coherence tomography/scanning laser ophthalmoscopy. Trans Am Ophthalmol Soc. 2007;105:121–9.
2. Govetto A, Lalane RA 3rd, Sarraf D, Figueroa MS, Hubschman JP. Insights into epiretinal membranes: presence of ectopic inner foveal layers and a new optical coherence tomography staging scheme. Am J Ophthalmol. 2017;175:99–113. https://doi.org/10.1016/j.ajo.2016.12.006.
3. Govetto A, Virgili G, Rodriguez FJ, Figueroa MS, Sarraf D, Hubschman JP. Functional and anatomical significance of the ectopic inner foveal layers in eyes with idiopathic epiretinal membranes: surgical Results at 12 Months. Retina. 2019;39(2):347–57.
4. Kim JH, Kim YM, Chung EJ, Lee SY, Koh HJ. Structural and functional predictors of visual outcome of epiretinal membrane surgery. Am J Ophthalmol. 2012,153(1):103–10.
5. Shimozono M, Oishi A, Hata M, et al. The significance of cone outer segment tips as a prognostic factor in epiretinal membrane surgery. Am J Ophthalmol. 2012;153(4):698–704.
6. Itoh Y, Inoue M, Rii T, Hirota K, Hirakata A. Correlation between foveal cone outer segment tips line and visual recovery after epiretinal membrane surgery. Invest Ophthalmol Vis Sci. 2013;54(12):7302–8.
7. Watanabe K, Tsunoda K, Mizuno Y, Akiyama K, Noda T. Outer retinal morphology and visual function in patients with idiopathic epiretinal membrane. JAMA Ophthalmol. 2013;131(2):172–7.

8. Spaide RF. Healing mechanisms after macular hole repair suggests process of foveation. Retina. 2023;43(4):539–46.
9. Doguizi S, Sekeroglu MA, Ozkoyuncu D, Omay AE, Yilmazbas P. Clinical significance of ectopic inner foveal layers in patients with idiopathic epiretinal membranes. Eye (Lond). 2018;32(10):1652–60.
10. Sato T, Mori R, Takahashi S, Yoshimura K, Hirata A, Manabe SI, Hayashi K. Retrospective comparison of visual prognosis after vitrectomy for idiopathic epiretinal membranes with and without an ectopic inner foveal layer. Ophthalmic Surg Lasers Imaging Retin. 2018;49(11):838–45.
11. González-Saldivar G, Berger A, Wong D, Juncal V, Chow DR. Ectopic inner foveal layer classification scheme predicts visual outcomes after epiretinal membrane surgery. Retina. 2020;40(4):710–7.
12. Alkabes M, Fogagnolo P, Vujosevic S, Rossetti L, Casini G, De Cillà S. Correlation between new OCT parameters and metamorphopsia in advanced stages of epiretinal membranes. Acta Ophthalmol. 2020;98(8):780–6.
13. Yanagida K, Wakabayashi Y, Usui Y, Umazume K, Yamamoto K, Kawakami S, Goto H. Ectopic inner foveal layer as a factor associated with metamorphopsia after vitrectomy for epiretinal membrane. Acta Ophthalmol. 2022;100(7):775–80.
14. Hubschman JP, Govetto A, Spaide RF, Schumann R, Steel D, Figueroa MS, Sebag J, Gaudric A, Staurenghi G, Haritoglou C, Kadonosono K, Thompson JT, Chang S, Bottoni F, Tadayoni R. Optical coherence tomography-based consensus definition for lamellar macular hole. Br J Ophthalmol. 2020;104(12):1741–7.
15. Govetto A, Dacquay Y, Farajzadeh M, Platner E, Hirabayashi K, Hosseini H, Schwartz SD, Hubschman JP. Lamellar macular hole: two distinct clinical entities? Am J Ophthalmol. 2016;164:99–109.
16. Govetto A, Hubschman JP, Sarraf D, Figueroa MS, Bottoni F, dell'Omo R, Curcio CA, Seidenari P, Delledonne G, Gunzenhauser R, Ferrara M, Au A, Virgili G, Scialdone A, Repetto R, Romano MR. The role of Müller cells in tractional macular disorders: an optical coherence tomography study and physical model of mechanical force transmission. Br J Ophthalmol. 2020;104(4):466–72.
17. Lu Y-B, Iandiev I, Hollborn M, et al. Reactive glial cells: increased stiffness correlates with increased intermediate filament expression. FASEB J. 2011;25:624–31.
18. Bringmann A, Iandiev I, Pannicke T, et al. Cellular signaling and factors involved in Müller cell gliosis: neuroprotective and detrimental effects. Prog Retin Eye Res. 2009;28:423–51.
19. Bringmann A, Syrbe S, Görner K, et al. The primate fovea: structure, function and development. Prog Retin Eye Res. 2018;66:49–84.
20. Govetto A, Sarraf D, Hubschman JP, Tadayoni R, Couturier A, Chehaibou I, Au A, Grondin C, Virgili G, Romano MR. Distinctive mechanisms and patterns of exudative versus tractional intraretinal cystoid spaces as seen with multimodal imaging. Am J Ophthalmol. 2020;212:43–56.
21. Rochon-Duvigneaud A. Recherches sur la fovea de la retine humaine et particulie ŕement sur le bouquet des cones centraux. Arch Anat Microsc. 1907;9:315–42.
22. Yamada E. Some structural features of the fovea centralis in the human retina. Arch Ophthal. 1969;82:151–9.
23. Gass JD. Müller cell cone, an overlooked part of the anatomy of the fovea centralis: hypotheses concerning its role in the pathogenesis of macular hole and foveomacualr retinoschisis. Arch Ophthalmol. 1999;117:821–3.
24. Syrbe S, Kuhrt H, Gärtner U, et al. Müller glial cells of the primate foveola: an electron microscopical study. Exp Eye Res. 2018;167:110–7.
25. Govetto A, Bhavsar KV, Virgili G, et al. Tractional abnormalities of the central foveal bouquet in epiretinal membranes: clinical spectrum and pathophysiological perspectives. Am J Ophthalmol. 2017;184:167–80.
26. Tsunoda K, Watanabe K, Akiyama K, Usui T, Noda T. Highly reflective foveal region in optical coherence tomography in eyes with vitreomacular traction or epiretinal membrane. Ophthalmology. 2012;119(3):581–7.

27. Crincoli E, Savastano MC, Savastano A, Caporossi T, Bacherini D, Miere A, Gambini G, De Vico U, Baldascino A, Minnella AM, Scupola A, DAmico G, Molle F, Bernardinelli P, De Filippis A, Kilian R, Rizzo C, Ripa M, Ferrara S, Scampoli A, Brando D, Molle A, Souied EH, Rizzo S. New artificial intelligence analysis for prediction of long-term visual improvement after epiretinal membrane surgery. Retina. 2023;43(2):173–81.
28. Mihalache A, Huang R, Ahmed H, Patil NS, Popovic MM, Kertes PJ, Muni RH. Pars plana vitrectomy with or without internal limiting membrane peel for epiretinal membrane: a systematic review and meta-analysis. Ophthalmologica. 2023. https://doi.org/10.1159/000534851.
29. Govetto A, Su D, Farajzadeh M, Megerdichian A, Platner E, Ducournau Y, Virgili G, Hubschman JP. Microcystoid macular changes in association with idiopathic epiretinal membranes in eyes with and without glaucoma: clinical insights. Am J Ophthalmol. 2017;181:156–65.
30. Iuliano L, Cisa di Gresy G, Fogliato G, Corbelli E, Bandello F, Codenotti M. Increased risk of postsurgical macular edema in high stage idiopathic epiretinal membranes. Eye Vis (Lond). 2021;8(1):29.

Macular Proliferative Vitreoretinopathy

Jose García Arumí, A. Luis Miguel Salazar, and Claudia Garcia Arumi Fusté

Abstract Proliferative vitreoretinopathy (PVR) is a disease characterized by the growth and contraction of cell membranes both on the retinal surface and intraretinal layers, being a post-surgical complication that can compromise vision permanently if not treated. Recent reports have showed that postoperative premacular membranes are a localized presentation of proliferative vitreoretinopathy. A specific subtype of this entity has been identified as macular proliferative vitreoretinopathy (mPVR), which etiology can be idiopathic or secondary to multiple surgical procedures. Short-term mPVR is a different entity from macular pucker in terms of rapid development, structural distortion, histopathological findings and visual compromise. OCT examination of eyes with mPVR shows hyperreflective membranes that are thicker than observed in ERM, sometimes doubling the thickness of the retina, with an important distortion and disorganization of retina layers; macular edema with cystic spaces is a common finding. Histopathological analysis shows some differences with epiretinal membranes (ERM). Idiopathic ERM are composed of myofibroblasts, glial cells, and fibroblasts, while PVR membranes are composed predominantly of retinal pigment epithelial (RPE) cells, glial cells, and myofibroblasts. Cell transdifferentiation into myofibroblasts represents an important process in pathogenesis of both entities, while RPE cells are more predominant in mPVR. Many intraocular and paraocular medical treatments have been attempted to treat mPVR, but none of them have been successfully reproduced or have led to a better visual outcome compared to surgical management. The first-line treatment is an early surgical peeling of the preretinal membrane altogether with the internal limiting membrane (ILM) of the posterior retina to release the traction and the consequent anatomical structural alteration that this entails. A delayed surgery may imply a permanent loss of vision. In those patients that have high risk of developing mPVR it is important to perform an ILM peeling up to the temporal vascular arcades after a staining with brilliant blue, as the ILM has been shown to act as an scaffold for membrane proliferation.

Present Address:
J. García Arumí (✉) · A. L. M. Salazar · C. Garcia Arumi Fusté
Department of Retina, Institut de Microcirugia Ocular, Barcelona, Spain
e-mail: jgarcia.arumi@gmail.com

A. L. M. Salazar
e-mail: salazar-luis@javeriana.edu.co

F. Patelli et al. (eds.), *Macular Surgery*, https://doi.org/10.1007/978-3-031-63508-3_6

Keywords Macular proliferative vitreoretinopathy · Membrane peeling · Retinal detachment · Macular pucker

1 Introduction

Proliferative vitreoretinopathy (PVR) is a vision threatening disease characterized by the growth and contraction of cell membranes both on the retinal surface and intraretinal layers, being a post-surgical complication that can compromise vision permanently if not treated. The presence of these membranes and subsequent fibrosis can be interpreted as an abnormal wound-healing response [1]. This contraction can lead to tractional retinal detachment, macular edema and atrophy [2]. Intraretinal fibrosis can prevent flattening of the retina even after removal of the membranes, increasing the risk of retinal detachment even after a surgical intervention. The incidence of PVR associated with postoperative vitrectomy is estimated to be between 5 and 10% and has not changed despite advances in vitreoretinal surgery [1–3], appearing frequently at the first 6 months after the intervention [3]. Additionally, there are risk factors that have been identified: pre-surgical PVR, aphakia, ocular hypotension, choroidal detachment, giant tears, extensive rhegmatogenous retinal detachment, chronic ocular inflammatory disease, retinal detachment associated with retinal diseases (such as stickler syndrome, Marfan syndrome). incomplete posterior vitreous detachment, high aqueous flare, and reoperations [4, 5].

Near to 77% of cases develop PVR within 1 month after retinal detachment surgery and 95% are found within 45 days [2, 6]. Anatomic success after PVR surgery have been reported to be around 45–85%; functional success after a PVR detachment surgery were 26–67% [2, 7].

Premacular membranes developing following pars plana vitrectomy (PPV) can cause significant anatomical and functional damage to the macula. Recent reports have shown that postoperative epimacular membranes may be a localized presentation of PVR [8]. For years, post-vitrectomy premacular fibrosis was categorized as part of macular pucker spectrum [9, 10]. Recently, few reports distinguished a unique subgroup with premacular fibrosisas macular PVR (mPVR) rather than ERM [2, 11]. mPVR was highly associated with retinal breakscompared to idiopathic ERM [12]. In this specific subtype of the disease most of the patients had previously primary repair of rhegmatogenous retinal detachment (RRD) before the development of mPVR; it can also be secondary to multiple surgical procedures such as: cataract extraction, trabeculectomy, scleral buckling, pars plana vitrectomy, laser, and cryoretinopexy; non-surgical causes have also been stated such as: blunt trauma, uveitis, diabetes, posterior vitreous detachment, retinal vascular diseases [13, 14]. In some case series, age, high myopia, and narrow retinal arteriolar diameter have been found to be factors associated with the presence of a concomitant epiretinal membrane [14]. In our experience mPVR is a different entity from macular pucker in terms of rapid development, structural distortion, and visual compromise. Patients with multiple previous retinal tears have an increased risk of developing mPVR.

2 Genetics

As part of the identification of risk factors leading to PVR genetic association studies have been performed. Single nucleotide polymorphism (SNP) in the TNF locus was associated with the formation of postoperative PVR in primary retinal detachment repair [15, 16].This increased risk have also been found in T309G polymorphism in the MDM2 gene, downregulating p53 suppressor pathway [17]; another polymorphisms associated with PVR formation are those in apoptosis mediators BAC and BCL-2 [18]. Patients with polymorphisms associated with PVR have more predisposition to develop postoperative mPVR.

3 Pathophysiology

Multiple studies have demonstrated the leading role of the retinal pigment epithelium (RPE) as the causative agent of mPVR, as well as retinal glial and inflammatory cells. Breakdown of the blood-retinal barrier induces an inflammatory reaction that drives a variety of cells to the retinal surface (RPE and glial cells), ending in the formation of fibrocellular membranes on both surfaces of the neuroretina. These fibrocellular membranes are composed of retinal pigment epithelium (RPE) cells, Müller cells, myofibroblast-like cells, microglia, astrocytes, ciliary body epithelial cells, hyalocytes, cellular immunity (macrophages, lymphocytes, and neutrophils) [11]. These cells transdifferentiate in a process known as epithelial-mesenchymal transition. As the differentiation ensues, mechanical stress and macrophages and glial cells secrete cytokines such as platelet-derived growth factor (PDGF), transforming growth factor alpha and beta (TGF-α and TGF-β), insulin-like growth factor 1 (IGF-1), vascular endothelial growth factor (VEGF), hepatocyte growth factor (HGF), epidermal growth factor (EGF), tumor necrosis factor alpha (TNFα), fibroblast growth factor (FGF) contributes to the growth and changes in the composition of mPVR. Some inflammatory cytokines associated with these changes are interleukin-1 (IL-1), IL-6, IL-10, interferon gamma (IFN-γ), and monocyte chemotactic protein 1 (MCP-1) [16]. RPE cells, hyalocites, glial cells and fibrocytes differentiate into contractile myofibrocytes that generate excessive amounts of collagenous extracellular matrix rich in actin filament bundles, generating tractional forces which, subsequently, can lead to the creation of tractional wrinkles, folds, tears, and retinal re-detachments. As this disease has acquired importance through the years, many studies have reviewed the composition of PVR membranes indicating that RPE has a primordial role in the pathophysiology. To our knowledge, mPVR develops via the migration of EPR and inflammatory cells to the retinal surface, into the virtual space between the remaining posterior vitreous cortex and internal limiting membrane.

Immunohistochemical analysis shows that cytokeratin-8, Emmprin, Ricinus communis agglutinin I and Ulex europaeus agglutinin I, are present in PVR membranes and are strongly associated with RPE structures [19]. Some studies have found biomarkers in subretinal fluid that could predict which patients can develop PVR; these biomarkers were CCL22, IL-3 and MIF [1]. For the authors and as many articles show, the retinal pigmented epithelium is one of the main cellular mediators of the inflammatory chain that leads the formation of PVR and mPVR. Idiopathic membranes are composed of myofibroblasts, glial cells, and fibroblasts, while PVR membranes are composed predominantly of EPR cells, glial cells, and myofibroblasts [12, 13, 19]. Cell transdifferentiation into myofibroblasts represents an important process in pathogenesis of both entities. To address future antifibrotic treatment strategies, we emphasize that both fibrotic diseases share distinct immunocytochemical and ultrastructural features.

4 OCT Findings

OCT examination of eyes with mPVR shows hyperreflective membranes that are thicker than observed in ERM, sometimes doubling the thickness of the retina (Figs. 1e, 2d and 3d), with an important distortion and disorganization of retina layers; and macular edema with cystic spaces is a common finding. They produce wrinkling of the inner retinal surface with confluent partial or full-thickness retinal folds (Figs. 2d, 4c and d). More advanced cases can develop subretinal bands, which appear as hyperreflective tubular structures [14].The presence of distinct fingerlike projections extending from the retinal surface to the plane of the membrane have been described to be highly correlated with the macular PVR, strongly related with retinal breaks.

Structural features of mPVR seem to differ to ERM. Previous reports using time-domain optical coherence tomography have indicated that ERM after retinal detachment repair seems to have a more focal adherence to the retinal surface than idiopathic ERM, which can be more globally adherent [20].

Membranes in mPVR are more prominent compared to idiopathic ERM. Additionally, SD-OCT demonstrates a significant decrease in the macular thickness postmembrane stripping (711–354 μm) which was inversely related to BCVA, emphasizing the importance of mPVR peeling to achieve a better visual prognosis [8, 21].

5 Prevention of mPVR

Prophylactic peeling of the internal limiting membrane (ILM) during surgery has shown to reduce the risk of developing postoperative PVR formation. Some baseline characteristics and degrees of surgical complexity may act as risk factors for membrane development. A metanalysis investigated the benefit of ILM peeling in patients without significant proliferative vitreoretinopathy (PVR) who underwent pars plana vitrectomy for RD repair. A literature search using PubMed and various keywords retrieved relevant papers from which data were extracted and analyzed

[22]. Finally, the results of 12 observational studies (3420 eyes) were summarized. ILM peeling significantly reduced the risk of postoperative ERM formation (RR = 0.12, 95% CI 0.05–0.28). The groups did not differ in final visual acuity (SMD 0.14 logMAR (95% CI – 0.03–0 to 31). The risk of RD recurrence (RR = 0.51, 95% CI 0.28–0.94) and the need for secondary ERM surgery (RR = 0.05, 95% CI 0.02–0.17) were also higher in the non-ILM peeling groups [23, 24]. In summary, prophylactic ILM peeling in retinal detachment with risk factors is important as the ILM has been shown to be an scaffold for membrane proliferation.

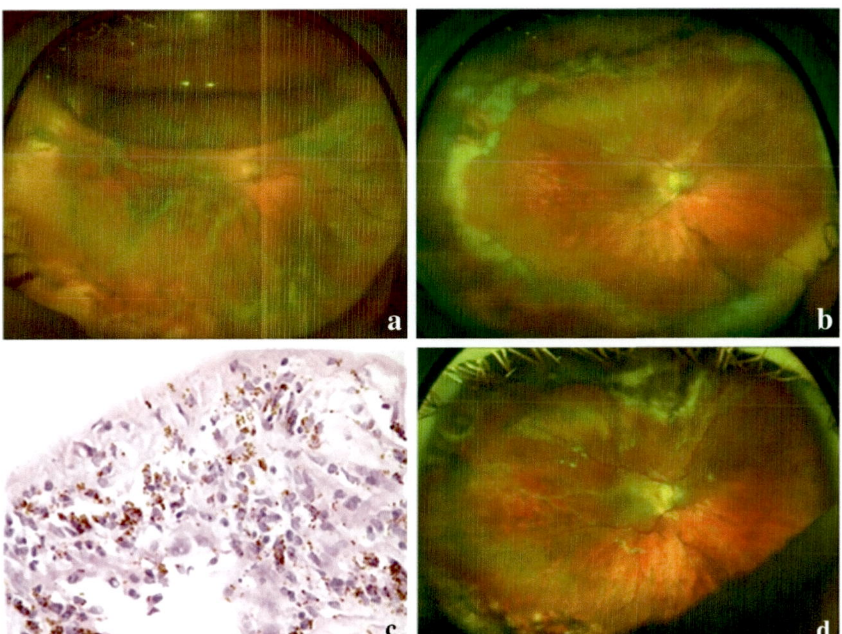

Fig. 1 21 y.o. patient who underwent scleral buckling surgery and cryotherapy abroad to treat RRD. She arrived to our institution 8 months after the procedure with a visual acuity of 20/500 and PVR (**a**). We performed an pars plana vitrectomy, ILM peeling, endophotocoagulation, and left silicone oil in the vitreous cavity (**b**). ILM was sent as pathology sample showing round shaped EPR-like cells with cytoplasmatic melanin inclusions (**c**). Four months later, the patient noted diminished visual acuity; ophthalmological exploration showed the formation of a macular PVR membrane (**d** and **e**). Fundus wide field optomap after removal of macular PVR **f**. We decided to do a new membrane peeling, having a final visual acuity of 20/100 with a residual macular edema (**g**)

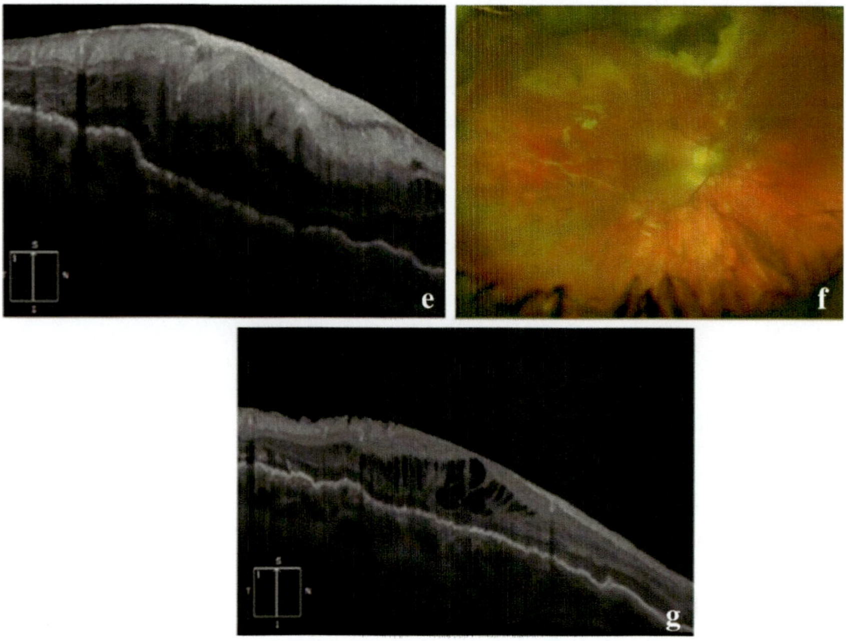

Fig. 1 (continued)

6 Treatment

Many intraocular and paraocular medical treatments have been attempted to treat macular PVR, but none of them have been successfully reproduced or have led to a better visual outcome compared to surgical management [25]. Studies using combined 5-fluouracil and heparin have shown no effect in the membranes caused by an established PVR. Oral colchicine did not show reduction in the incidence of developing PVR [26]; Thus, when identifying the onset of mPVR, the first-line treatment is surgical peeling of the internal surface of the retina to avoid tautness and the consequent anatomical structural alteration that this entails. The importance of a quick approach of mPVR must be outlined, because if not done promptly, the damage to the retina will be permanent even if a delayed surgery is performed. It is important to identify risk factors to plan ahead a preventive ILM peeling I order to avoid this complication.

Surgical treatment significantly restores macular anatomy and its function. Previous reports showed that epimacular membranes after retinal detachment repair have a focal adherence pattern rather than global adherence seen in idiopathic ERM patients [27].

The surgical approach that we propose is as follows:

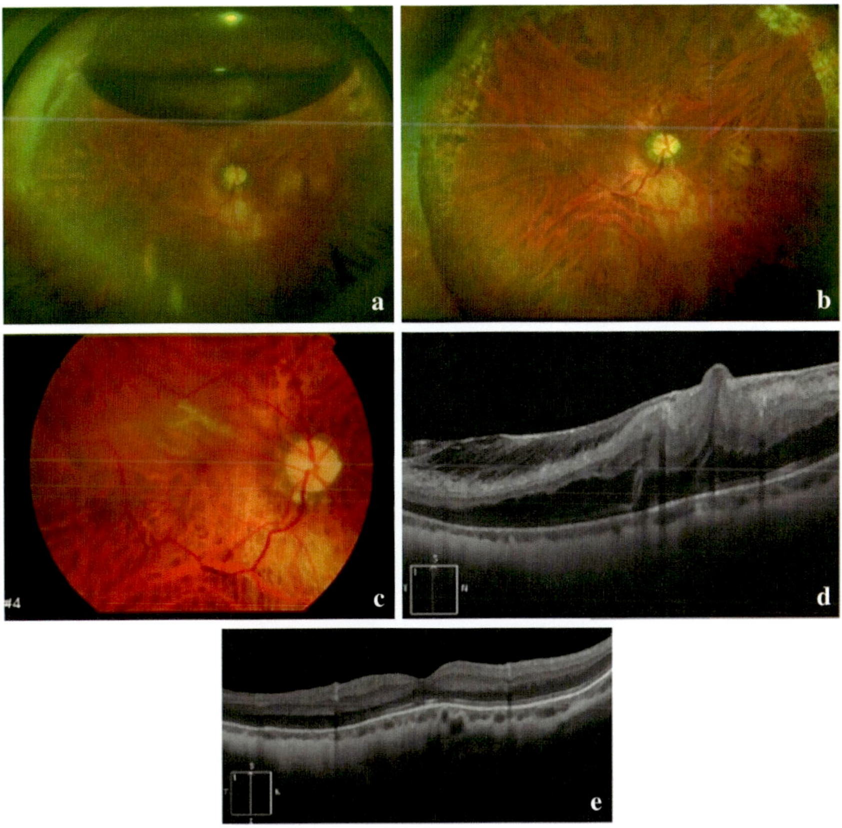

Fig. 2 35 y.o. male who had previous PPV and scleral buckling due to RRD; a month after the procedure he presented a new RRD (figure **a**). The visual acuity was 20/150. We decided to perform PPV and endolaser in the untreated lesions (figure **b**). A month later the patient developed a macular PVR (figures **c** and **d**), with almost full thickness retinal folds, and a multilayer epiretinal proliferative tissue, so we decided to perform the membrane peeling with shown results (figure **e**). The final visual acuity was 20/50

1. Dual staining with trypan blue and brilliant blue, to identify both epiretinal tissue and ILM. The staining must be complete in all the posterior pole to identify other PVR areas.
2. Membrane liberation shall be done with and end gripping or asimetrical Tano forceps, 23 or 25G, using a planoconcave precorneal lens or a 68° Wide field lens, beginning the dissection at the periphery of the membrane or at the ILM around the membrane, trying to perform a dissection of the ILM and the membrane at the same time. The traction must be tangential to the retina, not posterior-anterior, because the perpendicular traction may induce retinal tears in these high adherent membranes.

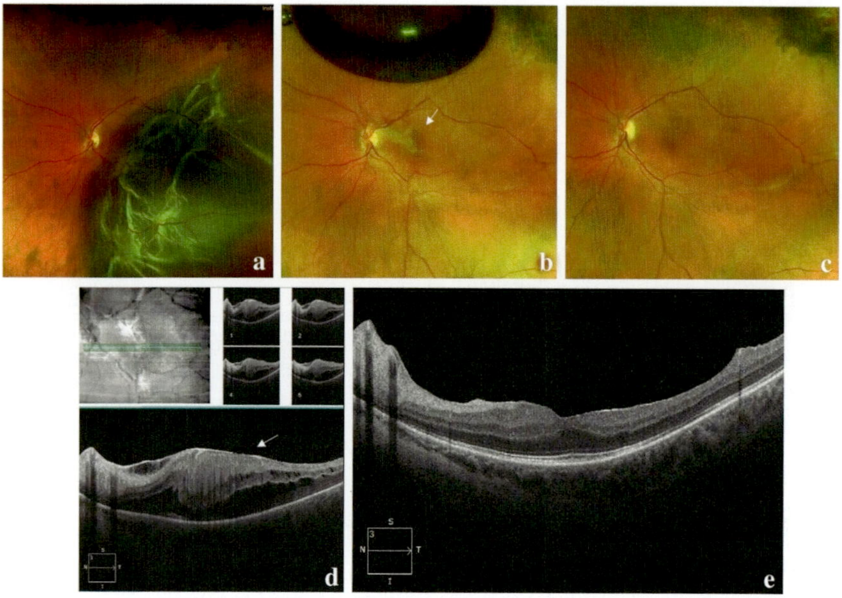

Fig. 3 67 y.o. women underwent pars plana vitrectomy for rhegmatogenous retinal detachment (**a**). Two weeks after surgical treatment, a whitish lesion (**b**) appeared over the macular surface (white arrow). OCT scan (**c**) showed a thickened membrane over the internal limiting membrane (ILM), with an important traction over the temporal vascular arcade. The visual acuity was 20/400. Retinal imaging after the procedure (ILM peeling) showed a normalization of the superior vascular temporal arcade, and the OCT scan confirmed an improvement of the macular structure (**d**). The final visual acuity was 20/25

3. If the dissection has not included both the membrane and ILM, re-staining with brilliant blue is crucial as it helps to identify the remnants of ILM that must be dissected.
4. After the dissection it is quite often to observe a whitening of the inner retina induced by the trauma of the dissection, it is important to not confuse this whitening with a remnant of the membrane. At the end of the dissection, it is important to check all the periphery searching areas of residual traction. Noair or gas endotamponade is necessary in cases of macular PVR without open retinal breaks.

Often, we observe mPVR in silicone oil filled eyes. It is true that membranes can be removed through the silicone oil, but the staining is more difficult and the visualization poorer. In these cases, we recommend removing the silicone oil, stain the membranes and remove them with a good visualization. If the retina remains attached without new holes, it is not necessary to refill the eye with silicone oil.

The visual outcomes are significantly reduced in cases of mPVR compared to idiopathic ERM (28). The presence of greater amounts of contractile elements in

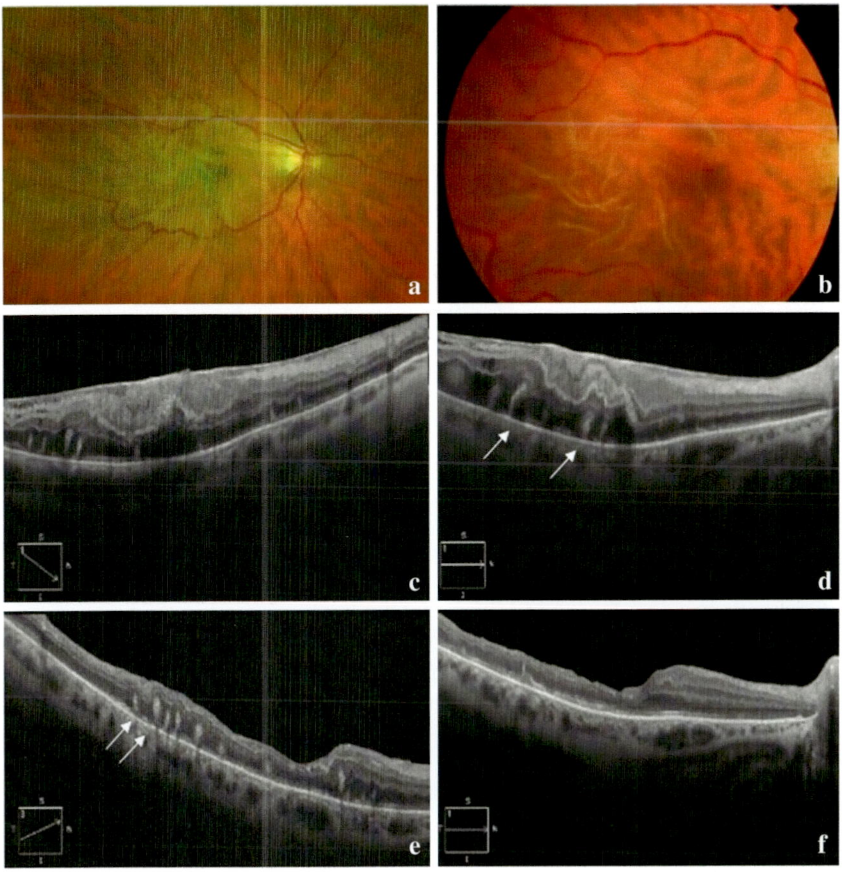

Fig. 4 54 y.o patient arrived at our service for a second opinion. He was treated with two sessions of photocoagulation in his right eye due to retinal tears, having a vitreous hemorrhage 10 months later which needed a PPV; during the procedure a superior RRD was discovered and treated. Two weeks later macular PVR was diagnosed (figures **a**, **c** and **d**). In the OCT (figures **c** and **d**) outer retinal folds were observed. Visual acuity was 20/800. We decided to perform mPVR peeling having the results shown: in the fundus retinography of figure b we can observe the persistent retinal folds in the immediate postoperative period, and the OCT of figures e and f show the persistence of the outer retinal folds. The final visual acuity was 20/100

mPVR leads to greater alteration in the underlying inner retinal structure, which may explain the greater impact on visual acuity (Fig. 5).

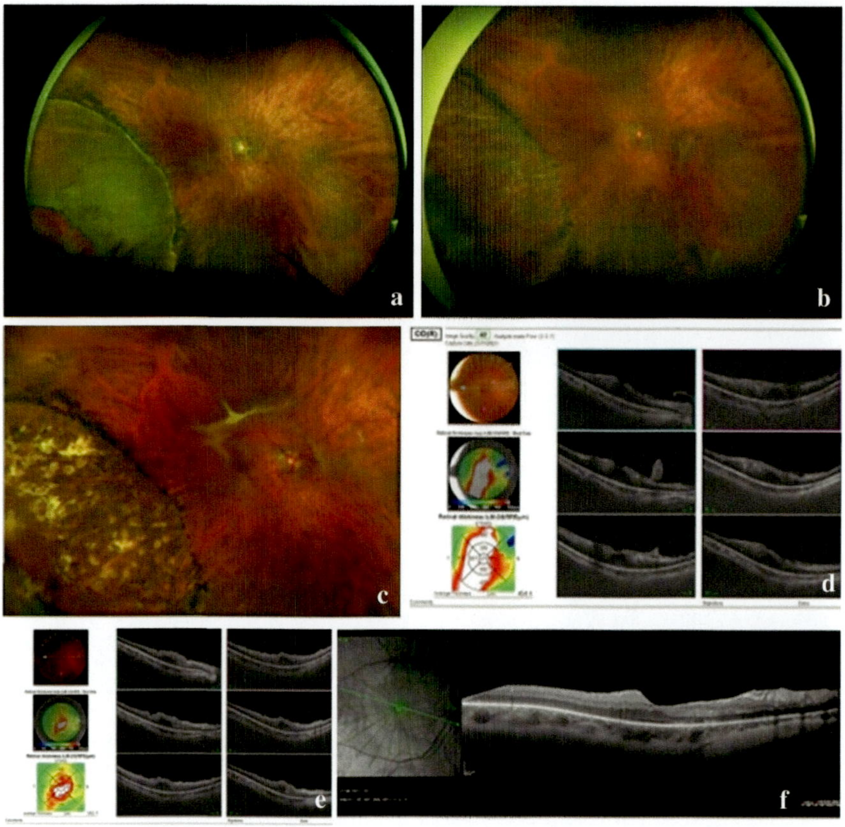

Fig. 5 Female patient that presented a chronic RRD on her right eye (**a**), with a BCVA of 0.3. PPV + ILM peeling was performed with a good visual outcome of 20/60 (**b**). A year later the patient developed mPVR both evident in fundus examination and SD-OCT (**c**–**e**). New PPV + Membrane extraction was performed with anatomical results as shown (**f**). Final visual acuity was 20/40

7 Conclusions

mPVR is a post-surgical pathology that should be evaluated in all postoperative patients after retinal procedures, as well as in those with proinflammatory baseline pathologies, because it may produce undesirable symptoms such as metamorphopsia and a noticeable reduction of the visual acuity. mPVR is a different entity from macular pucker in terms of rapid development, structural distortion, and visual compromise.

If mPVR is detected, it must be surgically intervened promptly in order to avoid permanent visual repercussions. Given the highly inflammatory nature of the disease, progress must be done towards the search for new coadjuvant anti-inflammatory agents in the treatment of this pathology that will lead to a better visual prognosis.

The importance of an early surgical intervention of this disease is the cornerstone of treatment.

We highlight the importance to do an ILM peeling that goes up to the vascular arcades, previous macular staining with both brilliant and trypan blue, in patients that have high risk of developing mPVR, like retinal detachments with multiple holes or eyes with chronic inflammation. The peeling should be done tangentially as perpendicular forces could risk macular rupture.

Clinical Pearls

- mPVR appears after vitreoretinal surgery (especially in the presence of retinal tears) and should be assessed both via clinical exam and multimodal imaging (OCT)
- Patient with multiple previous retinal tears have an increased risk of developing mPVR
- The eyes with polymorphisms associated with PVR have more predisposition to develop postop mPVR.
- As soon as de diagnosis is confirmed it must be surgically treated as it is a sight threating condition.
- The peeling should be done tangentially as perpendicular forces could risk macular rupture.
- in those patients that have high risk of developing mPVR it is important to perform an ILM peeling that goes up to the vascular arcades, previous macular staining with both brilliant and trypan blue.

References

1. Ricker LJAG, Kessels AGH, De Jager W, Hendrikse F, Kijlstra A, La Heij EC. Prediction of proliferative vitreoretinopathy after retinal detachment surgery: potential of biomarker profiling. Am J Ophthalmol. 2012;154(2):347-354.e2.
2. Idrees S, Sridhar J, Kuriyan AE. Proliferative vitreoretinopathy: a review. Int Ophthalmol Clin. 2019;59(1):221–40.
3. Coppola M, Marchese A, Cicinelli MV, Rabiolo A, Giuffrè C, Gomarasca S, et al. Macular optical coherence tomography findings after vitreoretinal surgery for rhegmatogenous retinal detachment. Eur J Ophthalmol. 2020;30(4):805–16.
4. Kon CH, Asaria RH, Occleston NL, Khaw PT, Aylward GW. Risk factors for proliferative vitreoretinopathy after primary vitrectomy: a prospective study. Br J Ophthalmol. 2000;84(5):506–11.
5. Asaria RH, Kon CH, Bunce C, Charteris DG, Wong D, Luthert PJ, et al. How to predict proliferative vitreoretinopathy: a prospective study. Ophthalmology. 2001;108(7):1184–6.
6. Pastor JC. Proliferative vitreoretinopathy: an overview. Surv Ophthalmol. 1998;43(1):3–18.
7. Quiram PA, Gonzales CR, Hu W, Gupta A, Yoshizumi MO, Kreiger AE, et al. Outcomes of vitrectomy with inferior retinectomy in patients with recurrent rhegmatogenous retinal detachments and proliferative vitreoretinopathy. Ophthalmology. 2006;113(11):2041–7.
8. Khateb S, Aweidah H, Halpert M, Jaouni T. Postoperative macular proliferative vitreoretinopathy: a case series and literature review. Case Rep Ophthalmol. 2021;12(2):464–72.

9. Appiah AP, Hirose T. Secondary causes of premacular fibrosis. Ophthalmology. 1989;96(3):389–92.
10. Muralidhar NS, Playfair TJ, Gregory-Roberts JC. Surgeryfor pre-macular fibrosis. Aust N Z J Ophthalmol. 1990;18(1):91–3.
11. Aweidah H, Khateb S. Rapid onset post-operative pre-retinal fibrosis is macular proliferative vitreoretinopathy (PVR) rather than epiretinal membrane (ERM)—a case series. Invest Ophthalmol Vis Sci. 2020;61(4246).
12. Tsotridou E, Loukovitis E, Zapsalis K, Pentara I, Asteriadis S, Tranos P, et al. A review of last decade developments on epiretinal membrane pathogenesis. Med Hypothesis Discov Innov Ophthalmol J. 2020;9(2):91–110.
13. Klein R, Klein BE, Wang Q, Moss SE. The epidemiology of epiretinal membranes. Trans Am Ophthalmol Soc. 1994;92:403–25 (discussion 425–430).
14. Sigler EJ, Randolph JC, Calzada JI. Comparison of morphologic features of macular proliferative vitreoretinopathy and idiopathic epimacular membrane. Retina Phila Pa. 2014;34(8):1651–7.
15. Rojas J, Fernandez I, Pastor JC, Garcia-Gutierrez MT, Sanabria MR, Brion M, et al. A strong genetic association between the tumor necrosis factor locus and proliferative vitreoretinopathy: the Retina 4 project. Ophthalmology. 2010;117(12):2417-2423.e2.
16. Wu F, Eliott D. Molecular targets for proliferative vitreoretinopathy. Semin Ophthalmol. 2021;36(4):218–23.
17. Pastor-Idoate S, Rodríguez-Hernández I, Rojas J, Fernández I, García-Gutiérrez MT, Ruiz-Moreno JM, et al. The T309G MDM2 gene polymorphism is a novel risk factor for proliferative vitreoretinopathy (Roemer K, editor). PLoS ONE. 2013;8(12):e82283.
18. Pastor-Idoate S, Rodríguez-Hernández I, Rojas J, Fernández I, García-Gutierrez MT, Ruiz-Moreno JM, et al. BAX and BCL-2 polymorphisms, as predictors of proliferative vitreoretinopathy development in patients suffering retinal detachment: the Retina 4 project. Acta Ophthalmol. 2015;93(7):e541–9.
19. Guenther SR, Schumann RG, Hagenau F, Wolf A, Priglinger SG, Vogt D. Comparison of surgically excised premacular membranes in eyes with macular pucker and proliferative vitreoretinopathy. Curr Eye Res. 2019;44(3):341–9.
20. Mori K, Gehlbach Pl, Sano A, Deguchi T, Yoneya S. Comparison of epiretinal membranes of differing pathogenesis using optical coherence tomography. RETINA. 2004;24(1). Disponible en: https://journals.lww.com/retinajournal/fulltext/2004/02000/comparison_of_epiretinal_membranes_of_differing.9.aspx
21. Yazici AT, Alagöz N, Celik HU, Bozkurt E, Alagöz C, Cakir M, et al. Idiopathic and secondary epiretinal membranes: do they differ in terms of morphology? An optical coherence tomography-based study. Retina Phila Pa. 2011;31(4):779–84.
22. Lamas-Francis D, Bande-Rodríguez M, Blanco-Teijeiro MJ. Primary ILM peeling during retinal detachment repair: a systematic review and meta-analysis. Sci Rep. 2023;13(1):3586.
23. Arias L, Padrón-Pérez N, Flores-Moreno I, Giralt L, Cobos E, Lorenzo D, et al. Internal limiting membrane peeling versus nonpeeling to prevent epiretinal membrane development in primary rhegmatogenous retinal detachment: a swept-source optical coherence tomography study with a new postoperative classification system. Retina Phila Pa. 2020;40(7):1286–98.
24. Aras C, Arici C, Akar S, Müftüoglu G, Yolar M, Arvas S, et al. Peeling of internal limiting membrane during vitrectomy for complicated retinal detachment prevents epimacular membrane formation. Graefes Arch Clin Exp Ophthalmol Albrecht Von Graefes Arch Klin Exp Ophthalmol. 2009;247(5):619–23.
25. Ahmadieh H, Feghhi M, Tabatabaei H, Shoeibi N, Ramezani A, Mohebbi MR. Triamcinolone acetonide in silicone-filled eyes as adjunctive treatment for proliferative vitreoretinopathy: a randomized clinical trial. Ophthalmology. 2008;115(11):1938–43.
26. Berman DH, Gombos GM. Proliferative vitreoretinopathy: does oral low-dose colchicine have an inhibitory effect? A controlled study in humans. Ophthalmic Surg. 1989;20(4):268–72.
27. Yamashita T, Uemura A, Sakamoto T. Intraoperative characteristics of the posterior vitreous cortex in patients with epiretinal membrane. Graefes Arch Clin Exp Ophthalmol Albrecht Von Graefes Arch Klin Exp Ophthalmol. 2008;246(3):333–7.

28. Katira RC, Zamani M, Berinstein DM, Garfinkel RA. Incidence and characteristics of macular pucker formation after primary retinal detachment repair by pars plana vitrectomy alone. Retina Phila Pa. 2008;28(5):744–8.

Macular Hole Classifications

Flavio A. Rezende and Bruna Gil Ferreira

Abstract Macular Hole classification has been for decades based on the rather impressive biomicroscopic work by Donald Gass. It was mainly created for pathophysiological purposes with an essential emphasis on the posterior hyaloid attachment at the macula and optic disc areas. The surgical approach for full-thickness macular hole (FTMH) was at its early inception. Twenty years later, with substantial improvements in imaging technologies, like spectral-domain (SD) optical coherence tomography (OCT), and surgical instrumentation and techniques, newer classifications were needed. The first meaningful one, based on SD-OCT, was proposed by the International Vitreomacular Traction Study (IVTS). They used the minimum hole width (currently named minimum linear diameter (MLD)) to classify eyes into small (< 250 μm), medium (≥ 250–400 μm), and large (> 400 μm). Pars plana vitrectomy (PPV) with wide (vascular arcade to arcade) internal limiting membrane (ILM) peeling and long-acting gas tamponade mainly became the gold standard. Holes ≤ 400 μm achieve nearly 100% closure rate with significant central vision improvement. But, for FTMH beyond 400 μm, closure rates after primary intervention drop down to an overall 80%. The Manchester Large Macular Hole Study was the first classification proposed for idiopathic FTMHs based on surgical results with primary PPV, ILM peel, longer-acting gas, and prone positioning. Although retrospective, with a relatively small number of eyes with FTMH > 400 μm and using only horizontal scans to measure MLD, they found a cutoff of 630 μm beyond which anatomical closure rates dropped to < 80%. More recently, the CLOSE Study Group introduced a more inclusive surgical classification for FTMHs > 400 μm with a significantly higher number of cases, using radial scans to determine MLD and other OCT biomarkers to stratify not only primary but also persistent and recurrent holes undergoing PPV with ILM peeling or other recently introduced surgical techniques. This chapter summarizes the evolution of classifications, didactyly dividing them in

F. A. Rezende (✉)
Centre Universitaire d'Ophtalmologie, Maisonneuve-Rosemont Hospital, University of Montreal, Montreal, QC, Canada
e-mail: frezendef@hotmail.com

B. G. Ferreira
Hospital Almodin, Maringá, PR, Brazil

F. Patelli et al. (eds.), *Macular Surgery*, https://doi.org/10.1007/978-3-031-63508-3_7

pre- and post-operative FTMH characteristics, and highlighting valuable features for daily clinical and surgical practice use.

Keywords Macular hole classification · Macular hole surgery · Gass classification · IVTS classification · Close study group classification · Large macular hole

Generally, classifications are used in medicine to transform general descriptions into a standardized nomination that can lead to a better understanding of the disease and its treatments. Classifications are also crucial in enhancing the accuracy of the diagnosis and facilitating research. This chapter aims to describe the historical progression of macular hole classifications. The authors aim to overview how the classifications have developed over the years, based on the technologies available, the development of the diagnosis processes, and most recently, the new surgical approaches of this relevant disease. For didactic purposes, we divided the macular hole classifications into two groups:

1. **Pre-operative hole characteristics**
2. **Post-operative hole characteristics**

1 Pre-operative Hole Characteristics

This first group can also be subdivided into pathophysiological- (pre- and post-OCT development) and treatment-based classifications.

1.1 Pathophysiological Classifications

Biomicroscopic Classification

One of the first and still primarily used worldwide macular hole classifications was proposed by Gass in 1988 and reappraised in 1995 [1, 2]. At this time, the technology available was the biomicroscopic examination and angiographic findings. This author based the classification on his biomicroscopic observations of how the disease developed and progressed. He observed and photographed the patients, following the natural history of the disease, to explain how the macular hole happened. Based on these observations, he proposed the classification to postulate a hypothesis concerning the pathophysiology of the disease.

Gass explained the macular hole formation based on the posterior vitreous separation from the macular and optic disc surfaces. Therefore, the author classified the disease into four stages in 1988 (Fig. 1) [1].

BIOMICROSCOPY CLASSIFICATION OF AGE-RELATED MACULAR HOLE			
		ANATOMIC INTERPRETATION	
STAGE	BIOMICROSCOPY FINDINGS	OLD	NEW
1A (Impending Hole)	Central yellow spot, loss of foveolar depression, no vitreofoveolar separation	Early serous detachment of foveolar retina	Same
1B (Impending or occult hole)	Yellow ring with bridging interface, loss of foveolar depression, no vitreofoveolar separation	Serous foveolar detachment with lateral displacement of xantophyll	SAME: for small ring For larger ring: central occult foveolar hole with centrifugal displacement of foveolar retina and xantophyll, with bridging contracted prefoveolar vitreous cortex. Cannot detect transition from impending to occult hole
2	Eccentric oval, crescent, or horse-shoe retinal defect inside edge of yellow ring	Hole (tear) in peripheral foveolar retina	Hole (tear) in contracted prefoveolar vitreous bridging round retinal hole, no loss of foveolar retina
	Central round retinal defect with rim of elevated retina		
	With prefoveolar opacity	Hole with operculum,(1) rim of retinal detachment	Hole with pseudo-operculum,(2) rim of retinal detachment
	Without prefoveolar opacity	Hole, no posterior vitreous detachment from optic disk and macula	Same
3	Central round ≥ 400 μm diameter retinal defect, no Weiss's ring, rim of elevated retina		
	With prefoveolar opacity	Hole with operculum, no posterior vitreous detachment from optic disk and macula	Hole with pseudo-operculum, no posterior vitreous detachment
	Without prefoveolar opacity	Hole, no posterior vitreous detachment from optic disk and macula	Same
4	Central round retinal defect, rim of elevated retina Weiss's ring		
	With prefoveolar opacity(3)	Hole with operculum and posterior vitreous detachment from optic disk and macula	Hole with pseudo-operculum and posterior vitreous detachment from optic disk and macula
	Without prefoveolar opacity	Hole and posterior vitreous detachment from optic disk and macula	Same

[1]Operculum contains foveolar retina.
[2]Pseudo-operculum contains no retinal receptors.
[3]Usually found near temporal border of Weiss's ring.

Fig. 1 Biomicroscopy classification was updated by Gass in 1995. The author classified the disease according to his observations of the biomicroscopy examination and angiogram. This table compares the previous classification from 1988 [1] to the new proposal in 1995 [2]

In 1991, Kelly and Wendel published their results on visual acuity recovery after pars plana vitrectomy (PPV) for stages 3 and 4 macular holes [3]. The authors reported excellent visual recovery after reattaching the retina around the macular hole, with 42% achieving improvement in central vision. Based on these new findings, Donald Gass updated his classification by dividing the first stage into 1A and 1B [2]. Gass's classification can be summarized as follows:

Gass Classification:

- Stage 1: Foveal Detachment

  Examination with a slit lamp shows a decreased or absent foveal depression, but there is no dehiscence. The patients complain of a recent decrease in visual acuity or metamorphopsia.

  – 1A: Impending Hole

    Contraction of the vitreous cortex causes foveolar detachment. In biomicroscopy examination can be seen as a yellow spot.
  – 1B: Occult Hole

    Further contraction of the posterior vitreous, with loss of the foveolar depression. During biomicroscopy examination is seen as a yellow ring with a bridging interface.

- Stage 2: Early Hole Formation

  One edge of the yellow ring develops full-thickness retinal dehiscence that enlarges as a can-opener mechanism. It initially forms a horse-shoe-shaped hole, then a round macular hole with an operculum attached to the posterior surface of the vitreous (in front of the hole).
- Stage 3: Fully developed Macular Hole with vitreofoveal separation.

  In fully developed macular holes $\geq$ 400 μm, in some patients, the operculum can be seen attached to the posterior vitreous, but the vitreous is still attached to the posterior pole.
- Stage 4: Macular Hole with Posterior Vitreous separation

  The stage 3 macular holes developed to stage 4 when there was a complete posterior vitreous detachment from the posterior pole with the presence of Weiss ring. According to Gass, only a minority of patients reached this stage.

Gass classification was very diffused worldwide; it provided insights into the clinical characteristics and helped physicians understand the natural process of macular hole formation. However, it lacked the detailed anatomic information necessary for treatment planning. Additionally, new imaging techniques have been developed, such as optical coherence tomography (OCT), which provided more features to develop further classifications.

The OCT technology enabled researchers to obtain high-resolution cross-sectional images of the retina, in vivo and non-invasive to the patients. This technology was a game-changer in the macular hole classification field. With this imaging tool, we could have a better understanding of the disease's anatomy and pathophysiology. The later classification systems that emerged after the OCT had much more detailed information regarding macular hole size, configuration, and vitreomacular abnormalities.

OCT-based classification systems enabled more objective and precise characterization of macular holes, contributing to the treatment decision-making process. Many classifications emerged, describing the anatomy of the macular hole and the post-treatment outcomes seen from the OCT. Three classifications became more relevant, first using time-domain (TD) and subsequently spectral-domain (SD) OCT characteristics (currently called biomarkers).

OCT-Based Classifications

(1) ***Gaudric*** [4]

In 1999, Alain Gaudric et al. published an updated classification for macular holes based on the TD-OCT findings. They observed and examined 76 patients who had macular holes in at least one eye. The patients were followed using: biomicroscopy, fundus photography, fluorescein angiography, and TD-OCT images (Fig. 2).

The main contribution of this classification was showing, through TD-OCT images, the relation between the posterior hyaloid to the central fovea and its critical role in forming a full-thickness macular hole.

Another significant contribution was showing that the central traction in the fovea caused a split between the inner and outer layers of the central fovea; the split developed further, creating an intraretinal cyst. With more traction, the roof of the cyst will open and then form the operculum, which can be seen attached to the posterior vitreous surface. This contradicted the idea from Gass [2] that there was a detachment of the central fovea prior to the formation of the macular hole.

Gaudric's Classification defines:

- Impending Macular Hole - Posterior vitreous causing intraretinal split
- Impending Macular Hole with intraretinal cyst
- Stage 2: Macular Hole - the cyst is opened to the vitreous cavity, but the operculum and the posterior vitreous are still attached to the inner layers of the retina
- Stage 3: Macular hole with detachment of the posterior vitreous from the macular area

(2) ***Duker*** [5]

Chan et al. introduced stage 0 to the Gass classification. They published this updated classification, also based on the TD-OCT observation of the vitreoretinal changes during the formation of macular holes.

This was a retrospective observational study that included 94 patients. The researchers included patients that had macular hole grade 2, 3, or 4; and had a normal biomicroscopically examination in the fellow eye, with no posterior vitreous detachment.

The stage 0 macular hole was defined as a clinically normal eye that presented with normal foveal contour and standard retinal thickness when seen on TD-OCT.

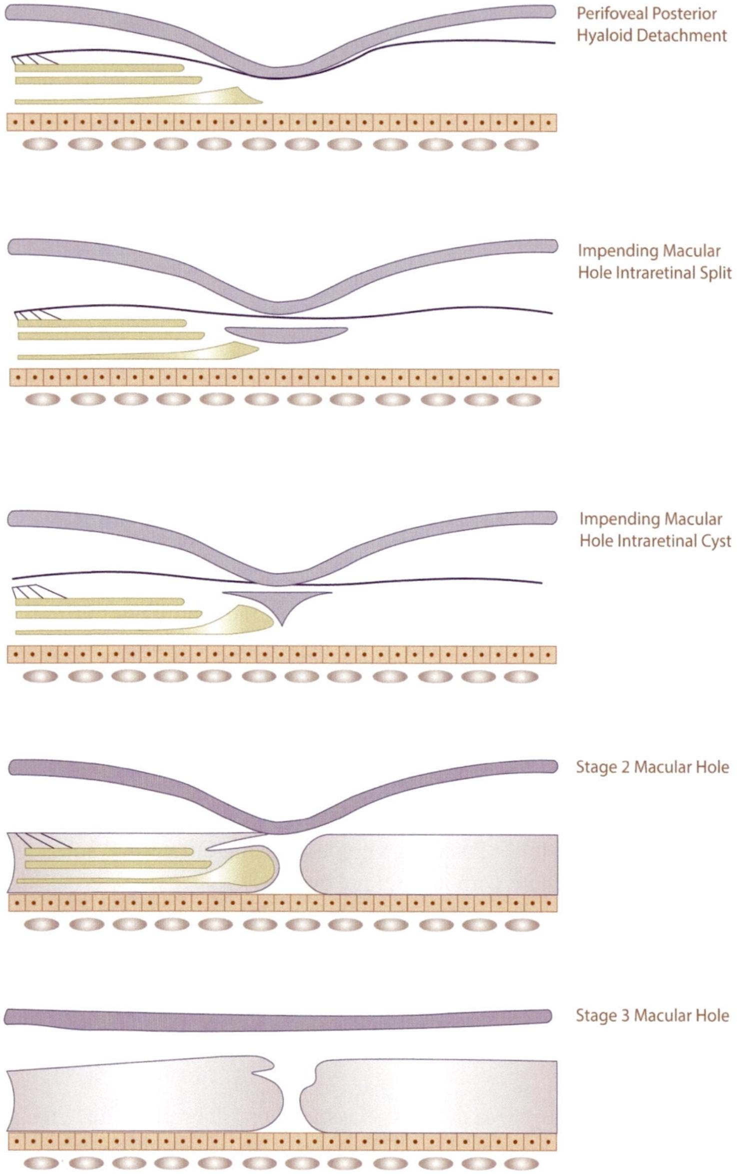

Fig. 2 Gaudric et al. classification used TD-OCT to evaluate how the posterior vitreous attachment played an essential role in the macular hole formation [4]

But the posterior hyaloid must be inserted on at least one side of the fovea, causing oblique traction.

Patients with stage 0 macular holes had approximately six times more chances of developing a macular hole compared to patients with no abnormalities seen on the OCT. These conclusions may offer physicians and their patient's valuable prognostic information; it aids patient counselling and shared decision-making with the patients.

The OCT technology benefited not only the understanding of the pathophysiology of macular holes but also provided important information about its healing process and outcomes after surgery.

Many authors have reported different features in OCT that led to a better understanding of the surgical outcomes and, furthermore, that could predict patients' visual recovery.

Then SD-OCT technology became more widely available as newer surgical techniques and adjuncts emerged. Classifications then evolved to rely on varied SD-OCT biomarkers and different treatment outcomes.

1.2 Treatment-Based Classifications

International Vitreomacular Traction Study (IVTS) Classification [6]

The first relevant treatment-based classification using SD-OCT imaging was proposed by the International Vitreomacular Traction Study Group Classification (IVTS) [6]. The IVTS group goals were to provide clinically valuable nomenclatures of the vitreomacular interface abnormalities (like vitreomacular traction (VMT), epiretinal membrane (ERM), and macular hole). This standardization allowed medical and surgical decision-making and subsequent cross-studies comparisons. Their initiative attempted to help determine the role of pharmacological vitreolysis treatment available at the time. They stated that the macular hole was an anatomical defect of neural tissue at the fovea and stratified treatment groups based on the minimum hole width (aperture size) measured by SD-OCT (Fig. 3). The minimum hole width (more recently renamed minimum linear diameter (MLD) [7]) is measured at the narrowest hole edge point in the mid retina with the SD-OCT caliper feature as a line parallel to the retinal pigment epithelium (RPE) (Fig. 3).

The IVTS classified the hole into:

- Small ($\leq$ 250 μm)
- Medium (>250 to $\leq$ 400 μm)
- Large (> 400 μm)

Manchester Large Macular Hole Study [7]

Ch'ng et al. in 2018 proposed a surgical classification based on outcomes of PPV, internal limiting membrane (ILM) peeling, and gas tamponade focusing on MLD > 400 μm macular holes. It was a retrospective interventional case series that included 258 eyes. Based on their results, the Small group from the IVTS remained unchanged.

CLASSIFICATION	SUBCLASSIFICATION	
Vitreomacular Adhesion	Size: Focal (≤1500 μm) or broad (> 1500 μm) Isolated or concurrent	
Vitreous Macular Traction (VMT)	Size: Focal (≤1500 μm) or broad (> 1500 μm) Isolated or concurrent	
Full-thickness macular hole	Size: Small (≤ 250 μm), medium (> 250 - ≤ 400 μm), or large (> 400 μm)	Status of the vitreous: With or without VMT Cause: Primary or Secondary

Fig. 3 The IVTS classification standardized the nomenclature of vitreomacular adhesion, traction, and full-thickness macular holes. Furthermore, this classification subclassified these pathologies into focal ($\leq$ 1500 μm) and broad (> 1500 μm); and the FTMH were divided into three categories: small ($\leq$ 250 μm), medium (> 250 μm and $\leq$ 400 μm) and large (> 400 μm)

They spread wider the Medium group to 250–650 μm and named Large all MLD beyond 650 μm (Fig. 4) [7].

OCT-Based Macular Hole Indexes

Using dense radial scans and the caliper function of commercially available SD-OCT machines, we can easily and reliably determine the MLD, base linear diameter (BLD), and height of macular holes (Fig. 5) [8]. It has been proposed that the MLD and BLD can indicate the tangential traction and that the height is a measure of antero-posterior traction and/or macular hole edge hydration and cystoid cavities presence. Based on these measurements, a few indexes were created to try to predict anatomical

IVTS - (MLD in μm)	MANCHESTER LARGE MACULAR HOLE STUDY (MLD in μm)
Small ≤ 250 μm	Small ≤ 250 μm
Medium > 250 - ≤ 400 μm	Medium > 250 - ≤ 650 μm
Large > 400 μm	Large > 650 μm

Fig. 4 The Manchester Study group updated the IVTS classification. This table shows the comparison between these two classifications

hole closure and improvement in central vision. Other more laborious methods of calculating macular hole area and volume can be done using additional software work. Until this isn't integrated into OCT machines, they remain less practical for clinical use. Here are some of the most used indexes:

- **Macular hole index (MHI)**: Height × BLD [8]
- **Diameter hole index (DHI)**: MLD × BLD [9]
- **Tractional hole index (THI)**: Height × MLD [9]

CLOSE Study Group Classification [10]

Based on the previous knowledge of all of the work mentioned above and considering the fact that many alternatives to wide ILM peeling surgical techniques have arisen in the last decade and that most studies excluded persistent/recurrent macular holes, we gathered an expert panel of experienced physicians that either introduced one of these newer techniques or were involved in previous macular hole studies and attempted to create a more inclusive, but relatively simple, SD-OCT classification.

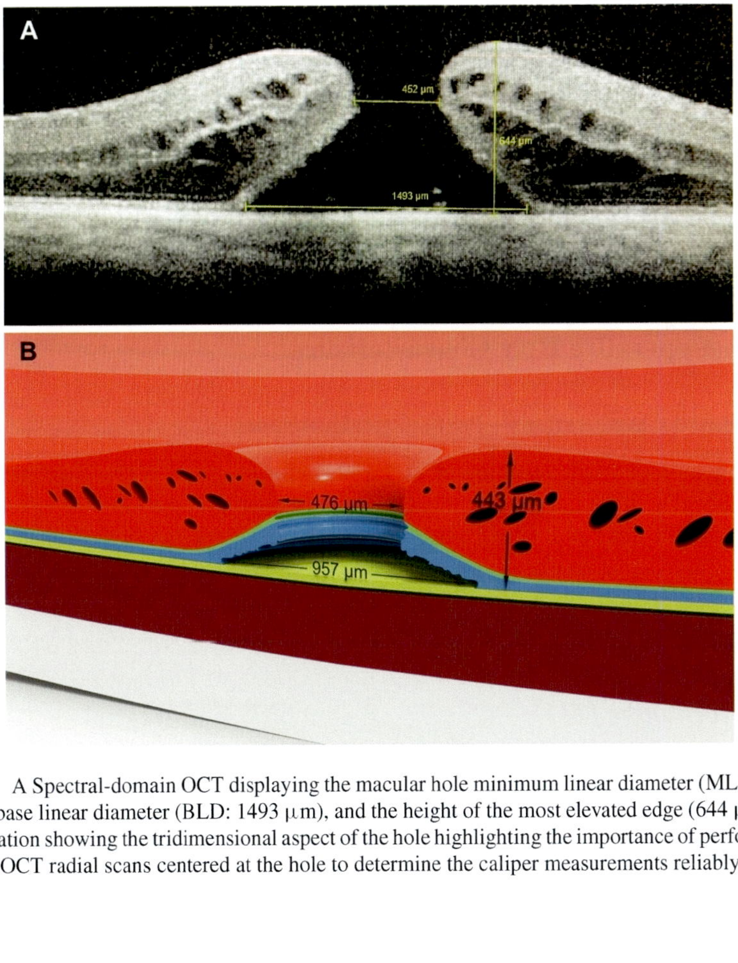

Fig. 5 A Spectral-domain OCT displaying the macular hole minimum linear diameter (MLD: 452 µm), base linear diameter (BLD: 1493 µm), and the height of the most elevated edge (644 µm). B Illustration showing the tridimensional aspect of the hole highlighting the importance of performing dense OCT radial scans centered at the hole to determine the caliper measurements reliably

Together we analyzed over 1000 cases of > 400 μm (MLD) that were either primary or failed (flat open or elevated open holes) previous interventions that underwent one of the following surgical techniques: wide ILM peeling, ILM flap, perifoveal hydro-dissection, human amniotic membrane graft (h-AM), or autologous retinal transplantation (ART) [10].

This new surgical classification stratified holes > 400 μm based on pre-operative MLD sizes plotted against type 1 hole closure and improvement in central visual acuity. The new MLD group's stratification and nomenclature were the following:

- **Large**: > 400 to ≤ 550 m.
- **X-Large**: > 550 to ≤ 800 m.
- **XX-Large**: > 800 to ≤ 1000 m.
- **Giant**: > 1000 μm.

Other relevant SD-OCT biomarkers were also recommended to be recorded in every case to allow further understanding of which technique is more likely to be successful in each clinical scenario. It also allows the calculation of the above-cited hole indexes. These biomarkers are:

- BLD (Base linear diameter)
- Height
- Hole edge configuration (elevated, flat, presence/amount of cystoid cavities)
- Presence of ERM (epiretinal membrane)/epimacular proliferation/VMT (vitreo-macular traction)

Figure 6 displays the evolution and comparison of the Gass, IVTS, and CLOSE classifications.

2 Post-operative Hole Characteristics

OCT-Based Classifications—Post-surgical outcomes

To allow a proper understanding of anatomical closure goals, a few classifications also evolved with the improvement in OCT imaging technology. More detailed visualization of the inner and outer fovea provided further comprehension of what should be aimed as macular hole healing patterns to achieve better functional outcomes. Here are the most significant closure pattern classifications.

2.1 Tornambe [11]

Tornambe was one of the first authors to study the anatomical outcomes after a vitrectomy for a macular hole. This classification focused on the post-operative appearance of the fovea endpoints (Fig. 7). In his published correspondence, he described three

FTHM STAGES BASED ON GASS (2)	INTERNATIONAL VITREOMACULAR TRACTION STUDY CLASSIFICATION (7)	CLOSE STUDY GROUP UPDATED CLASSIFICATION FOR FTMH BASED ON MINIMUM LINEAR DIAMETER (μM)	
Stage 0	VMA	VMA	
Stage 1: impending macular hole	VMT	VMT	
Stage 2: small hole	Small (≤250 μm) or medium (>250–≤400 μm) FTMH with VMT	Small	≤ 250 μm
Stage 3: large hole	Medium or large (>400 μm) FTMH with VMT	Medium	>250 to ≤400 μm
Stage 4: FTMH with PVD	Small, medium, or large FTMH without VMT	Large	>400 to ≤550 μm
		X-large	>550 to ≤800 μm
		XX-large	>800 to ≤1,000 μm
		Giant	>1,000 μm

Fig. 6 Table showing the comparison of Gass classification, IVTS classification, and Close study group

possible configurations (the imaging method used was not mentioned) as outcomes post-vitrectomy for macular holes.

- **Elevated/open (EO)**

  The borders of the hole remain elevated after surgery, and there is remaining fluid beneath the macular hole. This outcome indicates that the surgery failed, and visual acuity will not improve.
- **Flat/open (FO)**

  The borders of the macular hole become flat against the RPE, but there is no bond between them. The borders remain separated from each other. This outcome determines that there is still a retinal defect, but the author considered this endpoint as an anatomical successful surgery, although the visual acuity will rarely be better than 20/50.
- **Flat/closed (FC)**

  The borders of the hole are flat against the RPE but different from the FO; there is no separation between them; they are connected. Sometimes, a pinpoint defect may be visible.

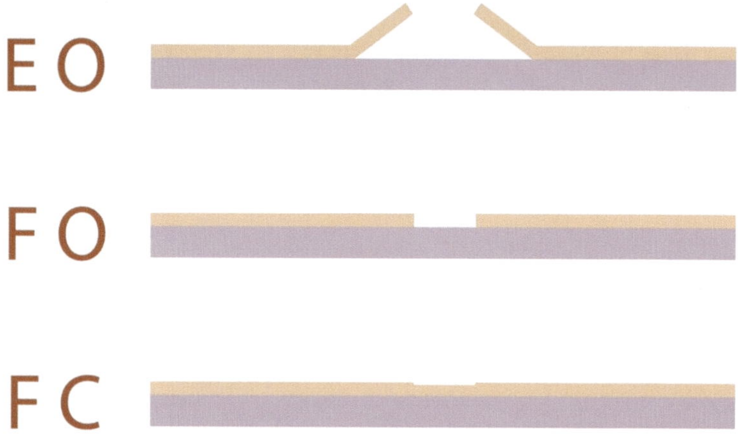

Fig. 7 Tornambe's classification defined three anatomical outcomes for macular holes after undergoing vitrectomy, as shown in the figure above. EO means elevated/open, FO means Flat/open, and FC means Flat/closed

This is the desirable endpoint to reach, and the author describes that this outcome should improve the visual acuity to 20/30 or better.

2.2 *Imai et al. [12]*

This classification was proposed by Imai et al. in 1999. The authors correlated the TD-OCT inner foveal contour configurations with visual recovery after macular hole repair with PPV and posterior cortical and ERM removal (no specific ILM peeling attempt).

This study included 33 eyes with idiopathic macular holes that underwent successful surgical repair. Patients were followed for six months, and macular OCT images were obtained during the follow-up. Postoperative success was determined as the edges of the macular hole appeared flat against the RPE.

The authors categorized the repaired holes into three categories (Fig. 8):

- **U-Type**

  The central area of the macular RPE was covered with retinal layers, and the fovea showed a circular surface that resembles the normal inner foveal depression (U shape). The biomicroscopy examination showed no evidence of a preexisting macular hole or a gentle circular contour on the eyes in this category.
- **V-Type**

  The RPE is completely covered by the retinal layers, but there is a notch in the central area with an extremely thin fovea. In the biomicroscopy evaluation, some

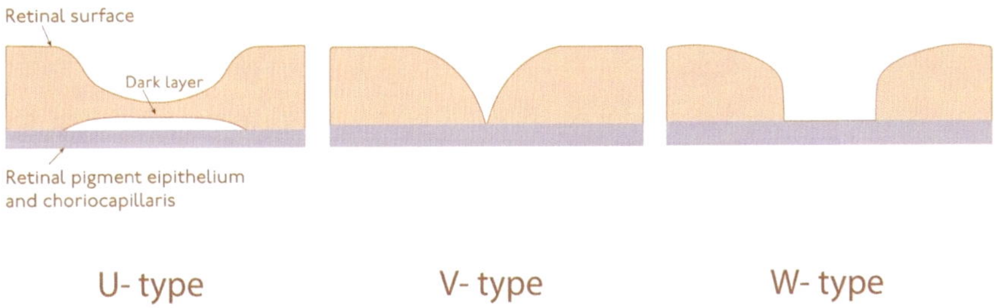

Fig. 8 Imai et al. schematic classification showing the different foveal contour patterns [12]

of the holes showed no evidence of previous hole, and some showed circular edges.

– **W-Type**

Retinal layers do not completely cover the RPE. The borders of the hole terminate abruptly on each side of a persistent central defect of the retina. In the ophthalmoscopic examination, the patients presented circular edges of the retinal defect, with depigmentation in all patients.

The authors of this study described that visual recovery was the best in the U-type, followed by the V-type, and the W-type (flat open from Tornambe's classification) was the one with the worst outcomes. They explained that the V-type patients probably had glial cells bridging the neurosensory retina and closing the hole; this was postulated to be responsible for the worse visual acuity recovery than the U-type closure. Patients with the U-type closure probably had fewer glial cells migrating into the hole. Therefore, there was a more complete approximation of the photoreceptors layer, which achieved better functional outcomes.

Finally, patients with W-type closure had the worst visual outcomes because they presented an incomplete approximation of the retinal layers leaving exposed RPE.

2.3 *Michalewska [13]*

The authors published this classification in 2008. The study aimed to use high-resolution SD-OCT to describe anatomical outcomes post-macular hole surgery.

The study included 68 eyes that underwent pars plana vitrectomy with ILM peeling with trypan blue staining. This classification was developed based on the previous inner foveal contour closure classification from the Imai et al. group [12].

- **Group I**: Foveal contour post-operative seen as U-shaped.
- **Group II**: Closure as V-shape contour of the fovea, with steep foveal contours.
- **Group III**: Closure of the macular hole formed an irregular contour.
- **Group IV**: Persistent neurosensory retinal defect in the fovea area, with flat cuffs and no subretinal fluid.

2.4 *Kang [14]*

Kang et al. developed a simplified SD-OCT-based classification evaluating the anatomical closure of macular holes. It was a retrospective series including 34 eyes undergoing pars plana vitrectomy, ILM peeling and fluid-gas exchange and anatomically successful macular hole closure. They divided the eyes in:

- **Type 1 Closure**: flat closed
- **Type 2 Closure**: flat open

Until then, type 2 closure with flat open macular holes was still considered a successful case. The further the technology evolved, and the more recent surgical techniques arrived, the target became type 1 closure. Currently, type 2 closure is considered a failed intervention, and other techniques may be attempted to convert a type 2 flat open into a type 1 flat closed hole.

2.5 *Rossi [15]*

Rossi et al. recently published a new macular hole closure pattern classification based on the integrity of the external limiting membrane (ELM) and ellipsoid zone (EZ) outer foveal layers. They included eyes operated with different PPV adjunct surgical techniques beyond ILM peeling, like inverted ILM flaps, use of adjuvants, h-AM graft and ART.

The authors defined macular hole closure as the condition of no bare RPE exposure to the vitreous cavity. Therefore, type 0 is considered a non-closed macular hole because of persistent post-operative exposed RPE. Type 1 and 2 are considered closed because there is tissue between the RPE and the vitreous chamber. Furthermore, type 1 differs from type 2, considering the type of tissue closing the macular hole. In type 1 closure, there is autologous tissue closing the macular hole, while in type 2, there is heterologous tissue closing the macular hole (Fig. 9).

- **Type 0**: Unsuccessful closure, there is bare RPE exposed to the vitreous cavity:
  - 0A—Borders are adherent to the RPE
  - 0B—Borders are elevated
  - 0C—Borders are edematous
- **Type 1**: Successful closure, constituted by autologous tissue
  - 1A—the presence of all retinal layers
  - 1B—interruption of external layers
  - 1C—interruption of internal layers
- **Type 2**: Successful closure, although there is heterologous tissue closing the gap in the retina (either ILM, human amniotic membrane or autologous retinal flap)

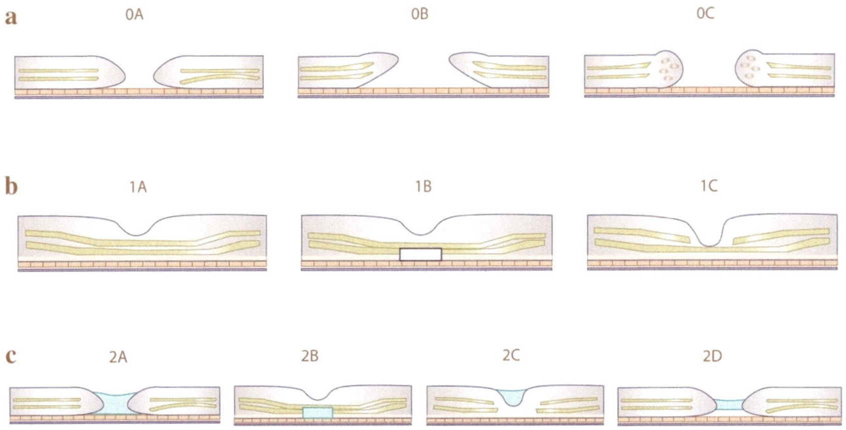

Fig. 9 Rossi et al. [15] schematic classification. Type 0 represents unsuccessful macular closure because there is a remaining gap between retinal tissue with exposure of the RPE. Type 1 represents successful macular closure with autologous retinal tissue. Type 2 represents successful closure, although heterologous tissue is closing the retinal gap (represented by the blue colour in the drawings)

- 2A—Dehiscence of internal and external retinal layers
- 2B—Presence of internal layers, but there is heterologous tissue in the external layers
- 2C—Reconstitution of external layers, but there is interruption of internal layers
- 2D—Bridging tissue reconstituting the anatomy, also called an "H-shaped" pattern.

Eyes with 1A and 1C closure patterns groups were the ones that achieved the best visual acuity recovery. Post-operative outer foveal integrity (ELM and EZ) provided the most successful outcomes in Type 1. Type 2 closure also demonstrated better visual recovery than Type 0 eyes, highlighting the importance of converting flat open into closed holes with adjunct techniques for larger or failed macular holes.

3 Future Aspects

In recent years, there has been a development in the ability of automated machine learning and artificial intelligence (AI) algorithms. These systems can potentially increase accuracy and efficiency when classifying macular holes based on OCT biomarkers and visual recovery.

We foresee in the near future even greater participation of these algorithms in developing more accurate classification systems, providing additional help in the decision-making process of which surgical technique is most suitable for each patient based on these newer classifications. One great advantage of these AI algorithms is the capability to consider a wide range of pre-operatory features that the human eye couldn't see. Therefore, these algorithms can analyze minor differences in the OCT and enhance the already existing classification systems. No macular hole should remain open…

Clinical Pearls (not essential)

- The importance of macular hole classification lies in its role in accurate diagnosis, pathogenesis understanding, disease monitoring, and utterly treatment selection based on evidence and research publications.
- Macular hole classification has changed throughout time, based on biomicroscopy, OCT, and most recently on surgical outcomes.
- The newer pre- and post-operative classifications should help the retina specialist in the decision-making process to determine which approach is more appropriate for each individual.
- Early staging systems provided the groundwork for more sophisticated and standardized classification systems to develop, including OCT findings and surgical outcomes.

References

1. Gass JDM. Idiopathic senile macular hole: its early stages and pathogenesis. Arch Ophthalmol. 1988;106(5):629–39.
2. Gass JDM. Reappraisal of biomicroscopic classification of stages of development of a macular hole. Am J Ophthalmol. 1995;119(6):752–9.
3. Kelly NE, Wendel RT. Vitreous surgery for idiopathic macular holes: results of a pilot study. Arch Ophthalmol. 1991;109(5):654–9.
4. Gaudric A, Haouchine B, Massin P, Paques M, Blain P, Erginay A. Macular hole formation: new data provided by optical coherence tomography. Arch Ophthalmol. 1999;117(6):744–51.
5. Chan A, Duker JS, Schuman JS, Fujimoto JG. Stage 0 macular holes: observations by optical coherence tomography. Ophthalmology. 2004;111(11):2027–32.
6. Duker JS, Kaiser PK, Binder S, de Smet MD, Gaudric A, Reichel E, et al. The International Vitreomacular Traction Study Group classification of vitreomacular adhesion, traction, and macular hole. Ophthalmology. 2013;120(12):2611–9.
7. Ch'ng SW, Patton N, Ahmed M, Ivanova T, Baumann C, Charles S, Jalil A. The Manchester large macular hole study: is it time to reclassify large macular holes? Am J Ophthalmol. 2018;195:36–42.
8. Kusuhara S, Escaño MFT, Fujii S, Nakanishi Y, Tamura Y, Nagai A, et al. Prediction of postoperative visual outcome based on hole configuration by optical coherence tomography in eyes with idiopathic macular holes. Am J Ophthalmol. 2004;138(5):709–16.
9. Ruiz-Moreno JM, Staicu C, Piñero DP, Montero J, Lugo F, Amat P. Optical coherence tomography predictive factors for macular hole surgery outcome. Br J Ophthalmol. 2008;92(5):640–4.
10. Rezende FA, Ferreira BG, Rampakakis E, Steel DH, Koss MJ, Nawrocka ZA, et al. Surgical classification for large macular hole: based on different surgical techniques results: the CLOSE study group. Int J Retina Vitreous. 2023;9(1):4.

11. Tornambe PE, Poliner LS, Cohen RG. Definition of macular hole surgery end points: elevated/open, flat/open, flat/closed. Retina. 1998;18(3):286.
12. Imai M, Iijima H, Gotoh T, Tsukahara S. Optical coherence tomography of successfully repaired idiopathic macular holes. Am J Ophthalmol. 1999;128:621–7. https://doi.org/10.1016/S0002-9394(99)00200-7.
13. Michalewska Z, Michalewski J, Cisiecki S, Adelman R, Nawrocki J. Correlation between foveal structure and visual outcome following macular hole surgery: a spectral optical coherence tomography study. Graefe Arch Clin Exp Ophthalmol. 2008;246:823–30. https://doi.org/10.1007/s00417-007-0764-5.
14. Kang SW, Ahn K, Ham DI. Types of macular hole closure and their clinical implications. Br J Ophthalmol. 2003;87(8):1015–9. https://doi.org/10.1136/bjo.87.8.1015. PMID: 12881347; PMCID: PMC1771782.
15. Rossi T, Bacherini D, Caporossi T, et al. Macular hole closure patterns: an updated classification. Graefe Arch Clin Exp Ophthalmol. 2020;258:2629–38. https://doi.org/10.1007/s00417-020-04920-4.

Use of the Inverted ILM Flap Technique for Macular Hole Closure

Zofia Anna Nawrocka and Jerzy Nawrocki

Abstract The Inverted ILM (internal limiting membrane) Flap Technique improved the closure rate not only of large full thickness macular holes but also of macular holes associated with different diseases, as pathological myopia, age related macular degeneration, diabetic retinopathy and others. This novel surgical technique allows to eliminate type 2 closure (flat margins of the macular hole, bare retinal pigment epithelium) from possible postoperative outcomes. Instead, some holes will be initially closed only with ILM (flap closure). Tissue regenerates with time and vision improves in this closure type. The only modification of the original Inverted ILM Flap Technique with results confirmed in a randomized study is the Temporal Inverted ILM Flap Technique. The technique consists of core vitrectomy, staining of the ILM with blue dye, peeling of the ILM from the temporal side of the fovea only and positioning it on the top of the fovea in an inverted upside-down fashion. The vitreous cavity is filled with air at the end of surgery. It is extremely important not to introduce the ILM into the hole, but only to gently cover it, in order to maintain a good functional outcome. Visual acuity improvement was reported to be superior to cases where the ILM was peeled in all indications. The continuous improvement of vision lasts at least twelve months after surgery.

Keywords Inverted ILM flap · Temporal flap · Macular hole · Vitrectomy · Recurrent macular holes · Flap technique

1 Epidemiology

Full thickness macular hole (FTMH), first described by Knapp in 1869 [1], is a round full-thickness opening in the fovea.

Z. A. Nawrocka (✉) · J. Nawrocki
Ophthalmic Clinic "Jasne Blonia", Rojna 90, 91-134 Lodz, Poland
e-mail: zosia_n@yahoo.com

J. Nawrocki
e-mail: jerzy_n@poczta.onet.pl

F. Patelli et al. (eds.), *Macular Surgery*, https://doi.org/10.1007/978-3-031-63508-3_8

FTMHs are reported in about 3.3/1000 cases [2]. More women are affected [3]. About 11–28% of patients have a bilateral disease [3, 4].

The etiopathogenesis of FTMHs is not completely understood. One of the main causes of FTMH formation is vitreomacular traction. However, FTMH formation was also reported in eyes with detached vitreous [5] or after vitrectomy [6]. Those cases might be partially explained by lower choroidal blood flow, which was observed in Swept-source optical coherence tomography angiography, (SS-OCTA) [7].

The hydration theory, proposed by Tornambe, explains that macular holes might be formed if fluid vitreous would soak into macular tissue. Gas used during surgery would enable the RPE pump to remove intraretinal fluid [8]. Another reason for FTMH formation might be involutional thinning or foveal degeneration.

Usually, macular holes tend to enlarge with time. Spontaneous closure, occurring more frequent in men, is a rare event [9].

2 Macular Hole Closure Types

2.1 U-shape, V-shape, Irregular and Type 2 Closure

For many years we were taught about four closure types: U-shape, V-shape, irregular and type 2 closure (Fig. 1). Best visual acuities were obtained in the U-shape closure, mostly resembling the normal fovea contour. Slightly worse in V-shape and irregular shape closures, which was probably associated with an increased number of photoreceptor and external limiting membrane defects.

2.2 Flat Open Macular holes

Another outcome, regarded for a long time as surgical success were flat open macular holes (type 2, type W closure). In this closure type the edges of the hole are adjacent, but the retinal pigment epithelium is still bare. Such patients did not experience vision improvement, but the holes did not further enlarge. This type is never observed if the Inverted ILM Flap Technique is performed.

2.3 Elevated Open Macular

Elevated open macular holes were always regarded as surgical failure.

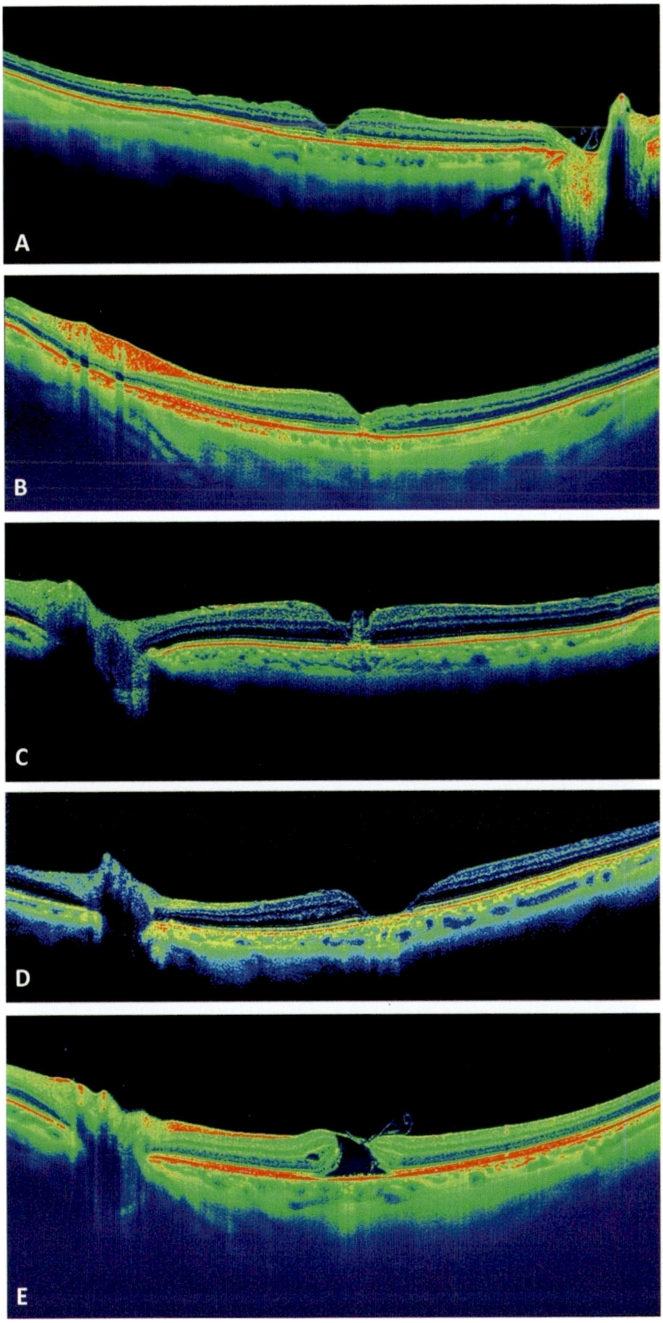

Fig. 1 Macular hole closure types. **a** U-type closure, **b** V-type closure, **c** irregular closure, **d** type 2 closure, **e** flap closure

2.4 The Flap Closure

Along with the introduction of the Inverted ILM technique a new closure type was distinguished (Fig. 1e). The flap closure represents an appearance, in which the hole is closed only with a thin flap of the ILM, which further leads to Muller cells proliferation and to restoration of other retinal layers with time.

2.5 Type 2 Closure

Type 2 closure was not reported to be a result of surgery with the use of the Inverted ILM Flap Technique. Probably eyes which would develop type 2 closure, tend to achieve the flap closure when the inverted ILM flap technique is used. Final vision is worse when compared to the U type or V type closure, but far better than the type 2 closure [10].

3 The History of the Inverted ILM Flap Technique

Despite the fact that ILM peeling was a gamechanger in full thickness macular holes surgery the results were still not satisfactory. The 90' were an era of search for different adjuvants to aid ILM peeling, especially in difficult cases. None of the substances proposed during this time period (tissue glue, autologous blood and others) resulted in replicable improvement of results.

The first surgery with the use of the Inverted ILM Flap Technique was performed in 2006 by Jerzy Nawrocki in a large, long-standing FTMH. The idea was initiated by precise analysis of all surgical videos performed by JN in that time period. The area of our special interest at that time were surgical failures and type 2 closures. In one case, in which a FTMH failed to close, during reviewing of the surgical video, JN had the idea that complete ILM peeling might have caused an unintentional peeling of a small part of retinal tissue. He had the feeling that if he did not peel the ILM completely, the hole would maybe close (Fig. 2).

Thus, he started to continue ILM peeling, but always to stop peeling at the margin of the macular hole, and to invert all flaps in a closing-flower like fashion.

His primary aim was not only to increase the success rate of FTMH surgery, but additionally to avoid type 2 closures.

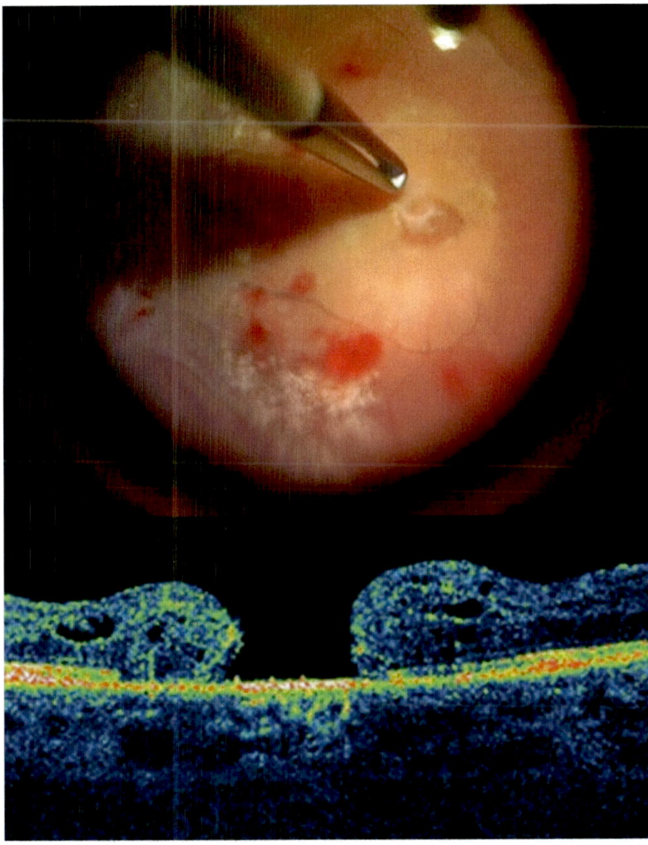

Fig. 2 Upper: intraoperative image of the patient who inspired JN to invent the inverted ILM Flap Technique. The tissue visible in the central part of the macular hole, was removed. When the surgery failed JN had the impression that leaving it intact might have facilitated the healing process. Lower: postoperative SOCT image of failed surgery

4 Inverted ILM flap Technique

4.1 Original Technique

In our first publication [11], we proposed the following steps of the inverted ILM flap technique (Fig. 3) and proved its almost 100% success rate in large full thickness macular holes.

- Core vitrectomy
- Trypan blue staining
- ILM peeling around the fovea with formation of several flaps, that were aimed to close the hole like a flower is closed after sunset.

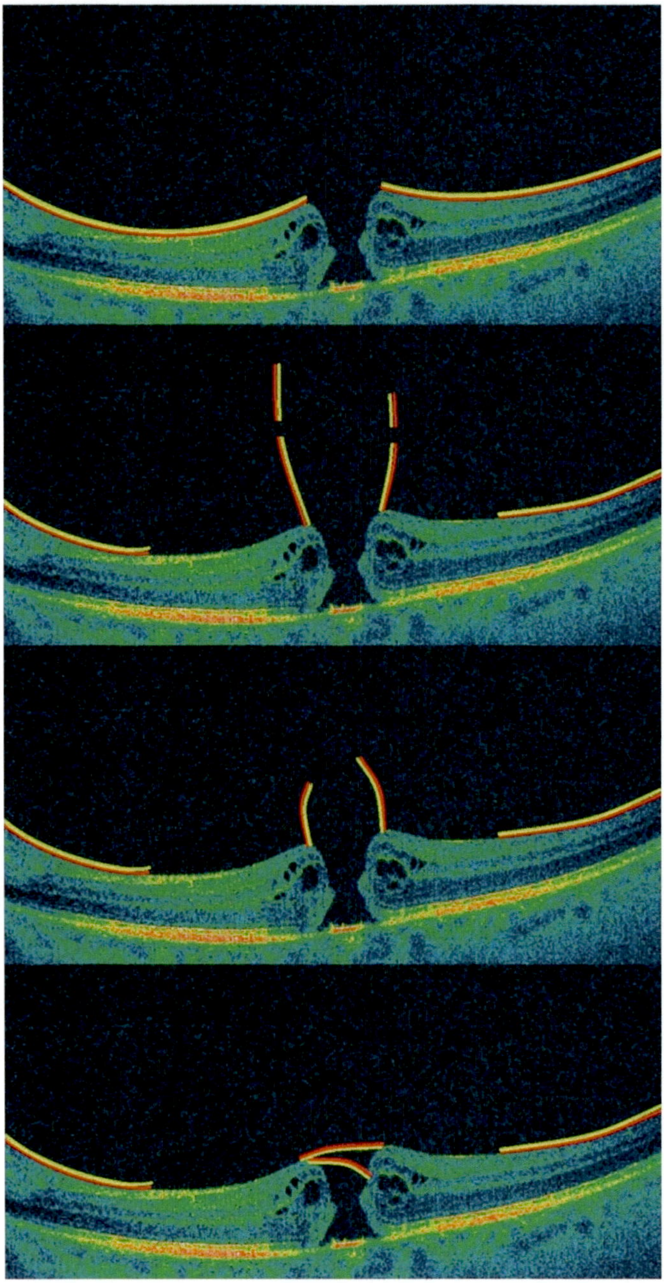

Fig. 3 Inverted ILM flap technique

- All flaps were shortened with a vitrectome.
- The flaps were never pushed inside, always positioned on the top of the macular hole.
- Air tamponade.

4.2 The Temporal Inverted ILM Flap Technique

Nowadays the authors technique of choice is the temporal inverted ILM flap technique [12] (Fig. 4).

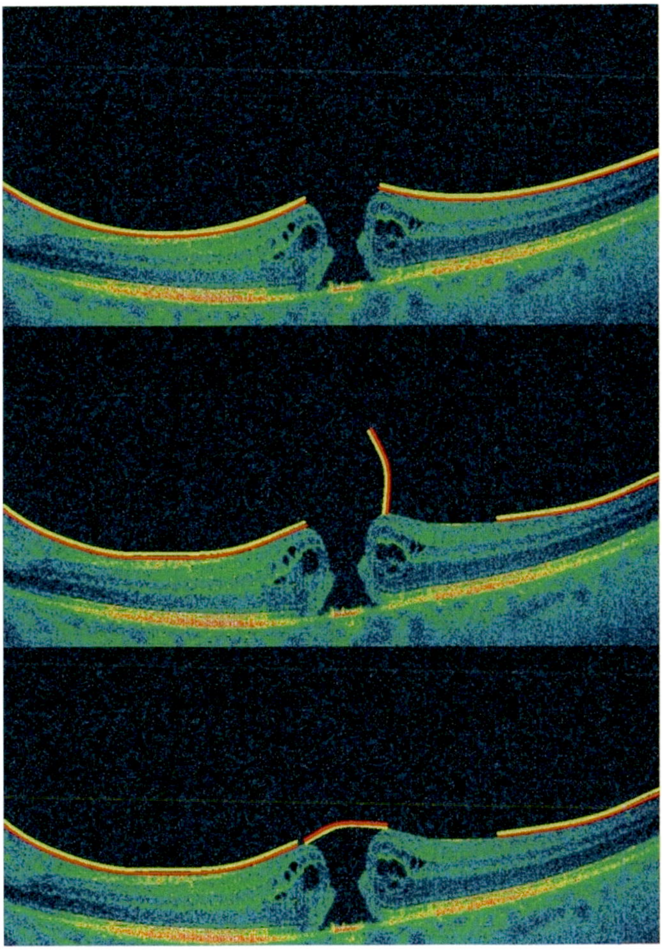

Fig. 4 Temporal inverted ILM flap technique

- Core vitrectomy
- Membrane blue staining
- ILM peeling only from the temporal side of the macular hole and gentle positioning of the flap on the top of the macular hole, never pushed inside.
- Viscoelastic positioned on the surface of the flap (Methylcellulose)
- Air tamponade.

The temporal inverted ILM flap technique is the only modification of the original method, which was compared to the original technique in a prospective randomized study. We proved that it is non-inferior in regard to anatomical and functional outcome to the original inverted ILM flap technique reported by our group. Moreover, it reduces defects of the nerve fiber layer on the nasal side of the fovea. We additionally observed that deep retinal vessels are altered in the area of ILM peeling and remain unchanged in the area, where no ILM removal was performed [13] (Fig. 5).

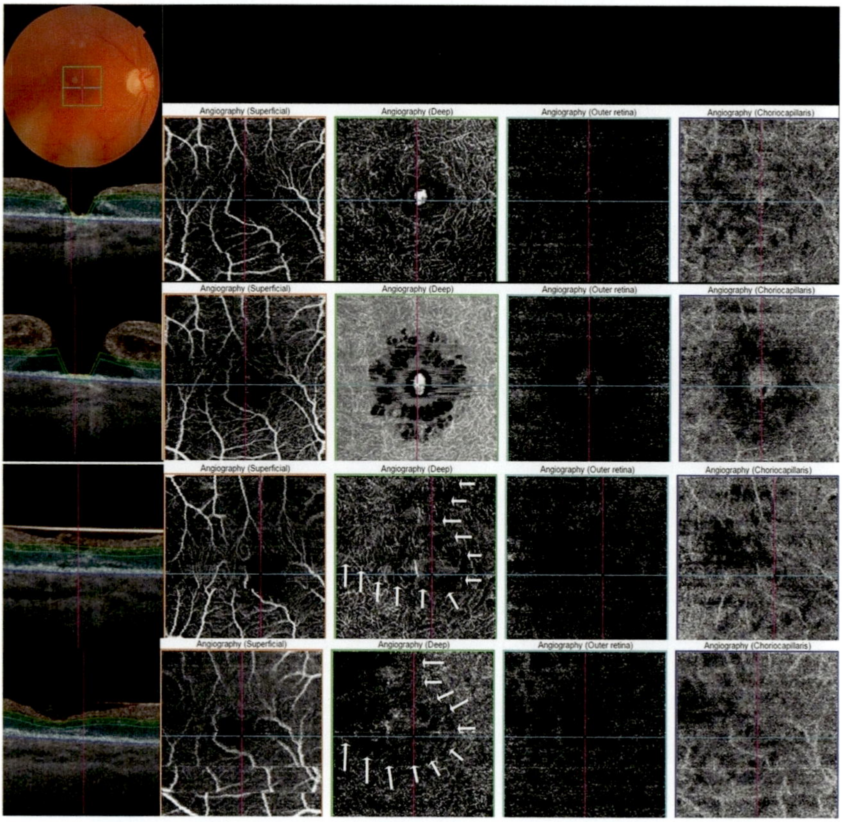

Fig. 5 SD-OCT and SS-OCT angiography of fovea healing 1 month and six months after surgery. The arrows present areas of ILM peeling corresponding to increased irregularities of vessels in the deep retinal vessels layer

4.3 *Modifications of the Original Technique*

1. Insertion technique. This is a method in which the flap is inserted inside the hole, instead of positioning it on the top. This technique should be avoided.

   It was confirmed that ILM finishing, tucking and massage is not necessary to obtain surgical success [14, 15]. Moreover covering the hole with the ILM is superior to pushing it inside in regard to final visual outcome [16].
2. Perfluorocarbon was also reported to enable the stabilization of the flap. In a comparative study the authors have proven better anatomical results in the ILM flap group stabilized with perfluorocarbon when compared to conventional peeling [17]. There is lack of comparative data to prove whether perfluorocarbon is superior to viscoelastic used by the authors of this chapter.
3. Choice of Tamponade. In the original technique air tamponade was used. Most later authors used SF6 in their studies. As the results are similar, probably it is not necessary to use longer-acting gasses.

   The authors of the current technique usually advise their patients to keep prone positioning for 3-5 days. However, it was also suggested by others that patients with a C3F8 tamponade and without positioning obtain results non-inferior to positioned patients [18].
4. Positioning. The authors of the current chapter usually advise patients to keep 3–5 days of prone positioning. However, there are reports stating that surgical success might be achieved even in large holes without positioning [18].

5 Mechanism of Action

ILM is a base membrane for Muller cells enabling cell proliferation [19]. We suggested in 2010 the possible mechanism of action of the inverted ILM flap technique is stimulation of Muller cell proliferation with its possible regrowth on the ILM serving as a scaffold. We observed photoreceptors reappearing in the foveal center and extrapolated that either happens secondary to redistribution of existing photoreceptors due to Muller cell gliosis or, what seemed highly improbable in those times, due to new photoreceptor formation [11] (Fig. 6).

Later, Shiode and coworkers, confirmed in non-human primates that the ILM serves in fact as a scaffold for the proliferation and migration of Muller cells and additionally may promote Muller cell activation [20]. Moreover, Morawski and coworkers confirmed with in vitro studies that regeneration is possible in adult retina when the inverted ILM flap technique is used [22].

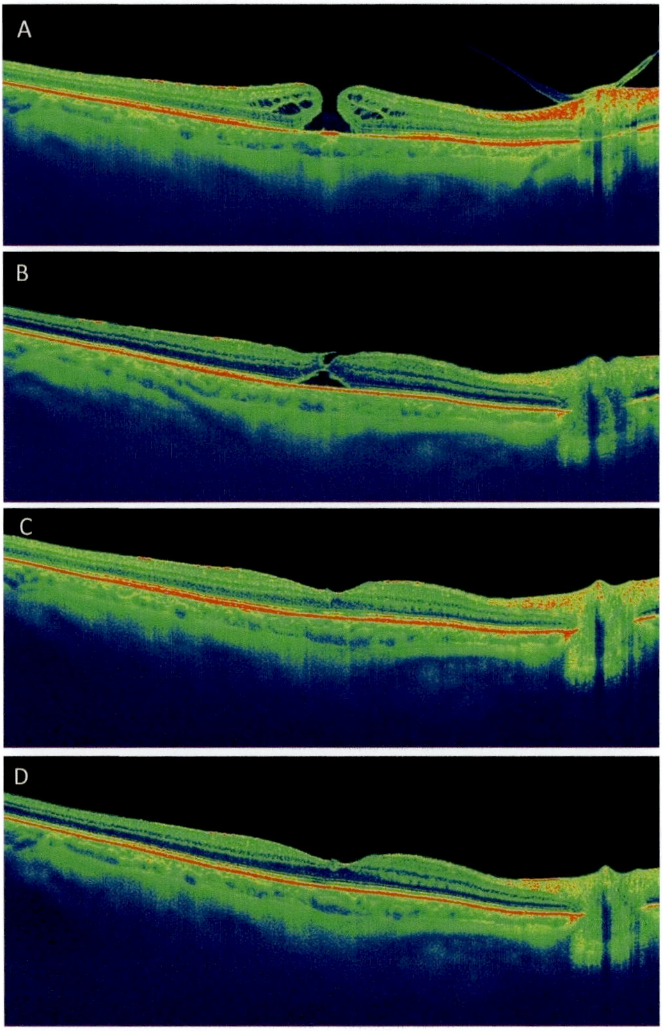

Fig. 6 **a** Full thickness macular hole in 71-year-old woman. **b** One week after surgery. **c** Five months after surgery. **d** Twelve months after surgery

6 Indications

6.1 Large, Long Standing Macular holes

The first described indication for the Inverted ILM Flap Technique is large, long standing macular holes. In a prospective, randomized clinical trial we reported that, 88% holes were closed in patients, in whom ILM peeling was performed and in

98% of patients treated with the Inverted ILM Flap Technique. Type 2 closure was observed in 19% of cases treated with ILM peeling and in none of the eyes treated with the Inverted ILM Flap Technique. Functional results correlated with anatomical outcome, showing inferiority of ILM peeling. This was confirmed by other comparative studies.

6.2 *Full Thickness Macular holes with myopia*

FTMHs associated with high myopia, with and without coexisting retinal detachment benefit from the inverted ILM flap technique. There are several studies comparing ILM peeling and the inverted ILM Flap in this indication. Mete and coworkers concluded that the odds ratio of the variable surgical technique indicated that the likelihood of surgical effectiveness was increased by 22.96 times when the Inverted ILM Flap Technique was performed [23]. Similarly, Rizzo presented a closure rate of 88.4% while using the inverted ILM Flap Technique, when compared to 38.9% closures with ILM peeling [24].

The functional results are better if the flap is positioned gently on the surface (as originally described by the authors) when compared to situations in which it was pushed inside the hole. It was true for high myopic macular holes which were, and which were not associated with retinal detachment [25]. Macular buckling was reported to be successful in retinal reattachment in myopic macular hole associated retinal detachment, but macular hole closure rates were difficult to estimate [26]. The hole closure rate of vitrectomy with ILM peeling was reported to be around 10–90% [27]. In one study it was reported there is no difference in final visual acuity between ILM peeling and the inverted ILM flap technique, which was probably associated with the fact, that drainage through the macular hole was performed during surgery [28]. Most other reports confirm a visual benefit with the inverted ILM flap technique [15].

6.3 *Full Thickness Macular holes Coexisting with Proliferative Diabetic retinopathy*

FTMHs coexisting with proliferative diabetic retinopathy have a similar appearance to myopic holes with a very high base diameter to minimum diameter ratio (1:10, when compared to 1:2 in idiopathic cases), which made them again a good candidate for the inverted ILM flap technique. It is important to note, that the closure begins in the inner retinal layers and if the hole is closed, the retina reattaches within several weeks or months [29] (Fig. 7).

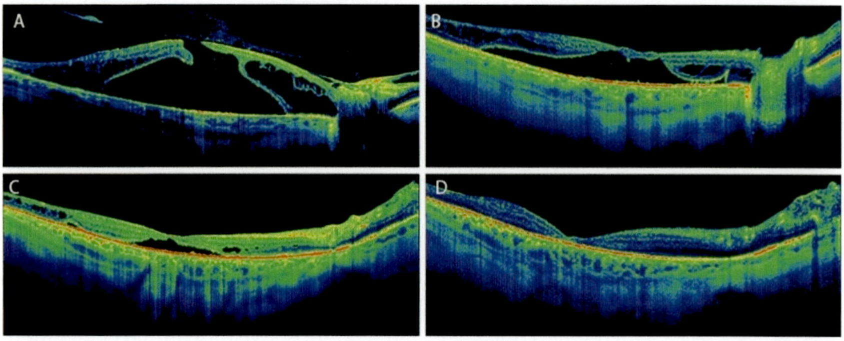

Fig. 7 **a** Full thickness macular hole in proliferative diabetic retinopathy. Minimum diameter is 507 μm. Maximum hole diameter is 5302 μm. The minimum to maximum diameter ratio is 1:10 which is much higher than in idiopathic macular holes. **b** One month after surgery, the MH was closed but subretinal fluid was still visible, and VA was 20/320 (1.2 logMAR; 0.063 Snellen). **c** Five months after surgery, VA was 20/320 (1.2 logMAR; 0.063 Snellen). **d** Twelve months after surgery VA was 20/500 (1.4 logMAR; 0.04 Snellen)

6.4 Full Thickness Macular holes Coexisting with Rhegmatogenous Retinal detachment

It was also confirmed that the inverted ILM flap technique was superior to ILM peeling in rhegmatogenous retinal detachment associated with full thickness macular holes [30, 31].

6.5 Full Thickness Macular holes Coexisting with Age Related Macular Degeneration

FTMHs in age related macular degeneration (dry and neovascular) are also successfully closed with the inverted ILM flap. Visual acuity improved significantly after surgery [32, 33].

6.6 Expanded Indications

Other indications include FTMHs in Coats disease, retinitis pigmentosa, trauma [34], uveitis [35] and others.

We suggested for many years that also small FTMHs might benefit from the inverted ILM flap technique due to the rare events of failure. In cases, in which the inverted ILM flap was used during the primary surgery, visual rehabilitation after second surgery is improved. Several authors now confirmed that also small macular holes are an indication to this surgery. They reported good anatomical and functional outcomes [24, 26]. The authors of this review perform vitrectomy with the inverted ILM flap technique in all eyes with a full thickness macular hole.

We also described its efficacy and long-term results in inserting the ILM flap into the optic nerve pit with associated maculopathy. In this method the flap is inserted into the optic disc pit and stuffed inside. It enables to achieve long-lasting improvement of anatomy and vision [37, 38].

7 Visual Acuity

Similarly, to the anatomical outcome, which is improved with the inverted ILM flap technique, also visual outcome is satisfactory. In our first study we reported that ILM peeling resulted in 20/38 (0.28 logMAR; 0.52 Snellen) and the inverted ILM flap in 20/29 (0.17 logMAR; 0.67 Snellen) visual acuity in large macular holes [11].

The functional results were also good in the first 44 eyes operated with the temporal inverted ILM flap technique. Mean visual acuity improved to 20/91 (0.66 logMAR 0.21 Snellen) at month three and to 20/50 (0.4 logMAR 0.4 Snellen) at month twelve postoperatively [12]. The temporal inverted ILM flap technique was described as non-inferior to the original technique and resulted in less retina nerve fiber layer defects.

The first metaanalysis performed on that subject confirmed that the inverted ILM flap technique is associated with anatomical and functional results superior to ILM peeling [39]. Recently, Kastl and coworkers achieved an improvement of visual acuity from 20/100 (0.7 logMAR; 0.2 Snellen) to 20/40 (0.3 logMAR; 0.5 Snellen) in FTMH 250-400um. They advise to use a single layered flap for small FTMHs, proving it is safe and effective [36].

When ILM peeling is used, both anatomical success and final visual outcome strongly depend on the size of the FTMH. This predictive factor lost its significance with the advent of the Inverted ILM Flap Technique, as almost all holes, irrespective the hole size and character might be closed [40].

Chou and coworkers, in a recent study, evaluated patients with small FTMHs. They concluded that vision improves faster in the inverted ILM flap group, which correlates with improved restoration of the external limiting membrane and interdigitation zone. This technique is also associated with significantly less postoperative gliosis [41].

There are few studies discussing microperimetry in eyes after the inverted ILM flap technique. In a study comparing 25 eyes treated with ILM peeling to 25 eyes treated with the inverted ILM flap technique, the authors realized, that in small macular holes, microperimetry was better in eyes, that underwent ILM peeling. That is contradictory to another study, proving that microperimetry is worse in ILM peeled areas when compared to areas, where the ILM is inverted upside down [42].

8 Epiretinal membrane Formation

We earlier reported a growing incidence of epiretinal membranes in cases, in which we did not peel the ILM completely in PVR retinal detachments [43]. Thus, in the early days of the Inverted ILM Flap Technique we were also a little concerned about the possibility of ERM formation. Thus, the initial technique consisted of peeling the ILM from all sides of the fovea. We additionally shortened the ILM from all sides. With the development of the technique, we started to peel the ILM only from the temporal side and to leave the unshorten piece of ILM on the top of the fovea. We performed a study, evaluating the visibility of ILM remnants. Our conclusion was that in idiopathic cases, in none of the analyzed cases ERM developed. Moreover, there were no differences in final visual acuity between eyes with and without ILM remnants visible in the SS-OCT [10]. However, the situation might differ in the rare cases of rhegmatogenous retinal detachment with coexisting FTMH. A group from Osaka reported histopathologically confirmed a case of ERM growth on the ILM Flap used in such a case. Visual acuity improved after ERM removal in their patient [44].

9 Repeated Surgeries

Even up to 44% of complicated FTMHs might remain open after vitrectomy with ILM peeling. The number is reduced to about 2–4% with the use of the inverted ILM flap technique.

Historically, when ILM peeling failed, further surgeries were frequently abandoned. Some surgeons used silicone oil during secondary intervention. It was also reported that enlarging the area of ILM peeling might be of some benefit [45]. Massage of the macular hole [46] usually associated with retinal pigment epithelium defects and low final vision, was never very popular.

The above-described methods were associated with limited success. Because of that during the last few years, several techniques, basing on the idea of the Inverted ILM Flap Technique, were developed in order to improve the outcome of repeated surgery after initial failure of ILM peeling.

If the ILM was peeled completely during the primary attempt, during secondary surgery different techniques might be used. An autologous ILM transplantation, described by Morizane and coworkers, is an elegant surgery [47] but complicated by the fact that ILM is thickest in the fovea area and thins to the periphery. This results in more challenging maneuvers if ILM is going to be harvested from besides the arcades. Morizane inserted the ILM Flap transplant under the edges of the macular hole. The authors of this chapter modified this technique by putting the harvested ILM on the top of the macular hole, which is in agreement with the general philosophy of the inverted flap technique. An additional challenge is to keep the harvested ILM on the top of the fovea during fluid air exchange.

Different other materials were used to close the hole, as anterior or posterior lens capsule [48], amniotic membrane [24] or autologous retinal transplant [49]. Visual acuity was reported to be higher with the use of anterior lens capsule, when compared to the posterior lens capsule. The functional outcome of repeated surgery with the use of amniotic membrane are dependent on its preparation and storage. Autologous retinal transplant is theoretically associated with a higher risk of retinal detachment. However good outcomes were reported in selected cases.

However, in the rare events of failure of the inverted ILM flap technique we might either reposition the flap or create another flap during repeated surgery [50]. The surgical technique is easier when compared to those described above and final anatomy and function are better (Fig. 8).

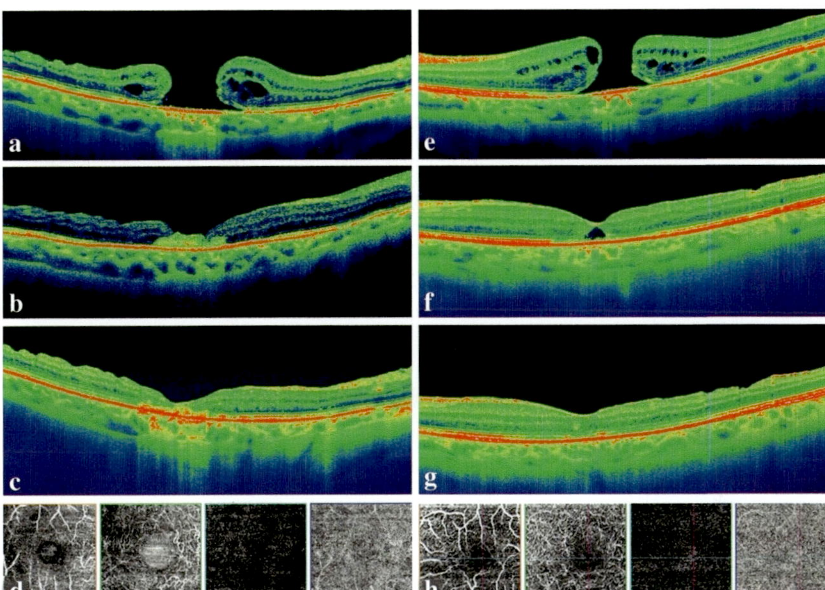

Fig. 8 Comparison of repeated surgery with an amniotic membrane and with a temporal inverted ILM flap. **a** Full thickness macular hole after primary vitrectomy and ILM peeling, performed in another clinic. **b** One month after vitrectomy with amniotic membrane. Visual acuity is 20/400 (1.3 logMAR; 0.05 Snellen). **c** Eighteen months after vitrectomy with amniotic membrane. Visual acuity is 20/400 (1.3 logMAR; 0.05 Snellen). **d** Swept source OCT angiography (SS-OCT A) of the same eye after eighteen months after vitrectomy with amniotic membrane. **e** Full thickness macular hole in the second eye of the same patient after primary vitrectomy with no peeling, performed in another clinic. **f** One month after vitrectomy with temporal inverted ILM flap. Visual acuity is 20/200 (1.0 logMAR; 0.1 Snellen). **g** Eighteen months after vitrectomy temporal with inverted ILM flap. Visual acuity is 20/32 (0.2 logMAR; 0.63 Snellen). **h** Swept source OCT angiography (SS-OCT A) of the second eye of the same patient after eighteen months after vitrectomy with inverted ILM flap

10 Clinical Pearls

1. Never insert the ILM into the hole
2. Viscoelastic material might facilitate maintaining the flap in position.
3. All full thickness macular holes might be treated with this technique.
4. Surgical failures are always due to returning of the flap to its original position on the surface of the retina. During repeated surgery performing the temporal inverted ILM Flap Technique again is easy and associated with satisfactory functional outcome.

11 Key Points

1. Inverted Flap is the method of choice in large and high myopic macular holes.
2. Type 2 closure was never observed after the inverted ILM flap technique.
3. Failure rate of the inverted ILM flap technique is about 4% and repeated surgery with the inverted ILM Flap Technique is simple and logic.
4. Improvement of visual acuity was reported to be quicker than with ILM peeling.

References

1. Knapp H. Ueber isolerte zerreissungen der aderhaut in folge von traumen auf dem augapfel. Arch Augenklinik. 1869;1:6–29.
2. Rahmani B, Tielsch JM, Katz J, Gottsch J, Quigley H, Javitt J, Sommer. The cause-specific prevalence of visual impairment in an urban population. Balt Eye Surv Ophthalmol. 1996;103(11):1721–6.
3. McCannel CA, Ensminger JL, Diehl NN, Hodge DN. Population-based incidence of macular holes. Ophthalmol. 2009;116(7):1366–9.
4. Niwa H, Terasaki H, Ito Y, Miyake Y. Macular hole development in fellow eyes of patients with unilateral macular hole. Am J Ophthalmol. 2005;140(3):370–5.
5. Smiddy WE. Macular hole formation without vitreofoveal traction. Arch Ophthalmol. 2008;126(5):737–8.
6. Medina CA, Ortiz AG, Relhan N, Smiddy WE, Townsend JH, Flynn HW Jr. Macular hole after pars plana vitrectomy for rhegmatogenous retinal detachment. Retina. 2017;37(6):1065–72.
7. Michalewska Z, Nawrocki J. Swept-source OCT angiography of full-thickness macular holes: appearance and artifact. Ophthalmic Surg Lasers Imaging Retin. 2018;49(2):111–21.
8. Tornambe PE. Macular hole genesis: the hydration theory. Retina. 2003;23(3):421.
9. Nawrocka ZA, Nawrocka Z, Nawrocki J. Spontaneous closure of full-thickness macular holes. Ophthalmologica. 2022;245(1):49–58.
10. Bonińska K, Nawrocki J, Michalewska Z. Mechanism of "flap closure" after the inverted internal limiting membrane flap technique. Retina. 2018;38:2184–9.
11. Michalewska Z, Michalewski J, Adelman RA, Nawrocki J. Inverted internal limiting membrane flap technique for large macular holes. Ophthalmology. 2010;117:2018–25.
12. Michalewska Z, Michalewski J, Dulczewska-Cichecka K, Adelman RA, Nawrocki J. Temporal inverted internal limiting membrane flap technique versus classic inverted internal limiting membrane flap technique: a comparative study. Retina. 2015;35:1844–50.

13. Michalewska Z, Nawrocki J. Swept source OCT angiography reveals ILM peeling alters deep retinal vasculature. Retina. 2018;S154–S160.
14. Casini G, Mura M, Figus M, Loiudice P, Peiretti E, De Cillà S, Fuentes T, Nasini F. Inverted internal limiting membrane flap technique for macular hole surgery without extra manipulation of the flap. Retina. 2017;37:2138–44.
15. Sasaki H, Shiono A, Kogo J, Yomoda R, Munemasa Y, Syoda M, Otake H, Kurihara H, Kitaoka Y, Takagi H. Inverted internal limiting membrane flap technique as a useful procedure for macular hole associated retinal detachment in highly myopic eyes. Eye. 2017;31:545–50.
16. Tao M, Wang G, Gou Y, Zhang M. Comparative study of conventional inverted ILM flap covering and ILM flap filling technique in idiopathic macular hole treatment: a meta-analysis and systematic review. J Ophthalmol. 2022;2022(19):4922616.
17. Pak KY, Park JY, Park SW, Byon IS, Lee JE. Efficacy of the perfluoro-N-octane-assisted single-layered inverted internal limiting membrane flap technique for large macular holes. Ophthalmologica. 2017;238:133–8.
18. Ruparelia S, Tuli R, Park JSY, Shoham-Hazon N, Berco E. Inverted internal limiting membrane flap technique without postoperative face-down positioning for macular hole repair. Retina. 2022;1(42):548–52.
19. Winter M, Eberhardt W, Scholz C, Reichenbach A. Failure of potassium siphoning by Müller cells: a new hypothesis of perfluorocarbon liquid-induced retinopathy. Invest Ophthalmol Vis Sci. 2000;41:256e261.
20. Shiode Y, Morizane Y, Matoba R, Hirano M, Doi S, Toshima S, et al. The role of inverted internal limiting membrane flap in macular hole closure. Invest Ophthalmol Vis Sci. 2017;58(1):4847–55.
21. Morawski K, Kocemba-Pilarczyk K, Zarzycka M, Dudzik P, Trojan SE, Laidler P. In vitro culture Muller cell model to study the role of inverted internal limiting membrane flap technique in macular hole closure. J Physiol Pharmacol. 2021;72(3).
22. Mete M, Alfano A, Guerriero M, Prigione G, Sartore M, Polito A, Pertile G. Inverted internal limiting membrane flap technique versus complete internal limiting Membrane removal in myopic Macular hole surgery. A comparative study. Retina. 2017;37(10):1923–30.
23. Rizzo S, Tartaro R, Barca F, Caporossi T, Bacherini D, Giansanti F. Internal limiting membrane peeling versus inverted flap technique for treatment of full-thickness macular holes: a comparative study in a large series of patients. Retina. 2018;38(1):S73–8.
24. Chatziralli I, Machairoudia G, Kazantzis D, Theodossiadis G, Theodossiadis P. Inverted internal limiting membrane flap technique for myopic hole: a meta-analysis. Surv Ophthalmol. 2021;66:771–80.
25. Ando F, Ohba N, Touura K, Hirose H. Anatomical and visual outcomes after episcleral macular buckling compared with those after pars plana vitrectomy for retinal detachment caused by macular hole in highly myopic eyes. Retina. 2007;27:37–44.
26. Kadonosono K, Yazawa F, Itoh N, Uchio E, Nakamura S, Akura J, et al. Treatment of retinal detachment resulting from myopic macular hole with internal limiting membrane removal. Am J Ophthalmol. 2001;131:203–7.
27. Baba R, Wakabayashi Y, Umazume K, Ishikawa T, Yagi H, Muramatsu D, Goto H. Efficacy of the inverted internal limiting membrane flap technique with vitrectomy for retinal detachment associated with myopic macular holes. Retina. 2017;37:466–71.
28. Michalewska Z, Nawrocki J. Fovea morphology after vitrectomy in eyes with full-thickness macular hole coexisting with diabetic retinopathy. J Vitr Retin Dis. 2020;9:53–9.
29. Jian Y, Nie L, Liu S, Jiang Y, Dou Z, Liu X, Yao X, Fu C. Comparison of internal limiting membrane peeling with the inverted internal limiting membrane flap technique for rhegmatogenous retinal detachment coexisting with macular hole. Retina. 2022;1(42):697–703.
30. Stappler T, Montesel A, Konstantinidis L, Wolfensberger TJ, Eandi CM. Inverted internal limiting membrane flap technique for macular hole coexistent with rhegmatogenous retinal detachment. Retina. 2022;1(42):1491–7.
31. Michalewska Z, Nawrocki J. Vitrectomy with the inverted internal limiting membrane flap technique in eyes with full-thickness macular hole and dry age-related macular degeneration. Eur J Ophthalmol. 2021;31:1320–5.

32. Nawrocka ZA, Nawrocka Z, Nawrocki J. Vitrectomy for full thickness macular hole developed during the course of anti-VEGF treatment of type 1 neovascular AMD. Eur J Ophthalmol. 2021;19(3):11206721211002123. Online ahead of print.
33. Abou Shousha MA. Inverted internal limiting membrane flap for large traumatic macular holes. Medicine (Baltimore). 2016;95: e2523.
34. Hirano M, Morizane Y, Kawata T, Kimura S, et al. Case report: successful closure of a large macular hole secondary to uveitis using the inverted internal limiting membrane flap technique. BMC Ophthalmol. 2015;15:83.
35. Kastl G, Heidenkummer P, Koss MJ. 360° inverted internal limiting membrane flap technique for idiopathic macular holes ≤ 250 μm, > 250 and ≤ 400 μm, and > 400 μm. Graefes Arch Clin Exp Ophthalmol. 2022;260:2183–90.
36. Nawrocki J, Boninska K, Michalewska Z. Managing optic pit. The right stuff! Retina. 2016;36:2430–2.
37. Michalewska Z, Nawrocka Z, Nawrocki J. Swept-source OCT and swept-source OCT angiography before and after vitrectomy with stuffing of the optic pit. Ophthalmol Retina. 2020;4:927–37.
38. Gu C, Qiu Q. Inverted internal limiting membrane flap technique for large macular holes: a systematic review and single-arm meta-analysis. Graefes Arch Clin Exp Ophthalmol. 2018;256:1041–9.
39. Narnaware SH, Bawankule PK, Bansal A, Chakraborty M, Raje D, Nagdeve R, Chivane A. Pre-operative optical coherence tomography predictors: do they hold any relevance in the era of inverted internal limiting membrane flap in large macular holes? Indian J Ophthalmol. 2022;70(5):1689–94.
40. Chou HD, Liu L, Wang CT, Chen KJ, Wu WC, Hwang YS, Chen YP, Kang EY, Chen YH, Yeung L, Lai CC. Single-layer inverted internal limiting membrane flap versus conventional peel for small- or medium-sized full-thickness macular holes. Am J Ophthalmol. 2022;235:111–9.
41. Kaluzny JJ, Zabel P, Kaluzna M, Lamkowski A, Jaworski D, Woznicki K, Zabel K. Macular sensitivity in the area of internal limiting membranePeeling in eyes after pars plana vitrectomy with the temporal Inverted internal limiting Membrane flap technique for a Full-thickness macular hole. Retina. 2021;41(8):1627–34.
42. Odrobina D, Bednarski M, Cisiecki S, Michalewska Z, Kuhn F, Nawrocki J. Internal limiting membrane peeling as prophylaxis of macular pucker formation in eyes undergoing retinectomy for severe proliferative vitreoretinopathy. Retina. 2012;32:226–31.
43. Kanda K, Nakashima H, Emi K. Macular pucker formation after inverted internal limiting membrane flap technique: two case reports. Am J Ophthalmol Case Rep. 2022;20(25):101282.
44. Moisseiev E, Fabian ID, Moisseiev J, Barak A. Outcomes of repeated pars plana vitrectomy for persistent macular holes. Retina. 2013;33(6):1137–43.
45. Alpatov S, Shchuko A, Malyshev V. A new method of treating macular holes. Eur J Ophthalmol. 2007;17(2):246–52.
46. Morizane Y, Shiraga F, Kimura S, Hosokawa M, Shiode Y, Kawata T, Hosogi M, Shirakata Y, Okanouchi T. Autologous transplantation of the internal limiting membrane for refractory macular holes. Am J Ophthalmol. 2014;157:861-869.e1.
47. Chen SN, Yang CM. Lens capsular flap transplantation in the management of refractory macular hole from multiple etiologies. Retina. 2016;36(1):163–70.
48. Thomas AS, Mahmoud TH. Subretinal transplantation of an autologous retinal free flap forchronic retinal detachment with proliferative vitreoretinopathy with and without macular hole. Retina. 2018;38(Suppl 1):S121–4.
49. Michalewska Z, Nawrocki J. Repeated surgery in primary failed vitrectomy for macular holes—a comparative study of primary classical ILM peeling vs. primary inverted ILM flap technique. Ophthalmic Surg Lasers Imaging. 2018;49(8):611–8.

Use of Amniotic Membrane for MH Closure

Stanislao Rizzo, Tomaso Caporossi, and Alfonso Savastano

Abstract In this chapter we shall analyze and focus our attention on the use of human amniotic membrane (hAM) when we are dealing with refractory macular holes or very large macular holes (diameter > 800 μm). In these cases, hAM can be very useful to achieve the closure of these holes, and different types of membranes can be used today according to the surgeons' choices and also the availability of tissues. We will examine several themes regarding the use of hAM in difficult cases and try to impart some technical advice to help manage hAM during vitrectomy. One of the main points to keep in mind is to have correct hAM management and surgical outcome, it is compulsory to have a specific equipment to perform this kind of surgery: some instruments cannot be exchanged with "similar" tools. Proper instruments, from the hAM preparation to its implant into the macular hole, *must be* available in order to carry out good quality and safe surgery. Another consideration worth making is that, despite the great anatomical success we can achieve using the hAM in refractory macular holes or very large macular holes, sometimes the visual acuity of this patients' eyes, may not be very satisfactory. Hence our main recommendation to use hAM only when strictly necessary, and when a previous vitrectomy has already failed in macular hole closure.

Supplementary Information The online version contains supplementary material available at https://doi.org/10.1007/978-3-031-63508-3_9.

S. Rizzo · T. Caporossi · A. Savastano (✉)
Catholic University Sacro Cuore, Rome, Italy
e-mail: alfonso.savastano@policlinicogemelli.it

S. Rizzo · A. Savastano
Ophthalmology Unit, Fondazione Policlinico Universitario A. Gemelli IRCCS, Rome, Italy

S. Rizzo
Consiglio Nazionale delle Ricerche, Istituto di Neuroscienze, Pisa, Italy

T. Caporossi
Vitreoretinal Surgery Unit, Isola Tiberina Gemelli Isola Hospital, Rome, Italy

F. Patelli et al. (eds.), *Macular Surgery*, https://doi.org/10.1007/978-3-031-63508-3_9

Keywords Human amniotic membrane · Vitrectomy · Vitreoretinal surgery · Macular surgery · Macular hole · Refractory macular hole · Macular hole recurrence · Persistent macular hole · Macular hole failure surgery

1 Introduction

Macular hole surgery has seen radical changes during the last decades. The introduction of human amniotic membrane (hAM) has, since its introduction in clinical practice (first described in 2019) [1], solved two main issues: refractory macular holes and very large holes (diameter > 800 μm). hAM has since been used in so many fields of vitreoretinal surgery [2]. Generally, for *refractory macular hole* we are referring to a macular hole failure closure of initial vitrectomy. Even if the peeling of the inner limiting membrane (ILM) and the inverted flap technique radically and positively changed the surgical outcomes of a macular hole greater than 400 μm, there are still difficult cases in which the macular hole relapses, or worse, it remains open after the surgery [3, 4]. On the other hand, the ILM peeling should be the surgical choice only for macular holes with a diameter greater than 400 μm, as the ILM removal can lead to worse visual acuity outcomes by comparison to eyes which had not the ILM removed [5, 6]. Keeping this concept in mind, we find it very useful to divide these conditions as follows:

- *Macular hole recurrence*: a macular hole that has been vitrectomized and after a period of closure, it relapses again.
- *Persistent / Refractory macular hole*: a macular hole that has been vitrectomized and the hole continues to remain opened.

In general, we use these two conditions in the context of **macular hole failure surgery**.

It is very important from the surgical viewpoint to have an indication regarding the ILM status. In fact, in both the above-mentioned cases (*recurrence* and *persistent/ refractory* macular holes) the ILM peeling, eventually carrying out an ILM inverted flap technique, is highly recommended. While in those cases in which the ILM has already been peeled, an alternative surgical choice has to be considered in order to achieve the macular hole closure. Moreover, the awareness of the ILM status, could be very important from a safety point of view. In fact, to peel the ILM usually vital dye is used to visualize the ILM itself. We know that the vital dyes can be toxic if applied onto a bare retina and are both useless and potentially harmful [7, 8].

Taking this into account, we will focus our attention on the surgical technique of using hAM in cases of *macular hole failure surgery* or in large macular holes that are usually considered already refractory at the diagnosis, due to their dimension [9].

2 hAM Preparation

One of the milestones of hAM use in vitreoretinal surgery is its preparation. The use of skin biopsy punches (Fig. 1) enables very small but perfect regular and circular hAM discs (from 1 mm up to 6 mm or even larger). Usually the Bank of Eyes (place where corneas and other human ocular tissues are stored and then distributed according to the demand) supplies the hAM in a vial with different storage liquids. The hAM is generally spread out (chorion side down) onto a sheet of tiny stiff plastic so that the hAM can be easily secured and prepared (Fig. 2). The typical procedure, is to carry out 2 or 3 punches of the hAM onto a soft material so that the circular blade of the skin biopsy punch can precisely cut both the hAM and the plastic sheet below. The discs obtained (hAM above and plastic below) are kept in the skin biopsy punch. At this stage the surgeon can directly observe the hAM discs in the punch. After tilting them, the last disc can be secured, and the hAM can be separated from the plastic disc below (Fig. 3). This maneuver can be easily performed using ILM forceps.

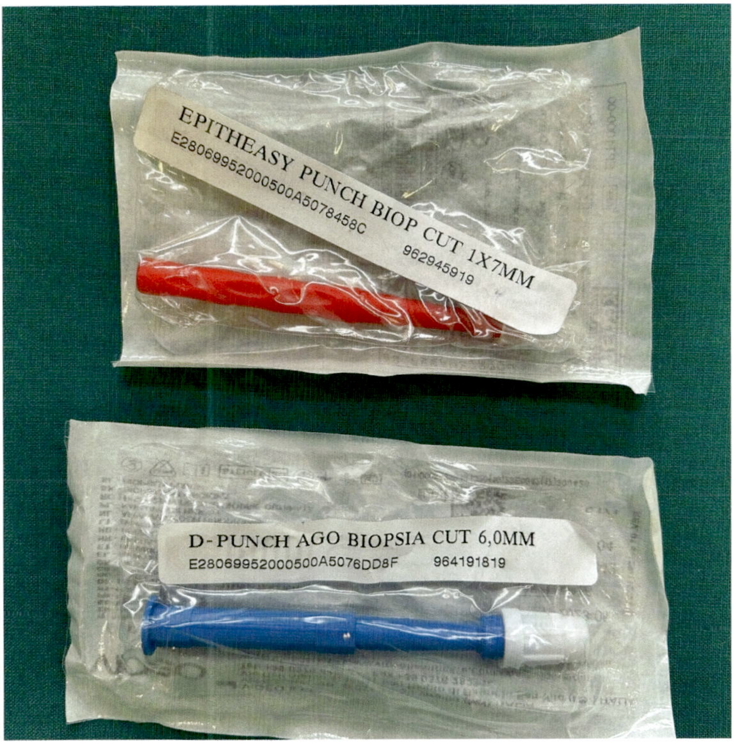

Fig. 1 Skin biopsy punches are generally used by dermatologists or plastic surgeons to perform skin biopsy

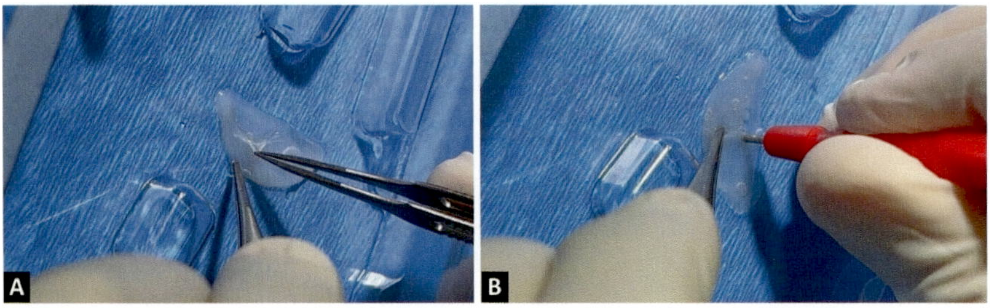

Fig. 2 A: Defrosted cryopreserved hAM laid on the plastic sheet support. B: Skin biopsy punch 1 mm used to obtain 3 lenticules of hAM. Full-video of hAM preparation is available on ….. (Video 1)

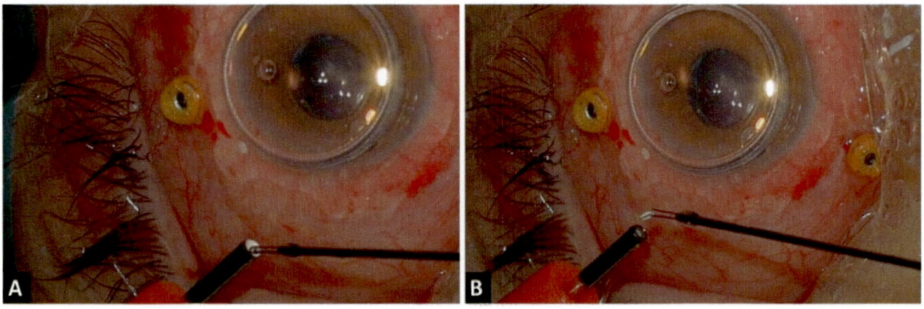

Fig. 3 A: How to secure a hAM lenticule; B: after first disc is secured using an ILM forceps while the second disc remains in the skin biopsy punch. This second one will be used only if something goes wrong using the first one

3 hAM Insertion into the Vitreous Chamber

Once the hAM has been prepared, the second step is its insertion into the vitreous chamber. Usually hAM diameter discs up to 3 mm are inserted into the vitreous chamber without any particular difficulties using the ILM forceps of the same diameter as the trocars. For larger hAM discs, a technique worth considering is to use a smaller Gauge (G) ILM forceps (i.e. 27G) so that the hAM tissue does not meet the resistance of the trocar. Trocar removal associated with opening the conjunctiva at the sclerotomy level, could be an alternative if small gauge forceps are not available. A technically difficult maneuver to perform, but very useful in cases of hAM discs greater than 4 mm, is to pull the hAM disc from one of the trocars, entering with the vitreal forceps from the opposite trocar (Fig. 4). A surgical recommendation worth keeping in mind using this last technique is that, if it is already known that a hAM disc diameter greater than 4 mm has to be used during the vitrectomy, trocars insertion at almost 180° at the beginning of the surgery, could be very useful to make this maneuver much easier.

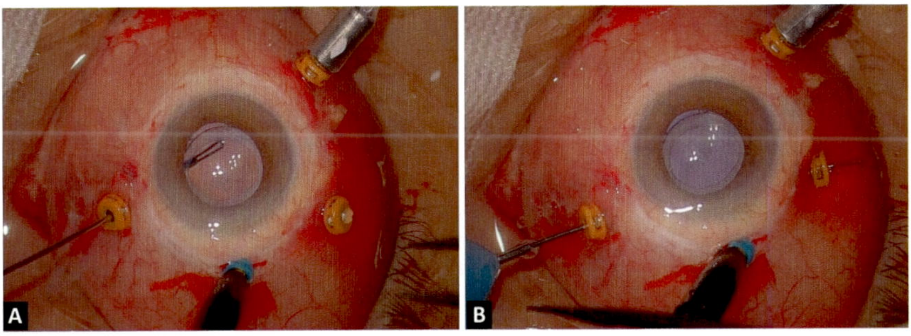

Fig. 4 Surgical technical maneuver we usually adopt to pull the hAM disc inside the vitreous chamber when a hAM disc greater than 4 mm is required. A: The 25G ILM forceps are introduced in the nasal trocar. B: The ILM forceps are pushed outside the temporal trocar ready to secure the large hAM disc

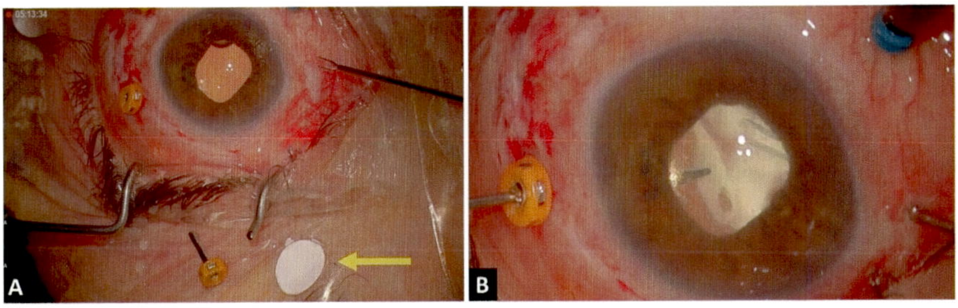

Fig. 5 A: 6 mm hAM disc (yellow arrow) has been prepared. In order to insert it into the vitreous chamber, the 23G trocar was removed. B: Bimanual technique to unfold the 6 mm lenticule at high magnification observation. Full-video of bimanual technique to spread the hAM lenticule is available on ….. (Video 2)

Once inside the vitreous chamber, the first action is to spread out the hAM disc, trying to unfold it as much as possible. This maneuver is supposed to be done *bimanually* so that while one forceps keeps the membrane stable, the other forceps can secure the opposite edge of the membrane and pull gently (Fig. 5).

4 hAM Placement into the Macular Hole

When the hAM is inserted into the vitreous chamber and after its initial stretching, it can be softly moved onto the retinal surface. One aspect to keep in mind is that the hAM lenticules tend to float on the balanced salat solution (BSS). For this reason, it is very important to spread out the hAM disc as soon as it has been introduced into the vitreous chamber in order to be able to distinguish the chorion side (*sticky side*) from the epithelial one (*smooth side*). Two very useful checks to make in order to be sure regarding the correct orientation of the hAM disc are:

- Observing the disc at high magnification, you should see some "filaments" coming out from chorion side, before carrying it close to the retina.
- The chorion side of the hAM disc tends to be "glued" to the branch of the forceps which it is in contact with.

Once the chorion side has been recognized, the surgeon can move the hAM disc close to the retinal surface. As soon as the chorionic side of the hAM touches the retinal surface, it rests on the retinal surface itself. If it does not, and the hAM disc tends to stay attached to one branch of your ILM forceps, be sure that you have correctly identified the chorion side. Sometimes the hAM lenticule goes upside down and its correct orientation could be difficult to detect.

Once the hAM lenticule is laid down onto the retinal surface, through gentle movements (a sort of *light massage*), it is positioned in the hole with its edge below the retinal ones. To do this, one of the ILM forceps branches can be used. Otherwise, a very useful instrument to carry out this maneuver is the Membrane Pik (with or without illumination).

This can also be used to perform a tiny lift of the retinal edges of the hole before putting the hAM disc underneath. Remember to take extra care when manipulating the retinal tissue close to the hole. Even minor damages to the retina in this area, can lead to severe negative consequences to the recovery of visual acuity.

Another consideration worth making is that, often, in highly myopic eyes, the low contrast, due to the rarefaction of retinal pigmented epithelium layer (RPE) associated with the thinning of the retina and choriocapillaris layers, makes the visualization of the hAM lenticule very difficult, once it has been laid down on the retinal surface. By coloring the hAM discs using a vital dye such as Trypan Blue and or Brilliant Blue G it can be easily visualized. This facilitation can be also used in cases of retinal detachment associated with a macular hole: the hAM disc can be put in the macular hole before injecting the heavy liquid inside, so that after the retinal applanation, the lenticule can be easily detected and nicely positioned (Fig. 6).

The last aspect to think carefully about, is the macular hole measurement before surgery. This can be thoroughly studied and documented using the caliper function within the modern optical coherence tomography (OCT) devices. In this way the surgeon already knows the correct size of the punch that is necessary to use in order to make hAM discs big enough to cover the whole hole. In fact, a larger than necessary hAM disc is difficult to manipulate, and it is very difficult to put under the retinal tissue (redundance of hAM tissue). Sometimes damage can be done on the retina and RPE by trying to put an oversized hAM disc below the retina. On the other hand, it is known that if the hAM disc is left upon the retina (difficulty to put it below the retina due to oversized punch hAM disc), the rate of hAM disc dislocation is much higher, unless silicone oil is used at the end of surgery as per endotamponade [10].

On the contrary, a small sized punched hAM disc, would leave portions of RPE and retina without hAM covering leading to a lack of the hAM bulking function.

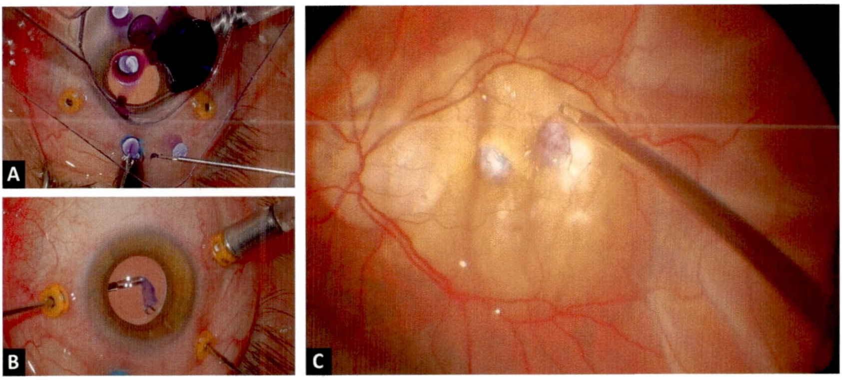

Fig. 6 Staining of the hAM using a vital dye. In this case we have used a combination of Trypan Blue / Brilliant Blue G and the hAM discs were immersed in the dye for 2 min. A: hAM disc separation from the plastic layer using ILM forceps. B: Stretching of the membrane once in the vitreous chamber. Note how the filaments coming out from the chorion side, allow the surgeon to understand the correct orientation of the lenticule (Video 2). C: Positioning of two different hAM discs under the retina. In this case the multiple macular holes in the eye were affected by high myopia and retinal detachment

In this case we suggest exchanging the small sized punched hAM disc for a proper sized one.

5 hAM Placement: Above or Below the Retina?

The maneuver to position the hAM lenticule in the MH is very important. What we usually do is to gently implant the hAM disc into the MH using the ILM forceps. One should spend more time trying to make sure that the hAM lenticule is not upside down once it has been secured. We identify the sticky stromal side as previously described (Fig. 5) and also try to put the stromal side in contact with the RPE and underneath the retina [11].

Sometimes the edge of MH is very adherent to the retina below. In these cases we usually perform a light lift of the edge of the MH using a Membrane Pik (with or without illumination) in order to create the space that allows the hAM lenticule to be nicely positioned below the retinal edges (Fig. 8). In other cases, when the macular hole is associated with a retinal detachment (silicone oil would be considered at the end of surgery) the hAM disc could be eventually left upon the retina. In this scenerio, it is advisable to keep the chorion side next to the retina due to the amount of growth factor it contains [12]. In this instance, a larger patch of hAM can also be used, unless it does not have to be inserted below the retina. The rate of dislocation and/or decentration of hAM using silicone oil as endotamponade at the end of vitrectomy is in most cases the same for both types of insertions (below or above the retina). On the contrary if gas is used as per endotamponade at the end of surgery, the rate of dislocation and/or decentration is much higher if the hAM disc is used epiretinal, regardless of the side of the hAM which has been put in contact with the retina [8].

6 hAM Cryopreserved or Lyophilized: Which One to Use?

There is little previous information in PubMed, however, from our experience both hAMs (cryopreserved and lyophilized) are a feasible alternatives for **macular hole failure surgery**. The approaches have similar anatomical and functional outcomes but the consistence and the behavior of the hAM tissue once in the BSS is very different [13–15]. The surgeon should be prepared for this physical difference and it should be taken into account that both cryopreserved and lyophilized hAMs work well in closing a refractory or large MH, when a correct and uncomplicated surgery is performed. In our experience, the lyophilized hAM is more difficult to cut (often the skin biopsy punch does not make a clear and neat cut), it is likely stiffer compared to the cryopreserved one and once inside the vitreous chamber, it tends to roll-up on itself with the chorion side inside the roll, making it more difficult to spread it out onto the retinal surface. This physical characteristic can be very difficult to handle, in particular if a hAM disc larger than 4 mm is used (Fig. 7). One of the main advantages of the lyophilized hAM is that its lifespan from preparation is almost 6 months. Moreover, it is not necessary to keep it in a low temperature freezer (cryopreserved hAM is usually stored at − 80 °C even if a recent study demonstrated that a temperature of − 28 °C it is likely to be as safe as a lower one) [16] so that can be easily stored and used when necessary. The cryopreserved hAM has to be ordered for that specific surgical time because once it has been defrosted, its lifespan is typically 1 week.

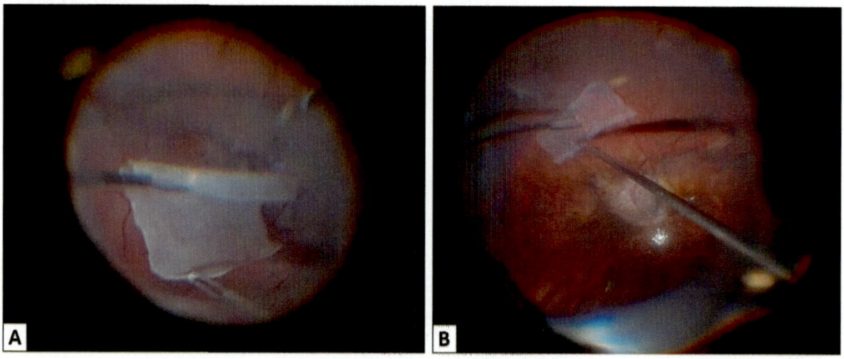

Fig. 7 Lyophilized hAM behavior once into the vitreous chamber. A: Shows how it tends to roll-up with the chorion side within the roll. Also, its greater stiffness can be observed by comparison with the cryopreserved hAM. B: Bimanual maneuver to spread out the lyophilized hAM using heavy liquid in a case of retinal detachment due to a large retinal break along the vascular arcade

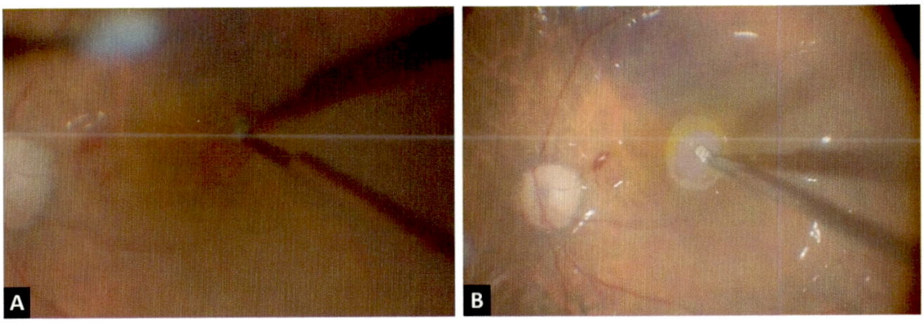

Fig. 8 A: Membrane Pik used to lift the edge of the macular hole. B: Membrane Pik used to insert the hAM under the retina (this last maneuver was carried using heavy liquid)

7 hAM Insertion Using Perfluoro Carbon Liquid: When and Why

hAM lenticules can be safely maneuvered when heavy liquid is used to flatten the retina in cases of retinal detachment related to a MH (Fig. 8B). In these cases, as already discussed, the use of membrane Pik can be more useful compared to condition in which the vitreal chamber is in BSS, because the hAM disc, once positioned close to the MH, has to be gently pushed below the retinal edges that "appear" heavier due to the weight of the perfluoro carbon liquid (PFCL) above. One factor that should be taken into account is that the hAM disc tends to float, with much more energy, once introduced into the PFCL bubble (Fig. 9).

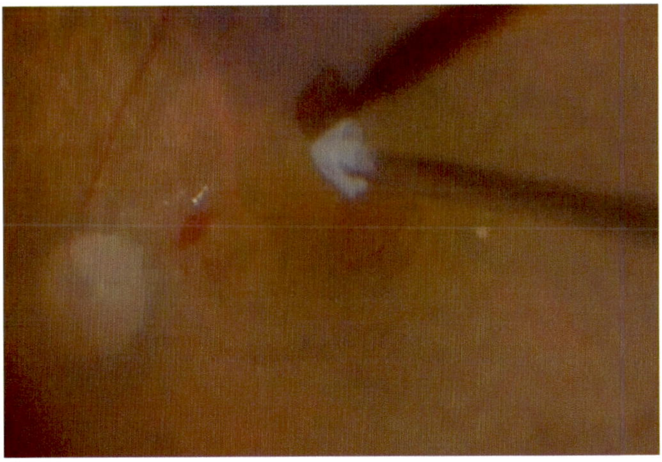

Fig. 9 Typical aspect of the hAM lenticule when it is introduced in a PFCL bubble: it is pushed against the forceps branches

8 Our Experience Using hAM and Our Resources in PubMed

In our experience, since hAM introduction in the clinical practice, we have reported several results among which were the closure of 8 *Persistent/Refractory macular holes* in 2018; the anatomical success was 100% (hAM disc was positioned under the retina) with a mid-term follow-up (6 months after surgery) using 20% sulfur hexafluoride (SF6) as per endotamponade in all cases [1]. Furthermore, we have treated thirty-six eyes of 36 patients affected by *Persistent/Refractory macular holes* who had already received vitrectomy with complete ILM peeling. 17 were male and 19 were female; the mean age was 66.3 ± 12.3 years (range 37–84 years). Also, in those cases we achieved the anatomical success of 100% MH closure rate with hAM disc positioned under the retina, with a mid-term follow-up of 6 months after surgery [17].

Several other surgical techniques have been proposed so far in order to solve the problem of **macular hole failure surgery** [18]. The ILM transplant for example (ILM taken close to the macular region) is a good "filling technique" but poor from a functional sight recovery standpoint, as it has been observed that the transplanted ILM created a sort of plug. We speculate that this is probably be due to the amount and quality of cells that are contained in the ILM used [19].

The use of autologous platelet concentrated or autologous whole blood has been reported to be an effective and safe surgical technique, with satisfactory anatomical and functional results after macular hole failure surgery. These hemoderivates, are likely to allow not only the anatomical closure but also seem to stimulate tissue regeneration [20, 21].

Another interesting surgical technique worth mentioning is the macular detachment injecting BSS below the macular area using a sub retinal injection needle (41G). The efficacy of this technique has been reported and highlights the risk of RPE damage, thus speculating the need to perform the retinotomy points outside the macula [22, 23].

9 Conclusions

Revising all the studies reported in PubMed so far, the hAM is, from an immunological point of view, completely inert. In fact, no greater rate of inflammation, endophthalmitis or post operative complications due to the use of hAM itself have been described or demonstrated [24].

The introduction of the hAM in our clinical practice has brought to a much higher rate of closure of *Persistent/Refractory macular hole* and *Macular hole recurrence*. Its safety, relatively simple use and availability have led to hAM use being one of the best surgical choices worldwide, when a vitreoretinal surgeon is dealing with **macular hole failure surgery**.

9.1 Clinical Pearls

- Bimanual technique should be preferred because it is easier to carry out such a delicate maneuver on both the hAM disc and retina.
- Use smaller gauge forceps for hAM disc insert into the vitreous chamber, if the disc "resists" the trocar during the insertion maneuver.
- Use PFCL only if necessary: hAM floats in PFCL (more difficult to maneuver)
- When possible, use the cryopreserved hAM because it is easier to deal with compared to the lyophilic one, as latter tends to roll-up on itself once inserted into the vitreous chamber.
- Use the hAM only when macular ILM around the hole is no longer available (the ILM has been already peeled during a previous vitrectomy)

References

1. Rizzo S, Caporossi T, Tartaro R, Finocchio L, Franco F, Barca F, Giansanti F. A human amniotic membrane plug to promote retinal breaks repair and recurrent macular hole closure. Retina. 2019;39(Suppl 1):S95–103. https://doi.org/10.1097/IAE.0000000000002320. PMID: 30312261.
2. Caporossi T, Tartaro R, Bacherini D, Pacini B, De Angelis L, Governatori L, Di Leo L, Oliverio L, Rizzo S. Applications of the amniotic membrane in vitreoretinal surgery. J Clin Med. 2020;9(8):2675. https://doi.org/10.3390/jcm9082675. PMID: 32824838; PMCID: PMC7463634.
3. Spiteri Cornish K, Lois N, Scott N, Burr J, Cook J, Boachie C, Tadayoni R, la Cour M, Christensen U, Kwok A. Vitrectomy with internal limiting membrane (ILM) peeling versus vitrectomy with no peeling for idiopathic full-thickness macular hole (FTMH). Cochrane Database Syst Rev. 2013;(6):CD009306. https://doi.org/10.1002/14651858.CD009306.pub2. PMID: 23740611.
4. Michalewska Z, Michalewski J, Adelman RA, Nawrocki J. Inverted internal limiting membrane flap technique for large macular holes. Ophthalmology. 2010;117(10):2018–25. https://doi.org/10.1016/j.ophtha.2010.02.011. Epub 2010 Jun 11. PMID: 20541263.
5. Al-Abdulla NA, Thompson JT, Sjaarda RN. Results of macular hole surgery with and without epiretinal dissection or internal limiting membrane removal. Ophthalmology. 2004;111(1):142–9. https://doi.org/10.1016/j.ophtha.2003.05.005. PMID: 14711726.
6. Morescalchi F, Costagliola C, Gambicorti E, Duse S, Romano MR, Semeraro F. Controversies over the role of internal limiting membrane peeling during vitrectomy in macular hole surgery. Surv Ophthalmol. 2017;62(1):58–69. https://doi.org/10.1016/j.survophthal.2016.07.003. Epub 2016 Aug 1. PMID: 27491476.
7. Hernández F, Alpizar-Alvarez N, Wu L. Chromovitrectomy: an update. J Ophthalmic Vis Res. 2014;9(2):251–9. PMID: 25279128; PMCID: PMC4181209.
8. Bracha P, Ciulla TA, Baumal CR. Vital dyes in vitreomacular surgery. Ophthalmic Surg Lasers Imaging Retina. 2018;49(10):788–98. https://doi.org/10.3928/23258160-20181002-07. PMID: 30395665.
9. Ullrich S, Haritoglou C, Gass C, Schaumberger M, Ulbig MW, Kampik A. Macular hole size as a prognostic factor in macular hole surgery. Br J Ophthalmol. 2002;86(4):390–3. https://doi.org/10.1136/bjo.86.4.390. PMID:11914205; PMCID: PMC1771090.

10. Garcin T, Gain P, Thuret G. Epiretinal large disc of blue-stained lyophilized amniotic membrane to treat complex macular holes: a 1-year follow-up. Acta Ophthalmol. 2022;100(2):e598–608. https://doi.org/10.1111/aos.14909. Epub 2021 May 16. PMID: 33998147.
11. Caporossi T, De Angelis L, Pacini B, Tartaro R, Finocchio L, Barca F, Rizzo S. A human Amniotic Membrane plug to manage high myopic macular hole associated with retinal detachment. Acta Ophthalmol. 2020;98(2):e252–6. https://doi.org/10.1111/aos.14174. Epub 2019 Jul 18. PMID: 31318489.
12. Kim TG, Do Ki K, Lee MK, So JW, Chung SK, Kang J. Comparison of cytokine expression and ultrastructural alterations in fresh-frozen and dried electron beam-irradiated human amniotic membrane and chorion. Cell Tissue Bank. 2019;20(2):163–72. https://doi.org/10.1007/s10561-019-09748-9. Epub 2019 May 6. PMID: 31062125.
13. Huang YH, Tsai DC, Wang LC, Chen SJ. Comparison between cryopreserved and dehydrated human amniotic membrane graft in treating challenging cases with macular hole and macular hole retinal detachment. J Ophthalmol. 2020;7(2020):9157518. https://doi.org/10.1155/2020/9157518. PMID: 32724671; PMCID: PMC7364261.
14. Rodríguez-Ares MT, López-Valladares MJ, Touriño R, Vieites B, Gude F, Silva MT, Couceiro J. Effects of lyophilization on human amniotic membrane. Acta Ophthalmol. 2009;87(4):396–403. https://doi.org/10.1111/j.1755-3768.2008.01261.x. Epub 2008 Oct 15. PMID: 18937812.
15. Niknejad H, Deihim T, Solati-Hashjin M, Peirovi H. The effects of preservation procedures on amniotic membrane's ability to serve as a substrate for cultivation of endothelial cells. Cryobiology. 2011;63(3):145–51. https://doi.org/10.1016/j.cryobiol.2011.08.003. Epub 2011 Aug 23. PMID: 21884690.
16. Witt J, Grumm L, Salla S, Geerling G, Menzel-Severing J. Cryopreservation in a standard freezer: − 28 °C as alternative storage temperature for amniotic membrane transplantation. J Clin Med. 2022;11(4):1109. https://doi.org/10.3390/jcm11041109. PMID: 35207382; PMCID: PMC8877302.
17. Caporossi T, Pacini B, Bacherini D, Barca F, Faraldi F, Rizzo S. Human amniotic membrane plug to promote failed macular hole closure. Sci Rep. 2020;10(1):18264. https://doi.org/10.1038/s41598-020-75292-2. PMID: 33106542; PMCID: PMC7588413.
18. Romano MR, Rossi T, Borgia A, Catania F, Sorrentino T, Ferrara M. Management of refractory and recurrent macular holes: a comprehensive review. Surv Ophthalmol. 2022;67(4):908–31. https://doi.org/10.1016/j.survophthal.2022.01.006. Epub 2022 Jan 31. PMID: 35101550.
19. Giansanti F, Tartaro R, Caporossi T, Bacherini D, Savastano A, Barca F, Rizzo S. An internal limiting membrane plug and gas endotamponade for recurrent or persistent macular hole. J Ophthalmol. 2019;7(2019):6051724. https://doi.org/10.1155/2019/6051724. PMID: 30956814; PMCID: PMC6431435.
20. Purtskhvanidze K, Frühsorger B, Bartsch S, Hedderich J, Roider J, Treumer F. Persistent full-thickness idiopathic macular hole: anatomical and functional outcome of revitrectomy with autologous platelet concentrate or autologous whole blood. Ophthalmologica. 2018;239(1):19–26. https://doi.org/10.1159/000481268. Epub 2017 Oct 20. PMID: 29050013.
21. Arias JD, Hoyos AT, Alcántara B, Sanchez-Avila RM, Arango FJ, Galvis V. Plasma rich in growth factors for persistent macular hole: a pilot study. Retin Cases Brief Rep. 2022;16(2):155–60. https://doi.org/10.1097/ICB.0000000000000957. PMID: 31895724.
22. Felfeli T, Mandelcorn ED. Macular hole hydrodissection: surgical technique for the treatment of persistent, chronic, and large macular holes. Retina. 2019;39(4):743–52. https://doi.org/10.1097/IAE.0000000000002013. PMID: 29303907.
23. Fotis K, Alexander P, Sax J, Reddie I, Kang CY, Chandra A. Macular detachment for the treatment of persistent full-thickness macular holes. Retina. 2019;39(Suppl 1):S104–7. https://doi.org/10.1097/IAE.0000000000002370. PMID: 30383713.
24. Jirsova K, Jones GLA. Amniotic membrane in ophthalmology: properties, preparation, storage and indications for grafting-a review. Cell Tissue Bank. 2017;18(2):193–204. https://doi.org/10.1007/s10561-017-9618-5. Epub 2017 Mar 2. PMID: 28255771.

Autologous Retinal Transplant for Macular Holes

Zujaja Tauqeer and Tamer H. Mahmoud

Abstract Macular holes are an anatomical defect that can result from the anteroposterior and tangential tractional forces that act on the fovea, ultimately causing it to dehisce from the underlying retinal pigment epithelium and causing a full-thickness retinal break between the two edges of the fovea. Idiopathic macular holes result from endogenic tractional forces acting on the retina. Secondary causes of macular holes include high myopia, trauma, macular schisis, and age-related macular degeneration. It can also result from sun or eclipse gazing, laser pointer use, and from anterior segment laser procedures. Macular hole surgery is a rapidly evolving branch of retinal surgery that has benefited from recent innovations in diagnostic imaging and surgical tools. Pars plana vitrectomy (PPV) alone improves the hole closure rate to 58% compared to natural history by removing anteroposterior vitreous traction from the fovea. Addition of the internal limiting membrane (ILM) peel improves success rate to over 90%. Certain features are associated with higher risk of surgical failure despite PPV with ILM peel and require nuanced approaches. These include using an inverted ILM Flap, a retracting door flap, or using Autologous Retinal Transplants.

Keywords Autologous retinal transplant · High myopia · Macular hole

1 Background on Macular Holes Development

The surgical repair of macular holes has only continued to improve since 1991 when vitrectomy surgery was officially proposed as a treatment for the repair of idiopathic macular holes [1]. To put the importance of surgical repair into perspective, consider that without surgery, only 11% of macular holes close [2]. With surgery? Over 75%. A

T. H. Mahmoud (✉)
Department of Ophthalmology, William Beaumont School of Medicine, Oakland University, Royal Oak, MI, USA
e-mail: tmahmoud@arcpc.net

Z. Tauqeer · T. H. Mahmoud
Associated Retinal Consultants, 3555 W. 13 Mile Road, Suite LL-20, Royal Oak, MI 48073, USA

F. Patelli et al. (eds.), *Macular Surgery*, https://doi.org/10.1007/978-3-031-63508-3_10

previously blinding condition had finally become treatable. With the advent of more modern approaches, macular hole closure rate now approaches or exceeds 90% [3].

To understand approaches to macular hole surgery, especially the techniques that have been developed to tackle the most complex cases, it is helpful to understand the etiologies and pathophysiology of how holes develop in the fovea. Idiopathic macular holes result from vitreoretinal tractional forces acting on the fovea. However, macular holes also result from secondary causes that have great implications for surgical decision-making. Some relevant causes of macular holes include high myopia, macular telangiectasia, and Alport's syndrome [4]. There are also iatrogenic causes of macular hole development including trauma, anterior segment laser use, laser pointer use, or sun/eclipse gazing [5–7]. The majority of cases of macular holes are idiopathic however, constituting between 80–90% of all cases [4, 8].

For idiopathic macular holes, the pathogenesis is contingent on the presence of vitreomacular adhesion in the fovea. Beginning in the 1960s, clinical and histopathologic studies began to highlight the relationship of the vitreous and the macula in eyes with macular holes [9, 10]. Several investigators concluded that traction, presumably anteroposterior forces, from the vitreous on the macula were important in the evolution of a macular hole [8].

Since then, we have had significant advancements in imaging techniques as well as experimental results showing that additional forces are at play. Namely, modern surgical approaches recognize the importance of tangential forces induced by any epiretinal membranes (ERM), as well as the physiologic internal limiting membrane (ILM), in the development of a macular hole through radial outward traction. The practical application of this is well-demonstrated by the fact that studies demonstrate significantly higher rates of macular hole closure with ILM peeling versus vitrectomy with no ILM peeling, and lower re-operation rates, even for higher stage of macular holes [3].

2 Background on Surgical Approaches to Macular Hole Repair

The surgical objective in macular hole repair is to relieve traction exerted by the vitreous or by epiretinal membranes to the central retina. Following on the heels of greater clinical and histopathologic understanding of macular hole development and progression, Gonvers and Machemer were the first to recommend vitrectomy, gas tamponade, and face down positioning for retinal detachments secondary to macular hole [11]. The modern approach in its current iteration as carried out by Kelly and Wendel in 1991 was predicated on removing the vitreous, including the posterior cortex, flattening the macular hole and the associated neurosensory macular detachment. With this method they achieved a 58% anatomic success rate as well as visual improvement of two or more lines in 42% of eyes. Their method essentially treated the macular hole like a retinal detachment arising from the macular hole. Because the classic teaching has always been that retina does not repair, the mechanism by which the macular hole is thought to overcome this phenomenon is possibly through glial cell proliferation and thus bridging of the foveal edges [12].

Membrane peeling has been variously described as removal of tractional membranes, manipulation of the foveal tissue, or retinal "scratching" or "shaving" [13]. The exact composition of the epiretinal tissue removed during surgery was not initially identified when membrane peeling came to the fore as a technique for macular hole repair. In the late 1990s, this "pre-retinal" vs internal limiting membrane removal for the treatment of macular hole with significant success was taken up with enthusiasm globally [14–17]. Subsequently, electron microscopy of epiretinal and internal limiting membrane tissue removed during surgery for idiopathic macular holes demonstrated cells with myofibroblastic differentiation on the ILM [18]. The hypothesis is that these cells contract on the surface of the ILM thus resulting in the formation and subsequent enlargement of macular holes, thereby being relevant to the surgical repair of them as well [13].

3 Playing with Grafts

In 2010, Michalewska et al. first reported on a technique where the ILM was not fully peeled, but rather used an adjunct to close the macular hole – an inverted ILM flap technique which resulted in an improvement of the postoperative closure rates and visual functions for large MHs with a minimum diameter > 400 μm [19]. After Michalewska et al.'s first report, there have been many studies on the inverted ILM flap technique with or without some modification [20–22]. Modifications of this technique include temporal inverted ILM flap, [23–25] ILM retracting door flap [26], pedicle ILM flap [27]), free ILM graft transposition with or without perfluoro-n-octane [28, 29], and double internal limiting membrane insertion (covering the macular hole with an inverted ILM flap with a free ILM graft on top) [30].

In addition, the inverted ILM technique was adopted for many other types of MHs other than large MHs, including myopic holes [31], and macular hole detachments [32]. This technique has also been modified to optic disc pit detachments and maculopathies [33].

While successful, one of the limiting factors with this technique is its applicability to very large or refractory macular holes. Due to the popularity of ILM peeling, other approaches are needed when the ILM has been completely removed during prior surgeries. Other non-peeling techniques described to attempt closure when reoperating on these patients include repeat fluid–gas exchange, endotamponade with silicone oil as opposed to gas, radial relaxing retinotomies on the macular hole margin, perifoveolar laser photocoagulation to form chorioretinal adhesions, addition of autologous blood to the autologous ILM flap, using other adjuvant blood components such as platelet-rich plasma, autologous anterior or posterior lens capsule flap, scleral shortening techniques, and the more recently introduced amniotic membrane as a scaffold to plug the hole.

The striking feature is that when large or complex holes close following the use of a free ILM patch or inverted ILM flap, the retina occasionally regains its laminar structure showing the hole is mostly "filled" with neurosensory retina rather than just plugged with basement membrane [34]. Nevertheless, studies of repair of large macular holes (>550 um) showed that even when very large holes were successfully closed, visual recovery was limited, potentially due to degenerative changes during the period the hole is open [35]. Understanding these drawbacks of existing techniques and the developments in grafting for macular holes leads us naturally to understanding the next major technical development in the field of macular hole repair surgery – the use of the autologous retinal free flap transplant.

4 The History and Development of ART

Despite the advances above, large and refractory macular holes remain difficult to repair with traditional surgical approaches when there is no more traction left to release or when available tamponade agents could not induce the hole to close. Moreover, even if a hole could be anatomically closed with adjunctive tissue scaffolds, visual prognosis remained sadly guarded because of the absence of neurosensory retina.

Into this lacuna came the technique of autologous retinal transplantation (ART), which enables closure by a third mechanism—providing a scaffold for cellular rehabilitation and inducing retinal tissue replacement of the degenerated gap to allow for possible visual recovery (Fig. 1).

The autologous retinal graft creates a barrier between the vitreous cavity and previously exposed subretinal space, allowing subretinal fluid to be removed by the retinal pigment epithelium (RPE) promoting MH closure [36–38]. Autologous retinal transplantation enables cellular rehabilitation in addition to tissue replacement. It is hypothesized that transplanted retinal photoreceptors could directly synapse with bipolar cells in the host area through ectopic synaptogenesis. Transplanted healthy photoreceptors may also promote cell–cell communication that rehabilitates damaged photoreceptors at the host site [39].

The retinal graft may also contain retinal progenitor cells (RPCs). Muller cell reconstitution or regeneration is thought to be a possible mechanism for successful macular hole closure and visual rehabilitation [25]. Müller cells harvested from post-mortem human retina samples were shown to demonstrate immortality and pluripotency in vitro with expression of neural stem cell markers [40, 41]. Fibroblasts have been induced into rod photoreceptor-like cells in vivo in mice into the subretinal space of rod degeneration mice has been demonstrated to produce partial restoration of the pupil reflex and visual function [42]. In addition, RPCs rehabilitate surrounding tissue through material transfer. In summary, ART replaces tissue and integrates healthy photoreceptors and potential RPCs, which may allow for structural and functional rehabilitation of surrounding retina [39] (Fig. 2).

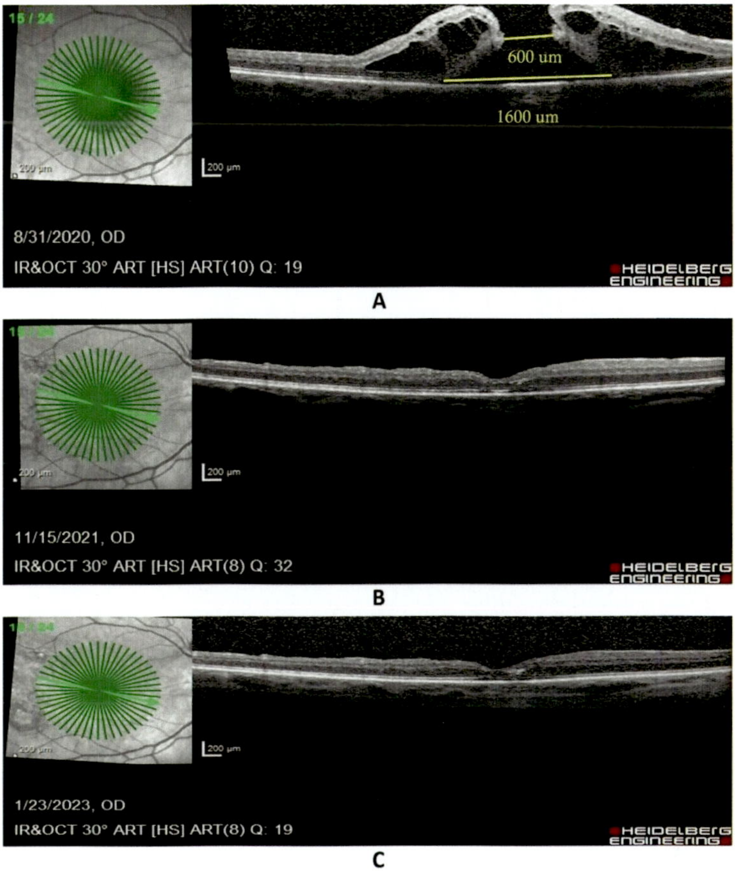

Fig. 1 A Pre-Operative OCT Scan of Patient with VA 20/400 following Failed ILM Peel with Gas Tamponade (Tamer H. Mahmoud, MD, PhD personal archive). B Post-Operative Macular Hole Repair with ART Showing Graft Placement and Reconstitution of Outer Retinal Layers at 1 Year and VA 20/60 (Tamer H. Mahmoud, MD, Ph.D. personal archive). **C** Post-Operative Graft Outer Retinal Preservation at 2.5 Years with VA 20/25 Following ART (Tamer H. Mahmoud, MD, PhD personal archive)

Thus the underlying hypothesis was that neurosensory retina would serve as an effective scaffold and progenitor for induction of glial cell proliferation that is the mechanism for macular hole closure as well as an effective sealant between the vitreous cavity and subsensory space, allowing for subretinal fluid to be pumped out further enabling closure of macular hole [36].

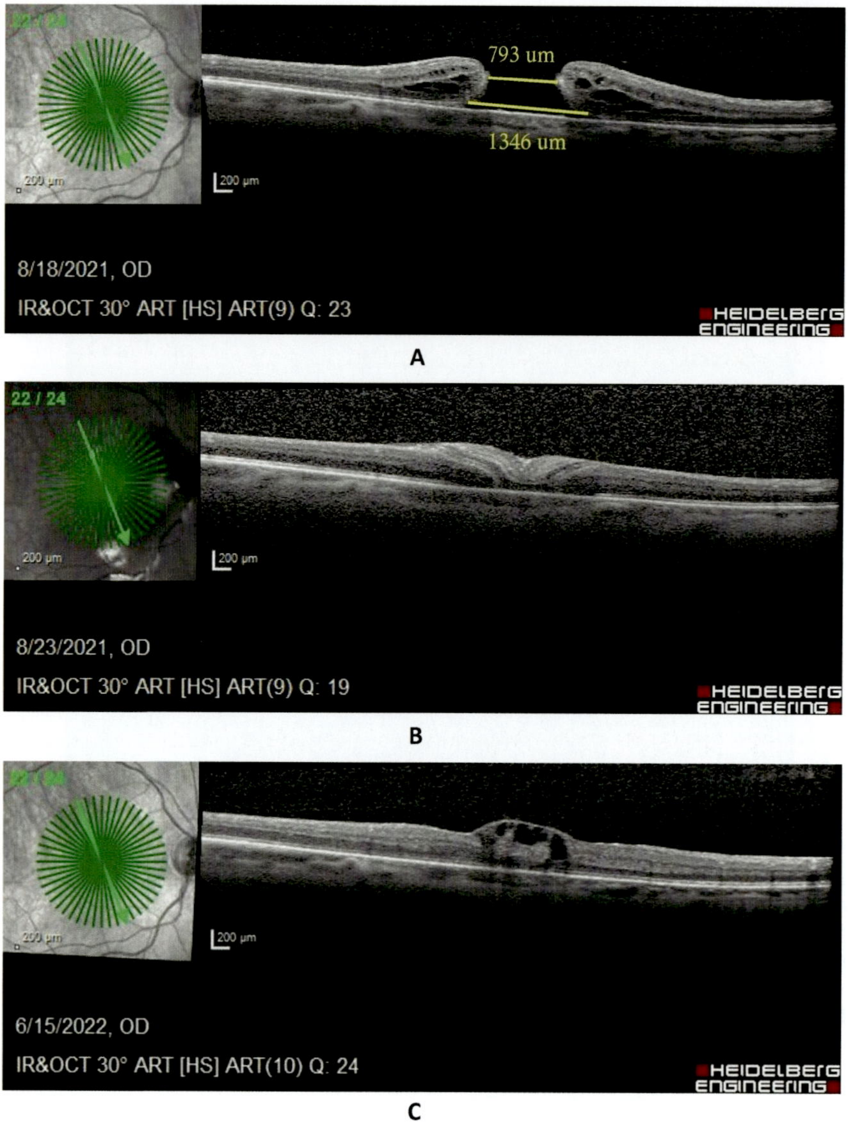

Fig. 2 A Pre-Operative OCT of Macular Hole with Resultant 20/200 vision (Tamer H. Mahmoud, MD, Ph.D. personal archive). B Day 5 Post-Operative OCT with Graft Under Perfluorocarbon Liquid (Tamer H. Mahmoud, MD, Ph.D. personal archive). C 10-Month Post-Operative OCT Demonstrating Partial Outer Retinal Integration with Inner Retinal Edema and VA 20/40 (Tamer H. Mahmoud, MD, Ph.D. personal archive)

5 Initial Description

In 2016, Grewal and Mahmoud described the seminal case of autologous neurosensory retina free flap transplantation for a patient with refractory myopic macular hole who had failed prior macular hole surgery with ILM peel, which had been complicated by post-operative retinal detachment. Intraoperatively, staining with indocyanine green showed peel of ILM tissue in the macula. Additional ILM could not be adequately harvested, nor was lens capsular tissue available given the patient was pseudophakic and status post Nd:Yag capsulotomy. Necessity being the mother of invention, neurosensory retina was harvested above the superotemporal arcade, using a bimanual approach with chandelier. The flap was 2-disc diameters in size, and it was positioned over the hole under perfluoro-n-octane. To avoid disturbing the free graft, a direct perfluoro-n-octane to silicone oil exchange was performed. The patient was positioned face down for 1 week post-operatively [36].

With respect to outcome, macular hole closure was achieved at 3-months follow-up with improvement in visual acuity from 20/200 pre-operatively to 20/80 at 3 months post-operatively. There was subjective improvement in distortion and scotoma size and objective improvement in mean retinal sensitivity on microperimetry from 7.5 dB at 1 week to 12.3 dB at 3 months postoperatively with progressive reduction of absolute scotoma [36]. That first ART patient is now eight years out from the ART repair with an improved VA to 20/50.

In a notable departure from other grafting techniques, the size and girth of retinal tissue used with this technique obviated the need to mechanically position it under the fovea to anchor it in place, which was needed when the graft was a thin lens capsular or ILM flap, thereby allowing the retinal graft to be left on the surface. This advantage minimizes potential iatrogenic trauma that could limit post-operative recovery.

6 Surgical Technique

Preoperative estimation of MH dimensions using spectral-domain OCT is essential to prepare an adequately sized graft (Figs. 1A and 2A). Of note, accurate measurements must account for true axial length and adjustment of OCT measurements as OCT measurements are typically proportioned to an assumed standard approximately 24 mm eye [43]. The intended retinal graft is oversized by about 1.2 to 1.5 times the original defect because of shrinkage of the retinal graft as the tissue integrates into the defect [39].

If the eye was not previously vitrectomized, a standard three-port pars plana vitrectomy is performed. A fourth port may be placed for chandelier illumination and bimanual maneuvers, depending on surgeon ease. Additional ILM peeling is often not helpful, particularly in eyes that have previously undergone ILM peeling. Light endodiathermy is applied to blood vessels at the edge of the chosen graft site to control intraoperative bleeding and to delineate the graft which is sized larger than the macular hole. The graft can be excised directly using vertical scissors or excised after induction of a focal retinal detachment with balanced salt solution infusion through a 41-gauge subretinal cannula. End-grasping forceps and curved or vertical scissors are helpful to cut the graft, leaving a graft hinge until the instillation of perfluorocarbon liquid so that the graft does not move with the ensuing fluid shifts. Once the hole and donor site are both covered, the residual graft hinge is severed, and the graft is transferred to the recipient site using end-grasping forceps or massaging across the retinal surface using a FINESSE Flex loop (Alcon) [39]. The retinal autograft site is then surrounded with multiple rows of barrier endolaser.

The graft can be placed on top of the hole, slightly overhanging the foveal edges around the hole, particularly nasally. Or it can be tucked temporal and left to hang over the nasal foveal retinal edge in anticipation of the post-operative temporal retinal shift. Both short-term perfluoro-n-octane tamponade and silicone oil tamponade have been used, as well as fluid-gas exchange with gas tamponade by different surgeons, with no difference in outcome [44].

The authors of the technique advocate the use of perfluorocarbon liquid before harvest of the flap because it is easier to stabilize the movement of the graft and maneuver it into position. Perfluorocarbon liquid can be left as a short-term tamponade, for 1 to 2 weeks, to allow for secure and accurate placement of the transplant in the macular hole, avoid any dislocation with exchanges of fluids and air, and to help achieve better functional results possibly because of better initial oxygenation to the retinal flap, especially in those chronic cases with underlying retinal pigment epithelium atrophy (Fig. 2B).

The most favored site for graft harvesting is superior for a better tamponade, and grafts are typically harvested posterior to the equator [44].

7 Outcomes

This technique for the most complex and challenging macular holes was studied in two large, multi-center cohorts.

The first study in 2019 was a multinational collaboration between 4 institutes in North America, Southern Europe, and Asia evaluating patients with full-thickness, refractory macular hole following vitrectomy with ILM peel who subsequently underwent ART and had greater than 6 months of follow-up [37]. These were challenging cases that, in addition to their prior surgical failure, also included exacerbating anatomic factors such as high myopia, macular-hole associated retinal detachment, proliferative vitreoretinopathy, Alport syndrome, macular telangiectasia, and pre-existing choroidal neovascular membranes. A significant proportion had a flat, open configuration on pre-operative OCT with dry, flat edges.

Out of 41 consecutive cases of autologous retinal transplantation, complete anatomic closure of the macular hole was achieved in 36 out of 41 eyes (87.8%). Moreover, 37% of eyes improved 3 or more lines demonstrating desirable visual improvement. By OCT, these patients had improved restoration of the ellipsoid zone and external limiting membrane showing some reconstitution of the retinal layers and thereby possibly enhanced prognosis for recovery. Visual improvement was observed in over half of the eyes that achieved successful anatomic closure, whereas no improvement was observed in the 5 eyes that did not achieve anatomic closure. Postoperative neurosensory retinal flap dislocation was seen in 2 cases.

Encouragingly, in the smaller subset of patients that did not achieve visual improvement despite anatomic closure and only maintained their pre-operative VA, they described a gradual but significant reduction of their central scotoma and reported that this reduction of the central scotoma helped them significantly with tasks at both distance and near.

Subsequently, a retrospective case series set out to evaluate outcomes when this technique was used as a *primary* treatment for previously untreated macular holes [44]. Up to this point, the cases of macular hole that were treated with the ART technique had undergone prior vitrectomy with ILM peeling. The seven cases under evaluation in this study had a minimum opening diameter of > 600 μm and a maximum basal diameter > 1000 μm and the holes had been present more than 1 year. All seven eyes treated achieved closure of the macular hole. One year post-operatively, average visual acuity improved significantly from 1.10 logMAR (Snellen equivalent 20/190) pre-operatively to 0.68 logMar (20/95 Snellen equivalent), with vision improving by more than 2 lines in 5 out of 7 eyes, and remaining unchanged in 2 out of 7 eyes.

Both studies demonstrated two vitally important facts. First, this technique provided hope regarding the potential for improvement in visual acuity and visual symptoms with closure of the macular hole with ART. Such hope did not exist for patients who had exhausted available surgical options. Secondly, it showed that reconstitution of the retinal layers was enhanced, by mechanisms as yet unknown.

Indeed, the 2020 study by Tanaka et al. deployed microperimetry evaluation to demonstrate light perception within the transplanted graft retina in the successful cases [45]. The degree of response in the grafted cases varied, and the response to light was weaker in cases where there was a less distinct ellipsoid line. The authors hypothesized that ellipsoid line integrity was likely a corollary to the degree of retinal pigment epithelium support and survival. Further multimodal testing with fluorescein angiography showed that transplanted retinal grafts took on blood supply from the choroid, which might explain why in cases of primary macular hole closure with ART, the grafts stayed in place more than 1 year after transplantation.

A short five years following the initial description of the technique, a robust multicenter consecutive case series was published to demonstrate outcomes of this technique in a mix of patients—primary macular holes, refractory macular holes, and combined macular hole-rhegmatogenous retinal detachments [44]. Surgeons across the world were invited to participate and submit any cases of ART for the above-mentioned indications. Thirty-three different surgeons around the world participated, sharing 130 unique cases, a testament to the growth and dissemination of the technique within 5 short years. The majority of cases were refractory macular holes (58%), then primary holes (27%), and then combined MH-RRDs (15%). The racial and ethnic backgrounds of the patients were diverse: 41% were White, 23% were Black, 19% were Asian, and 17% were Latino. Perfluorocarbon was used in nearly all the cases for harvesting and grafting the transplant. The final tamponade agent used at the end of the case was SO in 60% of cases, perfluoro-n-octane in 20% of cases, and gas in 20% of cases.

With respect to the results of the study, 85.7% of primary macular holes closed after ART surgery. For refractory macular holes, an even higher success rate of 88% closure was achieved with retinal transplantation. In macular hole retinal detachments, a 95% MH closure rate was observed after ART surgery.

For primary macular holes, the visual acuity gains were significant, from a mean VA of 1.090 logMAR (Snellen equivalent, 20/246) to 0.838 logMAR (Snellen equivalent, 20/138) after surgery. One-third of these patients gained 3 lines of vision, and 17% of them gained at least 5 lines of vision.

In the refractory MH group, the visual acuity gains were also significant, from a preoperative mean VA of 1.258 logMAR (Snellen equivalent, approximately 20/362), to 1.063 (Snellen equivalent, approximately 20/231) after surgery. Similarly in this group, over a third of patients achieved a 3-line gain in VA and 25% gained at least 5 lines of VA.

In the macular hole detachment group, visual acuity gains were also present, from a preoperative mean VA of 2.316 logMAR (approximately hand movements), to 1.403 logMAR (Snellen equivalent, 20/500) after surgery. The vast majority of patients achieved a 3-line gain of VA and 68% gained at least 5 lines of VA.

More recently, ART has been shown to provide robust anatomic and visual improvement in cases of Macular Telangiectasia (MacTel) type 2, a particular thorny problem in the field because of the small number of cases and the particularly recalcitrant nature of the disease which cause neurodegenerative changes in the macula leading to poor macular hole closure rates in this condition with existing techniques. Of 5 cases of MacTel treated with autologous retinal transplantation, all 5 achieved anatomic closure, as compared to the pre-existing estimates of 30% closure rate. And in contrast to the poor visual outcomes in prior studies, 25% of patients with MacTel macular holes achieved improvement in 2 lines of vision, although the majority remained stable [46].

8 The State of the Field

Autologous retinal transplantation was initially performed for closure of refractory myopic macular holes that did not resolve with peeling of ILM and where lens capsule (or other scaffold) was not available to harvest [36]. Today, the indications for ART have expanded to include use in any large hole refractory to conventional techniques [23], combined large macular hole-associated retinal detachments (with or without proliferative vitreoretinopathy) [24], large primary macular holes that would not close with traditional surgical approaches (e.g., high myopia–associated macular holes) [25], and large holes associated with other ocular (e.g., macular telangiectasia Type 2) or systemic conditions (e.g., Alport syndrome) [46, 47], optic pit maculopathies [48, 49], as well as degenerative atrophy from macular degeneration [50].

That 12% of patients in the global ART study reached 20/50 VA or better merits further exploration as to the role and potential of peripheral retina in acquiring macular resolution, which then could be a sign of hope for other macular diseases. Postoperative optical coherence tomography (OCT) scans in these studies have been critical to elucidating the potential physiologic mechanisms by which macular hole closure and visual recovery may be achieved. The scans illustrate bridging tissue in the junctional area of the retinal flaps, indicating integration of the retinal flap tissue. Although the mechanism of this microsurgical integration, partial outer retinal layer restoration, and the improved visual function are unclear, several hypotheses can be derived from experimental and animal work as well as multimodal imaging.

Foremost, establishment of vascular support to the transplanted retinal graft has been hypothesized as one factor promoting the success of macular hole closure and improvement in visual function. Using optical coherence tomography angiography (OCT-A) and early and late phase of fluorescein angiography, it has been demonstrated that there is partial vascularization and perfusion of the graft, specifically superficial and deep retinal capillary plexus. It is presumed that an ischemic drive, from hypoxic astrocytes, upregulates angiogenic mechanisms for vascularization and perfusion of the graft [51, 52].

Secondly, re-establishment of a viable ellipsoid zone has been shown to be important for visual recovery and for decreased risk of post-operative macular edema. It may be that the presence of macular edema shows a decreased pump function in the underlying retinal pigment epithelium or failure of vascular anastomosis between the host and graft retina. Or the macular edema itself may preclude the restoration of the ellipsoid zone. Morphological studies indicate that the outer retina is better preserved than the inner retina in the grafted retina, perhaps because of the integrity of the choroidal circulation which subserves the outer retina, as compared to the inner retina which is reliant on vascular anastomoses successfully being established between host and grafted retina and which are more vulnerable to metabolic stressors [53].

Lastly, it remains to be further elucidated how specific biochemical pathways produce recovery or regeneration of photoreceptor function. Immunohistochemical analysis of the peripheral human retina has shown cells positive for markers present in stem cells of neural origin (Pax6, Sox2, Nestin) and epithelial origin (ABCG2, N-cadherin). Cells with characteristics of neural progenitor or stem cells have been isolated from the neural retina. Müller glia isolated from the peripheral retina may be a source of producing cells with properties of rod photoreceptors in addition to producing neurotrophic growth factors as they traverse the scaffold of the transplanted or transposed tissue. Johnsen et al. showed that the neuroepithelial stem cells with Müller glia characteristics could respond to retinal injury by targeted migration into the vitreous, which has been seen in models of proliferative vitreoretinopathy (PVR). By using human enucleated eyes, vitreous samples from eyes with PVR, and a mouse model of PVR, they suggested that neural stem cells present in the Müller glia were quiescent in adult human peripheral retina and activated by retinal injury such as PVR. It could be that the autologous retinal transplant stimulates such processes [54].

In summary, mechanical scaffolding as well as stimulation of angiogenesis and neural stem cell potentiation are all thought to underlie the anatomic and visual recovery seen in macular hole repair with autologous retinal transplant. These mechanisms do not only provide rich avenues for further discovery as to the mechanisms by which peripheral retina can successfully be used to improve central vision loss from macular holes, but also methods for retinal regeneration and therapy for a wide variety of macular diseases.

References

1. Kelly NE. Vitreous surgery for idiopathic macular holes: results of a pilot study. Arch Ophthalmol. 1991;109(5):654. https://doi.org/10.1001/archopht.1991.01080050068031.
2. Parravano M, Giansanti F, Eandi CM, Yap YC, Rizzo S, Virgili G. Vitrectomy for idiopathic macular hole. Cochrane Eyes and Vision Group, ed. Cochrane Database Syst Rev. Published online May 12, 2015. https://doi.org/10.1002/14651858.CD009080.pub2
3. Spiteri Cornish K, Lois N, Scott N, et al. Vitrectomy with internal limiting membrane (ILM) peeling versus vitrectomy with no peeling for idiopathic full-thickness macular hole (FTMH). Cochrane Eyes and Vision Group, ed. Cochrane Database Syst Rev. Published online June 5, 2013. https://doi.org/10.1002/14651858.CD009306.pub2
4. Darian-Smith E, Howie AR, Allen PL, Vote BJ. Tasmanian macular hole study: whole population-based incidence of full thickness macular hole: Tasmanian macular hole study. Clin Experiment Ophthalmol. 2016;44(9):812–6. https://doi.org/10.1111/ceo.12801.
5. Kuhn F, Morris R, Mester V, Witherspoon CD. Internal limiting membrane removal for traumatic macular holes. Ophthalmic Surg Lasers. 2001;32(4):308–15.
6. Winslow RL, Taylor BC. Retinal complications following YAG laser capsulotomy. Ophthalmology. 1985;92(6):785–9. https://doi.org/10.1016/s0161-6420(85)33971-4.
7. Flaxel CJ, Adelman RA, Bailey ST, et al. Idiopathic macular hole preferred practice pattern®. Ophthalmology. 2020;127(2):P184–222. https://doi.org/10.1016/j.ophtha.2019.09.026.
8. Ho AC, Guyer DR, Fine SL. Macular hole. Surv Ophthalmol. 1998;42(5):393–416. https://doi.org/10.1016/s0039-6257(97)00132-x.
9. Aaberg TM, Blair CJ, Gass JDM. Macular holes. Am J Ophthalmol. 1970;69(4):555–62. https://doi.org/10.1016/0002-9394(70)91620-X.
10. Akiba J, Quiroz MA, Trempe CL. Role of posterior vitreous detachment in idiopathic macular holes. Ophthalmology. 1990;97(12):1610–3. https://doi.org/10.1016/S0161-6420(90)32368-0.
11. Gonvers M, Machemer R. A new approach to treating retinal detachment with macular hole. Am J Ophthalmol. 1982;94(4):468–72. https://doi.org/10.1016/0002-9394(82)90240-9.
12. Fekrat S, Wendel RT, La Cruz ZD, Green WR. Clinicopathologic correlation of an epiretinal membrane associated with a recurrent macular hole. Retina. 1995;15(1):53–7. https://doi.org/10.1097/00006982-199515010-00010.
13. Brooks HL. Macular hole surgery with and without internal limiting membrane peeling. Ophthalmology. 2000;107(10):1939–48. https://doi.org/10.1016/S0161-6420(00)00331-6.
14. Park DW, Sipperley JO, Sneed SR, Dugel PU, Jacobsen J. Macular hole surgery with internal-limiting membrane peeling and intravitreous air. Ophthalmology. 1999;106(7):1392–97; discussion 1397–1398. https://doi.org/10.1016/S0161-6420(99)00730-7
15. Olsen TW, Sternberg P, Capone A, et al. Macular hole surgery using thrombin-activated fibrinogen and selective removal of the internal limiting membrane. Retina Phila Pa. 1998;18(4):322–9. https://doi.org/10.1097/00006982-199807000-00005.
16. Eckardt C, Eckardt U, Groos S, Luciano L, Reale E. Entfernung der Membrana limitans interna bei Makulalöchern. Ophthalmol. 1997;94(8):545–51. https://doi.org/10.1007/s003470050156.

17. Smiddy WE, Pimentel S, Williams GA. Macular hole surgery without using adjunctive additives. Ophthalmic Surg Lasers. 1997;28(9):713–7.
18. Yooh HS, Brooks HL, Capone A, L'Hernault NL, Grossniklaus HE. Ultrastructural features of tissue removed during idiopathic macular hole surgery. Am J Ophthalmol. 1996;122(1):67–75. https://doi.org/10.1016/s0002-9394(14)71965-8.
19. Michalewska Z, Michalewski J, Adelman RA, Nawrocki J. Inverted internal limiting membrane flap technique for large macular holes. Ophthalmology. 2010;117(10):2018–25. https://doi.org/10.1016/j.ophtha.2010.02.011.
20. Yuan J, Zhang LL, Lu YJ, Han MY, Yu AH, Cai XJ. Vitrectomy with internal limiting membrane peeling versus inverted internal limiting membrane flap technique for macular hole-induced retinal detachment: a systematic review of literature and meta-analysis. BMC Ophthalmol. 2017;17(1):219. https://doi.org/10.1186/s12886-017-0619-8.
21. Mete M, Alfano A, Guerriero M, et al. Inverted internal limiting membrane flap technique versus complete internal limiting membrane removal in myopic macular hole surgery: a comparative study. Retina Phila Pa. 2017;37(10):1923–30. https://doi.org/10.1097/IAE.0000000000001446.
22. Rizzo S, Tartaro R, Barca F, Caporossi T, Bacherini D, Giansanti F. Internal limiting membrane peeling versus inverted flap technique for treatment of full-thickness macular holes: a comparative study in a large series of patients. Retina Phila Pa. 2018;38(Suppl 1):S73–8. https://doi.org/10.1097/IAE.0000000000001985.
23. Michalewska Z, Michalewski J, Dulczewska-Cichecka K, Adelman RA, Nawrocki J. Temporal inverted internal limiting membrane flap technique versus classic inverted internal limiting membrane flap technique: a comparative study. Retina Phila Pa. 2015;35(9):1844–50. https://doi.org/10.1097/IAE.0000000000000555.
24. Leisser C, Hirnschall N, Döller B, et al. Internal limiting membrane flap transposition for surgical repair of macular holes in primary surgery and in persistent macular holes. Eur J Ophthalmol. 2018;28(2):225–8. https://doi.org/10.5301/ejo.5001037.
25. Ho TC, Ho A, Chen MS. Vitrectomy with a modified temporal inverted limiting membrane flap to reconstruct the foveolar architecture for macular hole retinal detachment in highly myopic eyes. Acta Ophthalmol (Copenh). 2018;96(1):e46–53. https://doi.org/10.1111/aos.13514.
26. Finn AP, Mahmoud TH. Internal limiting membrane retracting door for myopic macular holes. Retina Phila Pa. 2019;39(Suppl 1):S92–4. https://doi.org/10.1097/IAE.0000000000001787.
27. Gekka T, Watanabe A, Ohkuma Y, et al. Pedicle internal limiting membrane transposition flap technique for refractory macular hole. Ophthalmic Surg Lasers Imaging Retina. 2015;46(10):1045–6. https://doi.org/10.3928/23258160-20151027-10.
28. Ozdek S, Baskaran P, Karabas L, Neves PP. A modified perfluoro-n-octane-assisted autologous internal limiting membrane transplant for failed macular hole reintervention: a case series. Ophthalmic Surg Lasers Imaging Retina. 2017;48(5):416–420. https://doi.org/10.3928/23258160-20170428-08
29. Morizane Y, Shiraga F, Kimura S, et al. Autologous transplantation of the internal limiting membrane for refractory macular holes. Am J Ophthalmol. 2014;157(4):861-869.e1. https://doi.org/10.1016/j.ajo.2013.12.028.
30. Chen SN, Yang CM. Double internal limiting membrane insertion for macular hole-associated retinal detachment. J Ophthalmol. 2017;2017:3236516. https://doi.org/10.1155/2017/3236516.
31. Kuriyama S, Hayashi H, Jingami Y, Kuramoto N, Akita J, Matsumoto M. Efficacy of inverted internal limiting membrane flap technique for the treatment of macular hole in high myopia. Am J Ophthalmol. 2013;156(1):125-131.e1. https://doi.org/10.1016/j.ajo.2013.02.014.
32. Baba R, Wakabayashi Y, Umazume K, et al. Efficacy of the inverted internal limiting membrane flap technique with vitrectomy for retinal detachment associated with myopic macular holes. Retina Phila Pa. 2017;37(3):466–71. https://doi.org/10.1097/IAE.0000000000001211.
33. Hara R, Tsukahara Y, Simoyama T, Mori S. Refined internal limiting membrane inverted flap technique for intractable macular detachment with optic disc pit. Case Rep Ophthalmol. 2017;8(1):208–13. https://doi.org/10.1159/000462956.

34. Wong D, Steel DHW. Free ILM patch transplantation for recalcitrant macular holes; should we save some internal limiting membrane for later? Graefes Arch Clin Exp Ophthalmol. 2016;254(11):2093–4. https://doi.org/10.1007/s00417-016-3462-3.
35. Yamashita T, Sakamoto T, Terasaki H, et al. Best surgical technique and outcomes for large macular holes: retrospective multicentre study in Japan. Acta Ophthalmol (Copenh). 2018;96(8):e904–10. https://doi.org/10.1111/aos.13795.
36. Grewal DS, Mahmoud TH. Autologous neurosensory retinal free flap for closure of refractory myopic macular holes. JAMA Ophthalmol. 2016;134(2):229. https://doi.org/10.1001/jamaophthalmol.2015.5237.
37. Grewal DS, Charles S, Parolini B, Kadonosono K, Mahmoud TH. Autologous retinal transplant for refractory macular holes: multicenter international collaborative study group. Ophthalmology. 2019;126(10):1399–408. https://doi.org/10.1016/j.ophtha.2019.01.027.
38. Chang YC, Liu PK, Kao TE, et al. Management of refractory large macular hole with autologous neurosensory retinal free flap transplantation. Retina Phila Pa. 2020;40(11):2134–9. https://doi.org/10.1097/IAE.0000000000002734.
39. Patel SN, Mahmoud TH, Kazahaya M, Todorich B. Autologous neurosensory retinal transplantation: bridging the gap. Retina Phila Pa. 2021;41(12):2417–23. https://doi.org/10.1097/IAE.0000000000003210.
40. Klassen H, Ziaeian B, Kirov II, Young MJ, Schwartz PH. Isolation of retinal progenitor cells from post-mortem human tissue and comparison with autologous brain progenitors. J Neurosci Res. 2004;77(3):334–43. https://doi.org/10.1002/jnr.20183.
41. Lawrence JM, Singhal S, Bhatia B, et al. MIO-M1 cells and similar muller glial cell lines derived from adult human retina exhibit neural stem cell characteristics. Stem Cells Dayt Ohio. 2007;25(8):2033–43. https://doi.org/10.1634/stemcells.2006-0724.
42. Mahato B, Kaya KD, Fan Y, et al. Pharmacologic fibroblast reprogramming into photoreceptors restores vision. Nature. 2020;581(7806):83–8. https://doi.org/10.1038/s41586-020-2201-4.
43. Scoles D, Mahmoud TH. Inaccurate measurements confound the study of myopic macular hole. Ophthalmol Retina. 2022;6(2):95–6. https://doi.org/10.1016/j.oret.2021.10.009.
44. Moysidis SN, Koulisis N, Adrean SD, et al. Autologous retinal transplantation for primary and refractory macular holes and macular hole retinal detachments. Ophthalmology. 2021;128(5):672–85. https://doi.org/10.1016/j.ophtha.2020.10.007.
45. Tanaka S, Inoue M, Inoue T, et al. Autologous retinal transplantation as a primary treatment for large chronic macular holes. Retina Phila Pa. 2020;40(10):1938–45. https://doi.org/10.1097/IAE.0000000000002693.
46. Park JG, Adrean SD, Begaj T, et al. Surgical management of full thickness macular holes in macular telangiectasia type 2. A global multicenter study. Ophthalmology. Published online September 2023:S0161642023006243. https://doi.org/10.1016/j.ophtha.2023.08.025
47. Hewson A, McAllister A, Reddie I. Autologous neurosensory retinal flap for closure of refractory macular hole in a patient with macular telangiectasia. Am J Ophthalmol Case Rep. 2020;18:100644. https://doi.org/10.1016/j.ajoc.2020.100644.
48. D'Souza P, Babu U, Narendran V. Autologous free internal limiting membrane flap for optic nerve head pit with maculopathy. Ophthalmic Surg Lasers Imaging Retina. 2017;48(4):350–3. https://doi.org/10.3928/23258160-20170329-11.
49. Temmerman IM, Mahmoud TH, Veckeneer MAH. Autologous neurosensory retinal transplant to treat refractory serous retinal detachment secondary to optic disk coloboma. Retin Cases Brief Rep. 2022;16(5):606–9. https://doi.org/10.1097/ICB.0000000000001031.
50. Parolini B, Grewal DS, Pinackatt SJ, et al. Combined autologous transplantation of neurosensory retina, retinal pigment epithelium, and choroid free grafts. Retina Phila Pa. 2018;38 Suppl 1(Suppl 1):S12-S22. https://doi.org/10.1097/IAE.0000000000001914
51. Tabandeh H. Vascularization and reperfusion of autologous retinal transplant for giant macular holes. JAMA Ophthalmol. 2020;138(3):305. https://doi.org/10.1001/jamaophthalmol.2019.5733.
52. Kitahata S, Inoue M, Yanagi Y, et al. Angiogenesis and anastomosis on graft retina after autologous retinal transplantation. Ophthalmol Retina. 2022;6(10):972–4. https://doi.org/10.1016/j.oret.2022.05.007.

53. Kitahata S, Inoue T, Nagura K, et al. Retinal morphologic features in patients with large macular holes treated by autologous neurosensory retinal transplantation. Ophthalmol Retina. 2023;7(5):406–12. https://doi.org/10.1016/j.oret.2022.12.004.
54. Johnsen EO, Frøen RC, Albert R, et al. Activation of neural progenitor cells in human eyes with proliferative vitreoretinopathy. Exp Eye Res. 2012;98:28–36. https://doi.org/10.1016/j.exer.2012.03.008.

Traumatic Macular Hole

Fabio Patelli, Mahmoud Leila, and Ehab N. El Rayes

Abstract Traumatic macular holes (TMH) are seen most commonly following blunt ocular trauma. The majority of TMHs develop immediately after trauma due to vitreous traction on the fovea associated with a rapid trampoline effect inflicted upon the globe or due to overstretching of the more elastic foveal area. Foveal microstructural OCT biomarkers and concomitant ocular pathologies secondary to trauma are significant riders that could affect the final visual outcome. Spontaneous closure of TMH is relatively more common compared to primary FTMH and warrants observation and monitoring of its development in selected cases. The size of the hole is an important factor in determining the optimal therapeutic intervention. Small TMHs $\leq 300\ \mu m$ can close spontaneously, while larger holes require surgery. Pars plana vitrectomy (PPV) and classic internal limiting membrane (ILM) peel could suffice in surgically naïve TMHs whose minimum linear diameter (MLD) is $\leq 500\ \mu m$. TMHs with larger MLD and recurrent cases require alternative surgical maneuvers.

Keywords Blunt ocular trauma · Traumatic macular hole · Secondary macular holes · Refractory macular holes · Multi-layer ILM plug technique

Supplementary Information The online version contains supplementary material available at https://doi.org/10.1007/978-3-031-63508-3_11.

F. Patelli
ASST Santi Paolo e Carlo Hospital, University of Milan, Milan, Italy
e-mail: fabio@patelli.it

M. Leila · E. N. El Rayes (✉)
Retina Department, Research Institute of Ophthalmology, Giza, Egypt
e-mail: erayes1@hotmail.com

F. Patelli et al. (eds.), *Macular Surgery*, https://doi.org/10.1007/978-3-031-63508-3_11

1 Pathogenesis

1.1 Epidemiology

A traumatic macular hole (TMH) is a full-thickness defect in the fovea from the internal limiting membrane (ILM) to the retinal pigment epithelium (RPE) that develops secondary to ocular trauma. The incidence of a TMH formation after ocular trauma is 9%. The vast majority of TMH cases are seen following blunt trauma rather than after open globe injury. The ratio is 9:1 [1].

1.2 Theories of Pathogenesis

The pathogenesis that leads to the formation of a TMH after blunt trauma is uncertain. In most cases, TMH develops immediately after trauma. A widely accepted theory entails a trampoline effect. Upon impact with a blunt object, there is a sudden shortening of the anteroposterior axis of the globe with subsequent expansion of the globe at the equator and flattening of the posterior segment. This is followed immediately by subsequent recoil to the baseline. This results in tangential traction by the relatively less mobile vitreous on the retinal surface, which snaps at the fovea, the thinnest point with a resultant full-thickness macular hole (FTMH) formation. The hole has a peculiar elliptical morphology and lacerated edges due to the uneven force inflicted on the foveal area by the blunt trauma [2, 3]. Rossi et al. [4] proposed that TMH following trauma is related to the differential elastic properties of the retina rather than to vitreous traction in the event of a trampoline effect. The avascularity of the fovea renders it relatively more elastic and, hence, more prone to deformation and rupture on extreme stretch than other parts of the retina. Less commonly, TMH has a delayed onset, which may be days or months after trauma. The purported mechanism is that blunt trauma causes dehiscence of the ILM with subsequent accumulation of fluid vitreous and hydration of the inner retina, cyst formation, and eventually a macular hole. [5, 6] In addition to direct trauma, TMH could develop through indirect mechanisms that include propagating mechanical shock waves following Nd:YAG iridotomy or head trauma [7]. In addition, TMH could develop secondary to degenerative changes that follow commotio-retinae affecting the macular area or sub-macular hemorrhage in shaken baby syndrome [8]. Obviously, open-globe injuries less commonly produce TMH because they entail sharp objects that penetrate the globe and cause extrusion of the intraocular contents rather than producing a compression force that requires an intact ocular wall. A TMH associated with open globe injury is usually caused by a direct puncture to the macular area [5].

1.3 *Factors Predicting the Visual Function After TMH Repair*

Foveal Microstructure Damage

The introduction of optical coherence tomography (OCT) particularly the ultra-high-speed models revolutionized our understanding of the foveal microstructure damage in cases of TMH and helped resolve the long-debated discrepancy of an anatomical success that is associated with less favorable visual outcome. In addition to baseline best-corrected visual acuity (BCVA), the baseline defect in the ellipsoid zone (EZ), and the macular hole height, which is defined as the vertical distance between the upper level of the hole edges and the junctional point of the detached photoreceptors and the RPE, are significant predictors of the postoperative visual outcomes. At baseline, a poorer BCVA and a lower macular height are associated with lower BCVA at 6 months after surgery. At baseline and 1 month after surgery, a larger EZ defect is associated with lower BCVA at 6 months after surgery [9, 10].

Ocular Co-morbidities

A TMH is associated frequently with other ocular morbidities caused by blunt trauma, which could compromise the final visual outcome of the patient. These morbidities could involve the anterior or posterior segments and include cataracts, sub-macular hemorrhage, traumatic optic neuropathy, rupture of Bruch's membrane that could involve the sub-foveal area, and rhegmatogenous retinal detachment (RRD) [10, 11]. Counseling the patient in the event of the presence of one or more of the aforementioned pathologies before surgical intervention for TMH is mandatory and defrays unrealistic expectations regarding the final visual outcome.

2 Management of TMH

2.1 *Observation for Spontaneous Closure: When is It Warranted?*

In contrast to primary FTMH, the incidence of spontaneous closure of a TMH is fairly high. The proportion is 10.7–44.4% compared to 2.7–6.2% for primary macular holes. The factors that herald spontaneous closure of TMH are small minimum linear diameter (MLD) $\leq$ 300 μm, absence of intraretinal cysts at the edges of the hole, and young age of the patient. The mechanism of spontaneous closure entails the proliferation of the glial cells at the edges and the bottom of the hole to bridge the full-thickness defect and eventually induce closure. Three prognostic factors combine in tandem to promote the closure of a traumatic FTMH. Firstly, a smaller MLD facilitates the approximation of the edges of the hole by the proliferating glial cells. Secondly, the absence of intra-retinal cysts at the edges indicates that there is no traction produced by the ILM, which if present would hinder the approximation of the edges. Finally, young age is associated with a more rigorous healing response than older age groups. Therefore, whenever one or more of these prognostic factors are present, it is prudent to observe a patient with a TMH as long as serial OCT examination demonstrates a reduction of the hole size and approximation of the edges. Spontaneous closure could take up to 12 months to fully ensue, however, waiting that long could risk irreversible damage to the photoreceptors. In pediatric patients during the amblyogenic period, early intervention is warranted to avoid the development of amblyopia. Therefore, surgical intervention is recommended if spontaneous closure is not completed within 3 months. [10, 12–15]

2.2 *Surgery for TMH*

Surgical intervention is indicated in cases where spontaneous closure is not likely to occur due to the large size of the hole at initial presentation, or whenever serial OCT scans reveal that the hole size is stationary or has increased.

Tailoring the Surgical Repair: Classic Surgical Approach

The classic surgical approach is adopted in small-sized TMH, typically whose MLD is $\leq$ 500 microns. It consists of pars plana vitrectomy (PPV) and peeling of epiretinal membrane (ERM) if present, ILM surgery, and gas tamponade. PPV and ERM peel eliminate the anteroposterior and tangential traction on the edges of the hole, respectively. Peeling the ILM will sheer off the footplates of Müller cells and induce a stimulus for glial cell proliferation to close the hole. In addition, ILM peel will increase the mobility of the edges of the hole to promote their approximation to close the hole. Gas tamponade will seal the hole and insulate it from the fluid currents in the vitreous cavity [16–19].

Surgery for Large-Sized Holes

In large-sized TMH whose MLD is $\geq$ 500 microns, the classic surgical technique invariably leads to inferior outcomes compared to those of small-sized TMH, with a higher incidence of failed closure, post-operative flat-open hole configuration, late re-opening, and less anatomical closure in terms of the failure of restoration of the EZ and the outer retinal layers continuity, namely the external limiting membrane (ELM) and the inner-segment/outer segment (IS/OS) junction layer and, hence worse visual outcome [20, 21]. Therefore, an alternative surgical technique that includes an additional scaffold effect is required to act as a platform for glial cell proliferation to bridge the gap between the edges. In surgically naïve TMH, this scaffold could be the ILM itself. Patients with recurrent TMH or those who had a failure of initial ILM surgery require alternative tissues to act as scaffolds. The most commonly used surgical techniques in large-sized TMH are as follows,

Surgical Techniques for the Initial Repair of TMH

Inverted ILM flap Technique

This technique was described by Michalewska et al. [22] in 2010. It entailed leaving remnants of the ILM attached to the margins of the macular hole instead of completely peeling the ILM. The ILM flaps were then inverted to cover the hole completely. The flaps were inverted upside down so that the vitreous side of the ILM faced the RPE. The rationale for this technique was that the remnants of the ILM that were left attached to the margins of the hole acted as a stimulus to incite glial cell proliferation and that the inverted flaps provided a scaffold for the proliferating cells to bridge the full-thickness defect. The authors used this technique in stage III and IV FTMH with a mean MLD of 759 μm. The authors reported a 98% closure rate and a flat-open closure in one eye.

Temporal Inverted ILM flap Technique

Michalewska et al. [23] introduced this technique in 2015. In this technique, the ILM is peeled only in an area approximately 2-disc diameters in size temporal to the macula, and the flap is left attached at the temporal margin of the hole and inverted to cover the hole. The authors demonstrated that similar anatomical and functional success rates could be achieved in large macular holes with a mean MLD of 544 μm using this technique compared to the classic inverted ILM flap technique while reducing the area of the peeled ILM and consequently surgical trauma in the form of dissociated optic nerve fiber layer (DONFL).

Authors' Approach for Large-Sized TMH: Multi-layer ILM Plug (MIP) technique [24]

We introduced the MIP technique in 2020 for large FTMH. The technique consists of creating multiple contiguous breaks in the ILM along 360° around the hole. The ILM breaks are initiated distally to the hole by a distance that is at least double its size using the Grieshaber FINESSE Flex Loop, Alcon, Geneva, Switzerland, or the Tano diamond-dusted scraper. The ILM breaks are joined using the Flex loop to form a rosette pattern ILM flap. The flap edges are elevated off the retinal surface and gently pulled centripetally toward the hole under PFCL until reaching the margins of the hole. The ILM flap is left tethered to the margins of the hole and then folded in multiple layers to cover the surface of the hole using the Flex Loop, Tano scraper, or vitreoretinal forceps to form a multi-layer plug. **Video, supplemental digital content 1**. It is important to avoid tucking the flap inside the hole to avoid damage to the RPE at its base. Finally, air/PFCL exchange is performed under low infusion pressure using passive suction over the optic nerve head to avoid displacing the flap, followed by air/sulfur hexafluoride (SF6) 20% exchange. Patients are asked to initially adopt a face-down position for at least 2 days and then a reading position for 3 more days. Three mechanisms in the MIP technique help close the hole in addition to relieving the anteroposterior traction on the margins of the hole by PPV. Firstly, the centripetal dragging effect produced by the Flex loop during reflecting the ILM flap towards the hole helps reduce the hole size. Secondly, the multilayer configuration of the ILM that forms the plug seals the hole effectively and renders the plug resilient to displacement intra- or post-operatively. Thirdly, the shearing of the footplates of Müller cells while peeling the ILM and the residual attachment of the ILM flap to the margins of the hole stimulate the proliferation of glial cells to close the hole. Finally, the undersurface of the multiple ILM flaps is laden with fragments of Müller cells that replenish the hole and induce glial cell proliferation. We published a prospective case series in 2022 including 15 eyes of 15 patients with different types of FTMH and a mean MLD of 702 μm. We had a 100%—hole closure rate, of which 93% was a U-type closure. The mean improvement of best-corrected visual acuity (BCVA) was 5 lines.

Surgery for Refractory TMH

Human Amniotic membrane (hAM) Graft

In patients who did not achieve hole closure following the MIP technique, or in whom the technique was not possible to execute, we perform repeat surgery using an amniotic membrane graft placed above the hole. The graft size should be at least double the MLD of the hole. The rationale for using hAM in macular hole surgery is based on experimental evidence that sub-retinal implantation of hAM promoted the proliferation of RPE cells. The growing cells demonstrated epithelial phenotypic features and produced growth factors capable of reproducing normal retinal homeostasis. In 2019, Rizzo et al. [25] demonstrated that sub-retinal implantation of hAM graft in a recurrent macular hole promoted the closure of the hole and restoration of the normal retinal layer stratification. In contrast to Rizzo et al. [25], we prefer an epi-retinal placement of the graft instead of tucking it inside the hole to avoid inadvertent damage to the RPE in the base of the hole Fig. 1.

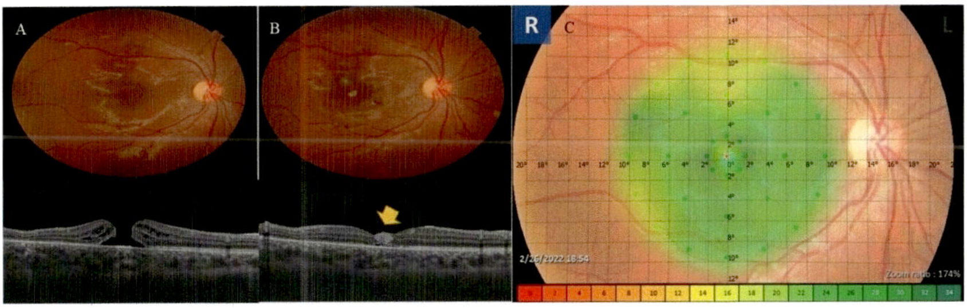

Fig. 1 A. The color fundus photo and the corresponding OCT scan of the right eye of a 38-year-old female show an FTMH. The patient previously had PPV and ILM peel for treating a traumatic FTMH that resulted in failed closure of the hole. B. The color fundus photo and the corresponding OCT scan of the same eye after repeat surgery using hAM graft. Note the hAM graft in situ (yellow arrow) and U-type closure of the hole. There is a residual localized sub-foveal neurosensory detachment. C. A microperimetry image of the right macula shows a stable fixation, which indicates improved macular sensitivity

3 Case Scenarios

Case 1. A 12-year-old boy presented with a history of blunt trauma to the left eye by a brick for 4 months. His BCVA was 3/60. His anterior segment examination was unremarkable. Fundus examination revealed an FTMH and diffuse RPE mottling covering an area of approximately 2-disc diameters (DD) around the hole. MLD by OCT was 648μm and the maximum diameter at the base of the hole was 3212 μm. The patient had PPV, MIP technique, and SF6 20% gas tamponade. One month post-operatively, OCT examination revealed U-type closure of the hole albeit foveal thinning and no restoration of the ELM and IS/OS layers. At the 6-month follow-up visit his BCVA improved to 6/60 with an approximation of the ELM and IS/OS ends on either side of the fovea albeit a persistent sub-foveal defect in both layers. Figures 2 and 3.

Case 2. A 28-year-old male presented with a history of blunt trauma to the right eye by a metal bolt for 8 months. His BCVA was 2/60. His anterior segment examination was unremarkable. Fundus examination revealed an FTMH. MLD by OCT was 731 μm and the maximum diameter at the base of the hole was 1187 μm. The patient had PPV, MIP technique, and SF6 20% gas tamponade. Oneweek post-operatively, OCT examination revealed U-type closure of the hole. His BCVA improved to 6/60 at the 1-month follow-up visit Fig. 4.

4 Clinical Pearls

- *Explore.* Frequently, a TMH is not an isolated event. Blunt ocular trauma is a pan-ocular event that dictates conducting a thorough full examination of the anterior and posterior segments of the eye to detect additional pathologies due

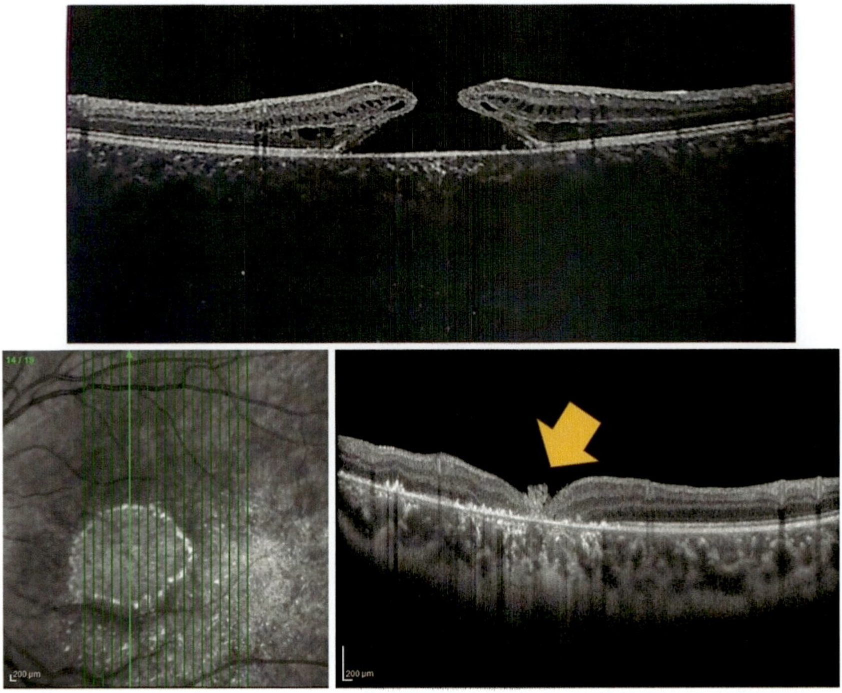

Fig. 2 Top. An OCT of the macular area of the left eye in a 5- line cross scan mode shows an FTMH with an MLD 648 μm. BCVA was 3/60. Bottom. An enhanced depth imaging (EDI)-OCT thickness map of the macular area of the same eye, 1 month after performing the MIP technique. Note the ILM plug (yellow arrow). The macular hole has closed in a U-type configuration

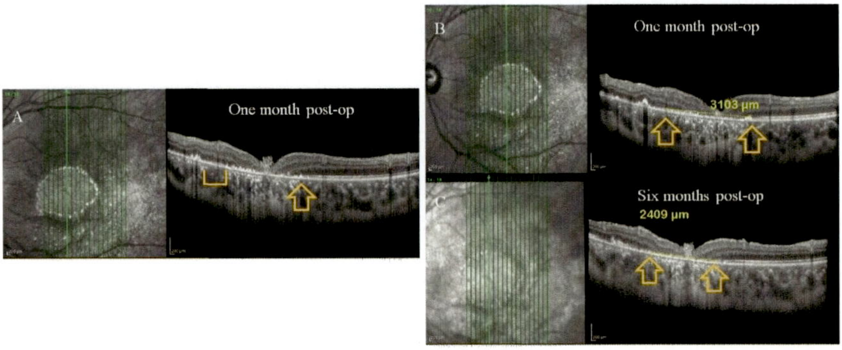

Fig. 3 A-C. Serial EDI-OCT thickness map of the macular area of the same eyefrom 1 to 6 months postoperatively. Note that at 1-month post-operative (A, B) there was still no restoration of the sub-foveal ELM and IS/OS layers. The yellow arrow marks the temporal end of the ELM and IS/OS layers, while the yellow bracket marks the only identifiable segment of the ELM and IS/OS layers in the nasal parafoveal area. The distance between the 2 ends is 3103 μm. At 6 months postoperatively (C), there is a gradual restoration of the ELM and IS/OS layers and a reduction of the distance separating them to 2409 μm (yellow arrows)

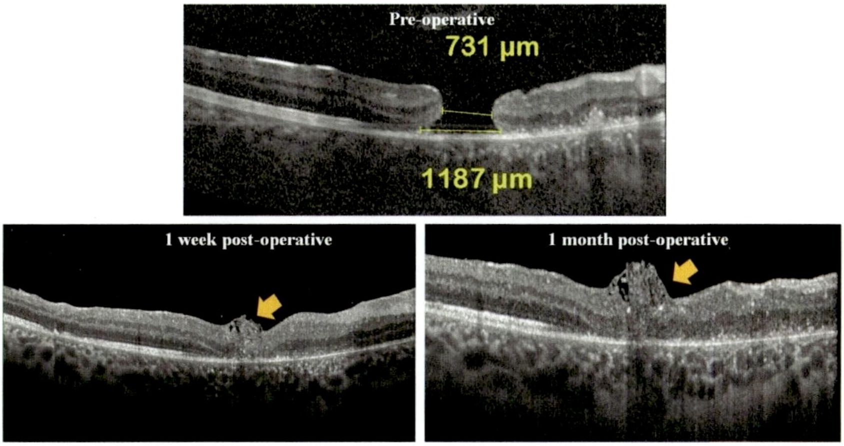

Fig. 4 Top. An EDI-OCT image in a radial scan mode of the right macula of a 28-year-old male shows an FTMH. Bottom. EDI-OCT images of the same eye 1 week (left) and 1 month (right) after PPV and MIP technique. Note the multi-layered ILM flap (yellow arrow) and the U-type closure of the hole. There was no restoration of the sub-foveal ELM and IS/OS layers

to trauma as a recession of the anterior chamber angle, cataract, retinal dialysis, or retinal detachment. The existence of one or more of these co-morbidities mandates tailoring a particular surgical plan that might not focus exclusively on the management of TMH.

- *Observe.* A TMH is known to undergo spontaneous closure. Therefore, once the diagnosis of a TMH is established, the patient must be observed for 3 months while performing serial OCT examination, particularly in young patients with a TMH whose MLD $\leq$ 300 µm, and in the absence of traction on the hole edges. The observation period should be interrupted whenever an OCT exam shows an enlargement of the hole size and surgery becomes the only viable option.
- *Counsel.* The patients or their parents should receive adequate explanation prior to proceeding to surgery to defray any unrealistic expectations regarding the surgical outcome, particularly in the presence of associated pathologies other than the TMH that could significantly compromise the final visual outcome as in a submacular hemorrhage, traumatic optic neuropathy, or choroidal rupture that bisects the fovea
- *Select.* The surgical procedure selected will depend on the size of the hole and should be based on the evidence provided by the literature. Macular holes with an MLD $\geq$ 500 µm are not expected to close using the classic ILM peeling procedure and are prone to an initial failure or late re-opening Fig. 5.

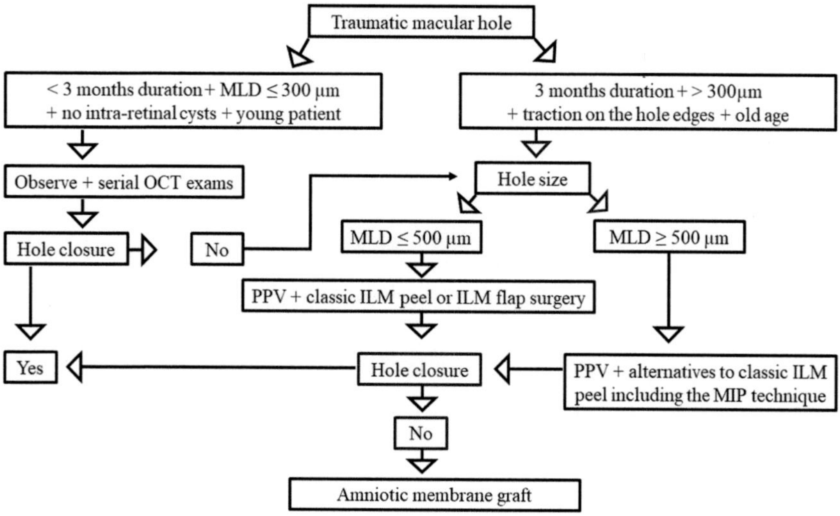

Fig. 5 A schematic diagram for the management of a TMH

References

1. Kuhn F, Morris R, Mester V, Witherspoon CD. Internal limiting membrane removal for traumatic macular holes. Ophthalmic Surg Lasers. 2001;32(4):308–15.
2. Johnson RN, McDonald HR, Lewis H, et al. Traumatic macular hole: observations, pathogenesis, and results of vitrectomy surgery. Ophthalmology. 2001;108(5):853–7.
3. Yanagiya N, Akiba J, Takahashi M, et al. Clinical characteristics of traumatic macular holes. Jpn J Ophthalmol. 1996;40(4):544–7.
4. Rossi T, Boccassini B, Esposito L, et al. The pathogenesis of retinal damage in blunt eye trauma: finite element modeling. Invest Ophthalmol Vis Sci. 2011;52(7):3994–4002.
5. Tornambe PE. Macular hole genesis: the hydration theory. Retina. 2003;23(3):421–4.
6. Huang J, Liu X, Wu Z, et al. Classification of full-thickness traumatic macular holes by optical coherence tomography. Retina. 2009;29(3):340–8.
7. Kunjukunju N, Navarro A, Oliver S, et al. Bilateral macular hole formation secondary to sclopetaria caused by shockwaves transmitted by a posterior vector: case report. BMC Ophthalmol. 2010;10:6. https://doi.org/10.1186/1471-2415-10-6.
8. Ou JI, Moshfeghi DM, Tawansy K, Sears JE. Macular Hole in the shaken baby syndrome. Arch Ophthalmol. 2006;124(6):913–5.
9. Wang M, Yu Y, Wang Z, Liang X, Liu W. Surgical treatment for traumatic macular holes: reconstructive changes in foveal microstructures and visual predictors analysis. Ophthalmologica. 2021;244(4):339–46.
10. Liu W, Grzybowski A. Current management of traumatic macular holes. J Ophthalmol. 2017;2017:1748135.
11. Weichel ED, Colyer MH. Traumatic macular holes secondary to combat ocular trauma. Retina. 2009;29(3):349–54.
12. Gao M, Liu K, Lin Q, Liu H. Management modalities for traumatic macular hole: a systematic review and single-arm meta-analysis. Curr Eye Res. 2017;42(2):287–96.
13. Menchini U, Virgili G, Giacomelli G, Cappelli S, Giansanti F. Mechanism of spontaneous closure of traumatic macular hole: OCT study of one case. Retina. 2003;23(1):104–6.

14. Miller JB, Yonekawa Y, Eliott D, Vavvas DG. A review of traumatic macular hole: diagnosis and treatment. Int Ophthalmol Clin 2013 Fall;53(4):59–67.
15. Chen H, Chen W, Zheng K, et al. Prediction of spontaneous closure of traumatic macular hole with spectral domain optical coherence tomography. Sci Rep. 2015;21(5):12343. https://doi.org/10.1038/srep12343.
16. Kelly NE, Wendel RT. Vitreous surgery for idiopathic macular holes. Results of a pilot study. Arch Ophthalmol. 1991;109(5):654–9.
17. Wendel RT, Patel AC, Kelly NE, et al. Vitreous surgery for macular holes. Ophthalmology. 1993;100(11):1671–6.
18. Eckardt C, Eckardt U, Groos S, et al. Entfernung der Membrana limitans interna bei Makulalöchern Klinische und morphologische Befunde. Ophthalmologe. 1997;94:545–51.
19. Smiddy WE, Feuer W, Cordahi G. Internal limiting membrane peeling in macular hole surgery. Ophthalmology. 2001;108(8):1471–6.
20. BEAVRS Macular hole outcome group. Factors affecting anatomical and visual outcome after macular hole surgery: findings from a large prospective UK cohort. Eye (Lond). 2021;35(1):316–25.
21. The Manchester Large Macular Hole Study. Is it time to reclassify large macular holes? Am J Ophthalmol. 2018;195:36–42.
22. Michalewska Z, Michalewski J, Adelman RA, Nawrocki J. Inverted internal limiting membrane flap technique for large macular holes. Ophthalmology. 2010;117(10):2018–25.
23. Michalewska Z, Michalewski J, Dulczewska-Cichecka K, Adelman RA, Nawrocki J. Temporal inverted internal limiting membrane flap technique versus classic inverted internal limiting membrane flap technique: a comparative study. Retina. 2015;35(9):1844–50.
24. El Rayes EN, Leila M, Stavrakas P. Multi-layer internal limiting membrane plug technique for management of large full-thickness macular holes. Int J Retin Vitr. 2022;8:80.
25. Rizzo S, Caporossi T, Tartaro R, et al. A Human amniotic membrane plug to promote retinal breaks repair and recurrent macular hole closure. Retina. 2019;39(Suppl 1):S95–103.

Myopic Traction Maculopathy

Giacomo Panozzo and Giovanni Bellisario

Abstract Myopic Traction Maculopathy (MTM) can be considered an "umbrella" term under which different kinds of myopic maculopathies can be located. All of them are caused by the interaction of tractional forces. MTM is one of the possible manifestations of pathologic myopia. Knowing the physiopathology of a high-myopic eye is essential in order to achieve the best management of the related conditions.

Keywords Degenerative Myopia · Myopic Maculopathy · Myopic Traction Maculopathy · Vitrectomy

1 Myopia, a Different World

Myopia is a common eye disorder characterized by a mismatch between the refractive power of the eye and the corresponding axial length. As result, the focal plane of the image is located in front of the retina. The retina and the sclera are strictly involved: concurrently to the eye development, the sclera axially elongates the eye to properly locate the focal plane on the retinal surface.

Myopia is a complex disease with a multi-factorial etiology, where both genetics and environment play a major role. In many species, it is well demonstrated that a dopamine-based light-dependent local signaling process is beside the development of an emmetropic eye.

A great number of animal studies reports that although genetics determine myopic susceptibility, the eye growth is finally affected by environmental factors. Thus, several risk factors have been highlighted (near work, ambient lighting, higher education, scholastic performance, lack of open-air activities, urbanization and more), and

G. Panozzo (✉)
Casa di Cura S. Francesco, Verona, Italy
e-mail: g.panozzo@iol.it

G. Bellisario
Ophthalmology Unit, Department of Neurosciences, Biomedicine and Movement, University of Verona, Verona, Italy

F. Patelli et al. (eds.), *Macular Surgery*, https://doi.org/10.1007/978-3-031-63508-3_12

different strategies improved in the attempt of managing the development of myopia to a higher stage.

High variability of the prevalence of myopia can be observed in different ethnic and geographic populations. The reported prevalence rates of myopia in the United States are 20–50%, while in some parts of Asia 80–90%. Usually, myopia is classified in non-pathologic and pathologic.

Non-pathologic myopia accounts 95% of cases, the refractive error is low-to-moderate (< 6.00 D of SE or an axial length < 26.5 mm), the onset is in childhood with a stabilization in the second decade of life; the eye is normally developed, but the refractive power and the axial length are not correlated.

Pathologic or degenerative myopia (PM) appears earlier in the childhood and worsens faster; it is defined as a form of high myopia (HM, such as a refractive error > 6.00 D of SE or an axial length > 26.5 mm) associated to degenerative changes in the sclera, choroid and retina.

1.1 The Role of the Sclera in Pathologic Myopia

The main structural change in the myopic eyes is axial elongation; changes in scleral composition and biomechanics contribute to determine changes in the scleral shape.

The human sclera is made of fibrous connective tissue: fibroblasts and myofibroblasts are surrounded by extracellular scleral matrix.

Collagen is the major component of the matrix; thus, its microstructural arrangement determines the biomechanical properties of the sclera.

In an emmetropic eye, type I collagen is the most represented subtype (in humans it represents the 90%) and plays a major role in the scleral architecture; usually, the scleral collagen is arranged in multilayered sheets of lamellae, whose orientation and thickness vary depending on the location among the globe.

Proteoglycans, and their glycosaminoglycans (GAG) side chains, have a marginal impact on sclera's weight, though they play an important role in the viscoelastic behavior of the sclera. The most frequent GAGs are dermatan sulfate and chondroitin sulfate.

In a myopic environment both the ECM and the cellular population of the sclera show great changes (discussed later), contributing to determine the peculiar scleral shape.

Posterior staphyloma

The typical degenerative process that characterizes PM is staphyloma. One of the most updated, though not comprehensive, definition of staphyloma was proposed by Spaide R. F. et al. as "an outpouching of the wall of the eye that has a radius of curvature that is less than the surrounding curvature of the wall of the eye". The term "posterior pole staphyloma" refers to the staphyloma that involves both the macula and the optic nerve, and it is based on the first classification proposed by Curtin B.

J. in 1977:ten different types of posterior staphyloma were described (five primary and five compound forms, based on their funduscopic appearance).

A better insight and classification of the staphyloma were possible by matching the results of multi-modal imaging techniques, such as three-dimensional magnetic resonance imaging (3D MRI), optical coherence tomography (OCT) and wide-field fundus imaging, overcoming the limitation of ultrasonography (US) in analyzing larger staphyloma.

In such a way, Ohno-Matsui K. et al. developed a new classification of posterior staphylomas: wide macular, narrow macular, peripapillary, nasal, inferior and other staphylomas. Furthermore, they evaluated the role of staphyloma in the development of myopic maculopathies: its presence is correlated to the development of diffuse chorioretinal atrophy and mCNV, while asymmetric staphyloma is frequently seen in eyes developing MTM.

Posterior staphyloma is the major anatomic feature predisposing high myopic eyes to the development of tractional maculopathies .

2 The Rising of a New Concept: The Myopic Maculopathy (MM)

2.1 *Clinical Features and Classification*

Since 1970s, several attempts were made to reach a comprehensive classification of the pathological processes affecting an eye with pathologic myopia (PM). Both the retinal periphery and the macular area are affected by PM.

The key-clinical aspects of the myopic maculopathy are:

- consequences of tractional stress (VMT, MH, schis-like lesions);
- choroidal neovascularization;
- different patterns of chorioretinal atrophy (tessellated fundus, diffuse atrophy, patchy atrophy, and lacquer cracks) and anomalies in the choriocapillaris or in the Bruch's membrane (macular-Bruch membrane holes)

In 2015 Ohno-Matsui K. et al. proposed a classification, the META-PM (Table 1), based on fundus photographs, aiming to reach reproducibility in diagnosing and staging the pathology.

Indeed, in 1970 Curtin and Karlin have already described aspects of myopic maculopathy basing on the characteristic fundus changes: chorioretinal atrophy, central pigment spot ("Fuchs' spot"), lacquer cracks, posterior staphyloma, and optic disc changes.

Table 1 META-PM classification proposed by Ohno-Matsui K. et al. in 2015

I. Myopic macular lesions
Tessellated fundus (category 1) Well-defined choroidal vessels that can be observed clearly around the fovea as well as around the arcade vessels
Diffuse chorioretinal atrophy (Category 2) Yellowish-white appearance of posterior pole. When present, further estimate size and extent using disc area as a relative size unit
Patchy chorioretinal atrophy (category 3) Well-defined, grayish-white lesions in the macular area or around the optic disc
Macular atrophy (category 4) Well-defined, grayish-white or whitish, round chorioretinal atrophic lesion in the foveal region; May appear around a regressed CNV (Fuchs' spot)
II. "Plus" lesions of the myopic macular lesions
Lacquer cracks Yellowish linear lesions in the macula. Often crisscross over the underlying choroidal vessels. Newly developed lacquer cracks may be seen with hemorrhage
Choroidal neovascularization (CNV) Lesion associated with choroidal neovascularization and exudation, hemorrhage or serous retinal detachment at the posterior pole
Fuchs' spot Pigmented grayish-white scar of myopic CNV without associated exudation, and sometimes associated with pigmentation
III. Posterior staphyloma
Local bulging of the sclera at the posterior pole of the eye, that has a radius of less than the surrounding curvature of the wall of the eye: • Macula involved: wide (Curtin's type I), narrow (Curtin's type II), and inferior (Curtin's type V) • Macula not involved: peripapillary (Curtin's type III), nasal (Curtin's type IV) and inferior (Curtin's type V) • Others (Curtin's type VI–X and any posterior staphyloma that cannot be classified into Curtin's I–X)

Avila et al. in 1984 proposed a scale of macular changes including:

- Tessellation (M1),
- posterior staphyloma (M2),
- lacquer cracks (M3),
- focal choroidal atrophy (M4),
- large geographic atrophy (M5).

Hayashi et al. in 2010 described thoroughly different myopic maculopathy lesions, proposing a pattern of progression for each of them.

Trying to overcome limitations of the previous classifications, but encompassing both (Avila et al. and Hayashi et al. classifications), the META-PM was developed to obtain a systematic description of MM features in the most reliable, reproducible (inter- and intra-observer agreement) and accessible way (fundus photography); thus, allowing an easier diagnosis and classification of the myopic maculopathy.

Five "categories" were identified:

- No myopic retinal lesions (Category 0),
- Tessellated fundus only (Category 1),
- Diffuse chorioretinal atrophy (Category 2),
- Patchy chorioretinal atrophy (Category 3),
- Macular atrophy (Category 4).

Furthermore, three "plus" lesions were identified, which were not included among the other categories since they can develop from—and coexist with—each category; they are:

- lacquer cracks (Lc),
- myopic CNV,
- Fuchs' spot (Fs).

Basing on long-term clinical observation, the progression from Category 1 to 3 was associated with the increasing risk of developing myopic CNV and macular atrophy. Finally, slightly changes to the Curtin classification of posterior staphyloma were introduced, although it wasn't included in any categories since considered an independent morphological aspect.

It was reported a relatively high intra-observer agreement and acceptable inter-observer agreement adopting this classification system; this was a major goal for META-PM classification.

In an era characterised by the limited availability of OCT or fluorangiography in the non-referral centres, the adoption of the funduscopic appearance as diagnostic and classification parameter has allowed a wider clinical use of that classification; on the other hand, the spectrum of changes detectable only by OCT was totally excluded. Myopic Traction Maculopathy (MTM), as well as dome-shaped macula (DSM) and different stages of CNV were absent in META-PM classification of MM, weakening the possibility of its comprehensive use in the clinical practice.

That's why, in 2019 Fang Y. et al. conducted an observational retrospective study to establish an OCT-based classification of myopic maculopathy, including MTM and DSM. Their purpose was to overcome the limitations of the META-PM classification through the adoption of the OCT technology as diagnostic tool (more reliable and standardize); furthermore, they analyze the choroidal thickness (CT) for each "category" of MM lesions identified by META-PM classification.

A continuous, although not homogenous, reduction of CT leads and diagnostically characterized—the worsening of the MM. CT was found almost halved in all locations with the progression from "no maculopathy" to "tessellated fundus". Later, the ophthalmoscopic finding of diffuse chorioretinal atrophy develops initially around the optic disc (PDCA—peripapillary diffuse choroidal atrophy) and is accompanied by a CT reduction confined to the nasal location.

A value of CT < 56.5 μm at 3000 μm nasal from the fovea, predicts the progression from tessellated fundus to PDCA.

The progressive reduction of subfoveal CT is found when the atrophy enlarges to cover the entire posterior pole (MDCA—macular diffuse choroidal atrophy).

A value of CT < 62 μm at subfoveal, predicts the progression from PDCA to MDCA.

The progression from diffuse CA to patchy atrophy was no longer characterized by a further decrease in CT but—coherently with previous swept source—OCT analyses—to a new development of Bruchs membrane (BM) hole. It was hypothesized that those holes in the macular BM may be accounted to an enlargement of lacquer cracks, or to a vulnerability of BM in already advanced atrophic region.

The final stage "macular atrophy" was the result of an enlargement of the patchy atrophy, or the last evolution of a myopic CNV.

Furthermore, the value of CT < 56.5 μm at 3000 μm nasal from the fovea in conjunction to/or alternatively to the presence of Bruch membrane (BM) defects (Lacquer cracks and patchy atrophy) establishes the passage from "high myopia" to "pathologic myopia". Finally, subfoveal CT was found as significantly correlated to axial length and age, as well as to CNV, MTM and DSM (all these MM aspects were counted in the classification).

In 2019 Ruiz-Medrano J. et al. proposed a new, more comprehensive classification system (the ATN classification) to encompass all the possible manifestations of the myopic maculopathy.

The spectrum of alterations determining a "maculopathy" in a myopic eye can be outlined in three main areas: atrophic lesions, tractional lesions and neovascular lesions.

Basing on these categories, the new ATN classification identifies (Table 2):

A—atrophic-MM, T—tractional-MM, N—neo-vascular-MM

The purpose of our chapter is to analyze the tractional myopic maculopathy, its pathogenesis, clinical manifestations, hence its management strategies and surgical treatment.

A large part of our knowledge on myopic maculopathy derives from the in-vivo information provided by diagnostic instruments, histological studies, animal models, as well as from experiences in surgical treatments of high myopic eye. The role of novel diagnostic technologies was pivotal in the enhancements of our insight in physio-pathological basics of traction maculopathy.

3 The Advent of the OCT Technology: A New Gold Standard for Retinal Imaging

In the pre-OCT era, very few instruments were available to study a myopic eye, its particular aspects and the eventual onset of complications; the magnitude of the disease was often detected only at his most dramatic- and final-stage: posterior retinal detachment with macular hole. Slit lamp examination, fundus camera photography, A-scan or B-scan ultrasonography were the most diffused and used tools in the

Table 2 ATN classification proposed by Ruiz-Medrano et al. in 2019

Atrophic MM	
A0	No myopic retinal lesions
A1	Tessellated fundus only
A2	Diffuse chorioretinal atrophy
A3	Patchy chorioretinal atrophy
A4	Complete macular atrophy
Neovascular MM	
N0	No mCNV
N1	Macular Lc
N2a	Active CNV
N2b	Scar or Fuch's spot
Tractional MM	
T0	No macular schisis
T1	Inner or outer foveoschisis
T2	Inner + outer foveoschisis
T3	Foveal detachment
T4	Full-thickness macular hole
T5	Macular hole + retinal detachment

retinal examination. Laser photocoagulation, and its blenching effect on the treated retina, was proposed as a useful technique to differentiate retinal detachment from retinoschisis; it was soon archived due to the lack of specificity.

With the advent of the OCT technology, it became possible to early detect macular abnormalities and to gain insight to the physio-pathological processes that lead to MTM.

By the end of the 90s, several studies agreed that myopic macular holes can be complicated by the development of extensive retinal detachment. In 1985, Green highlighted a particular histopathologic aspect of the peripheral retina called "stretch schisis"; no internal membranes or focal inner retinal traction were detected in these areas. Formerly in 1938, Rochon-Duvigneaud reported similar findings in the posterior pole.

In 1999 Michael Ip et al. first reported the role of the OCT technology in the differential diagnosis of retinal detachment and retinoschisis. They described retinoschisis as a splitting of the neurosensory retina, with a thin band of moderately reflective tissue over the more reflective RPE band; retinal detachment as a full-thickness separation of the moderately reflective neurosensory retina from the underlying high reflective RPE band.

The demonstration of the utility of OCT imaging in this field helped to overcame other less accurate diagnostic procedures (e.g.: laser photocoagulation, visual field test, B-Scan echography, etc.) and turned-on the attention on other retinal pathology that could benefit from tomographic technique.

In 1999 Takano M. et al. applied the new OCT technology to evaluate retina tomographic aspects in patients with severe myopia and posterior staphyloma. They moved from the observation that idiopathic macular hole in emmetropic patients is rarely associated with retinal detachment; in high myopic patients with posterior staphyloma macular hole is usually associated with retinal detachment. First, they observed that retinoschisis or retinal detachment is quite frequent among high myopic patients with posterior staphyloma (34%). They adopted the above-mentioned imaging criteria to differentiate retinoschisis from retinal detachment and postulated that in severe myopic eye, retinal detachment and retinoschisis can develop inside macular area even without a preexisting macular hole; thought MH can develop in the macular area in case of preexisting RD or retinoschisis.

Since the surgeons experienced the presence of a large liquefied lacuna and preretinal vitreous cortex in the posterior staphyloma, they suggested to proceed the investigation of the vitreoretinal interface in order to understand macular holes' pathogenesis in high myopic eyes.

The OCT technology played a pivotal role, since it enhanced and integrated histological studies of the morphological appearance of the posterior staphyloma.

In myopic eyes, indeed, several characteristics and abnormalities can be found, especially in that interested by degenerative myopia; both the anterior and the posterior retina are affected. The choroid, the retina, and the vitreoretinal interface in degenerative myopia can often assume characteristic and confounding features (i.e., tigroid fundus, thin retina, areas of choriocapillaris atrophy, retinal pigment epithelium hypopigmentation and/or hyperpigmentation, posterior staphyloma, etc.). The cross-sectional images of retinal structure obtained with the first available OCT technologies, allowed a better study of the posterior vitreoretinal anatomy in eyes with high myopia and the detection of subtle macular changes.

In 2004 Panozzo e Mercanti firstly proposed to unify all the pathologic features generated by tractions in the myopic environment under the name of "myopic traction maculopathy" (MTM), with the purpose of achieving a better insight of the disease's genesis. In an OCT-based study, they analyzed non symptomatic degenerative myopic eyes to reveal the potential presence of early—and otherwise undetectable—epiretinal traction or retinal abnormalities. These early stages of MTM, indeed, are almost invisible to the commonly available diagnostic techniques and tools (e.g. biomicroscopy, stereoangiography, ultrasonography), that usually allowed a late detection of the most advanced stages of MTM.

As already demonstrated by Gallemore et al., the OCT is much more sensitive than biomicroscopy in detecting subtle internal retinal changes through cross-sectional images with a high spatial resolution.

According to Panozzo et al, almost half of the eyes analyzed showed a form of macular traction (either tangential-ERM- or anteroposterior-VMT) beside the typical myopic staphyloma. Up to one third of eyes had a form of retinal damage such as macular retinoschisis, alone or associated with other lesions. Only few eyes with macular changes had only a staphyloma condition, the majority of them showed association with epiretinal traction.

These findings led to speculate that epiretinal tractions probably play a major role in the development of retinal damage, eventually enhanced by the presence of staphyloma and retinal stretching due to progressive scleral elongation.

4 Myopic Traction Maculopathy (MTM): Pathogenesis

The development of tractional forces leading to MTM takes place in the post equatorial area. In a study of Henaine-Berra et al. it was estimated the prevalence of macular anatomic abnormalities in high myopic eyes: it was of 22.41% in eyes with pathologic myopia and of 53.65% in eyes with posterior staphyloma.

The macular damage can be accounted to the interaction of different elements, alone or variably associated: the epiretinal membrane (ERM) and the foveal vitreoretinal adhesion (vitreomacular traction, VMT) generate forces acting in different directions, in a contest already characterized by the presence of posterior staphyloma and by the progressive global scleral stretching.

Schematically, in a contest of degenerative myopia (with a posterior staphyloma) the posterior retinal environment is characterized by a condition of general instability mainly accountable to the interaction of two forces:

(1) an internal/centripetal traction and tangential force, caused by epiretinal membranes (ERM), vitreomacular traction (VMT) and incomplete posterior vitreous detachment (PVD);
(2) an external/centrifugal traction, caused by staphyloma and progressive scleral stretching.

Thanks to its unique multi-layer anatomy, the retina presents different stiffness values, thus different reactions to tractional stress. Under these forces the retina does not detach or rip, but is stretched in opposite directions since a "point of break"—reached when the intrinsic elasticity of the tissue is overcome—represented by the so-called "schisis": the opening of the neurosensory retina into two or more layers, usually involving the foveal region (foveoschisis), that happens either at the level of the fiber layers (inner and outer plexiform layers) or at the level of the basement membrane of the Muller cells, the ILM.

It's important to underline that, though generally called "schisis", the MTM appearance is determined by opening and stretching—but not by rupture and separation—of the retinal layers; the cystoid edema aspect shown by MTM on OCT b-scan (a retinal thickening in the macular area with cystic cavities) is the result of that trac tion. For that reason, the substantial integrity of the retinal "wiring" network grants the maintenance of a fairly good visual acuity. In Fig. 1 are shown some examples of eyes under MTM condition, with the typical schisis-like thickening of the macula, with an excellent BCVA.

Physiopathologically, three main elements must be considered: the elastic properties of different retinal components, the staphyloma and the vitreoretinal adhesion. An overview is shown in Fig. 2.

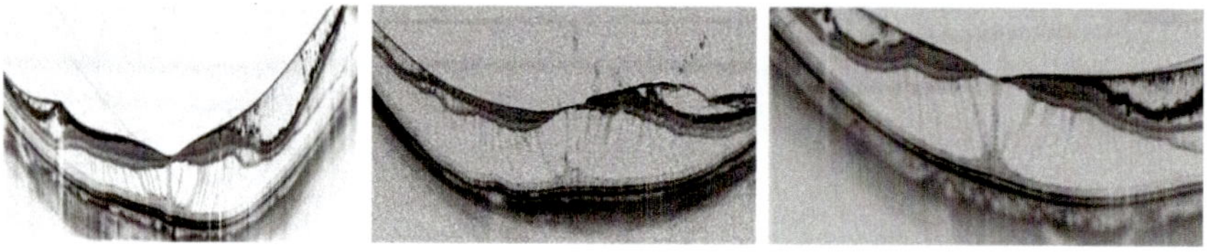

Fig. 1 Some examples of eyes with MTM preserving good visual acuity (BCVA): 20/25 (on the left), 20/25 (in the middle) and 20/20 (on the right). Archive of Panozzo G.

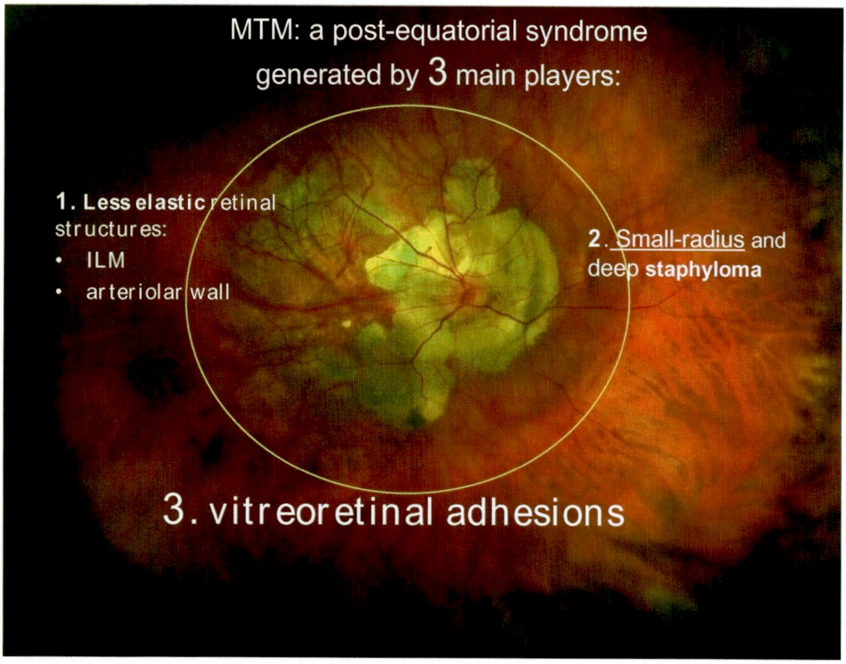

Fig. 2 An overview of pathologic mechanisms leading to the development of MTM. Archive of Panozzo G.

4.1 *The Elastic Properties of Retinal Tissues*

**Internal limiting membrane and vitreoretinal interface*

Basing on surgical experience, in 2003 Ferenc Kuhn evoked a role for the internal limiting membrane (ILM) in the genesis of retinal detachment (RD) in myopic eyes with staphyloma; in particular, the ILM's rigidity was accounted as responsible for the retinal detachment. ILM was found strongly attached to the retina at the edge of the staphyloma and in the foveal region, while bridged in a "contact-less" way over the detached retina (the concept of MTM as a retinoschisis was not already diffused, nor diagnostically distinguishable from a RD, ndr). The evidence of the RD's resolution after vitrectomy and ILM removal, helped to put in discussion the well-established idea that whole-retinal inelasticity was the main responsible for RD in eyes with staphyloma. Or, at least, it helped to hypothesize a possible difference in the behavior of the inner retinal membrane from the rest of the neuroretina.

Later on, in 2009 Mark Johnson strengthened the idea that different stiffness of the inner-compared with the outer retina-in the concavity of the staphyloma must be accounted as causative for the "schisis-like thickening" of the retina. These differences in elastic properties of the retina were supposed to be related to a combination of cortical vitreous remnants after PVD, ERM, relatively non-distensible ILM and inner retinal blood vessels.

A great effort was conducted to analyze the cellular composition and biomechanical properties of the actors involved in the MTM genesis: the ERM/ILM complex and the vascular structures. Useful information about mechanical properties of retinal tissues derives from both surgical experiences and imaging findings.

In the 1980s studies have reported the presence of RPE cells, macrophages, fibrocytes, fibrous astrocytes, and myofibroblast—like cells in the epiretinal membranes obtained during surgery for different vitreo-retinal pathologies.

In 2000, Ishida S. et al. ultra-structurally analyzed the epiretinal membrane obtained during surgery for macular hole retinal detachment in high myopic eyes. The ERM resulted composed by cortical vitreous—containing newly-formed collagen—and fibrous astrocytes as the most represented cellular type. A great emphasis was posed on the role of collagen neo-synthesis, probably led by astrocytes, which was supposed to be responsible for vitreous aggregation and tangential traction on the posterior retina.

In 2005 Bando H. et al. underwent transmission electron microscopic study on specimens of internal limiting membrane (ILM) peeled off after vitrectomy for foveoschisis and macular hole. It was demonstrated that collagen fibers were still present on the ILM in foveoschisis, as well as some cellular debris and fibrous glial cells. The collagen size and aggregation suggested a possible in situ production accountable to fibroblast-like cells and fibrous glial cells.

In 2017, a similar analysis conducted by Yokota R. et al. adopted the transmission electron microscopy (TEM) to study ILM's composition in eyes with MTM. The results—coherently with previous studies—confirmed the presence of glial cells, RPE-like cells and myofibroblast-like cells, all located at the vitreoretinal interface adherent to the ILM. Hence, the collagen neo-synthesis was confirmed by the presence of thick collagen fibers sandwiched with native collagen fibers and compact fibrous long-spacing collagen (FLSC). Finally, was highlighted the ability of glial cells to penetrate and pass through the thickness of ILM, and to proliferate on the vitreoretinal interface. Considering that in high myopic eyes (especially if associated with posterior staphyloma) a vitreoschisis can develop in the macular area, the posterior wall of this "schisis" remains well attached to the ILM. This posterior wall of the schisis' chamber plays a dual function: as a "merger zone" with the ILM and the basement membranes produced by the proliferation of glial and RPE-like cells; as an anterior–posterior and tangential traction on the retina.

Finally, in 2018 Chen L. et al. conducted a multi-modal advanced study to elucidate the morphology, composition, and biomechanical contribution of the ILM to the pathogenesis of MF. Some remarkable results must be reported. TEM microscopy showed a reduced ILM thickness in MF patients. It was already demonstrated that choroidal thickness in highly myopic patients is thinner, and is negatively correlated with age, refractive spherical equivalent and axial length in high myopia. Similarly, the scleral thickness in the posterior pole is reduced in high myopia. They speculated a similar mechanism for the ILM thinning, such as a result of biomechanical stretching induced by excessive axial elongation. Abnormalities in ILM's morphology were confirmed by TEM and SEM imaging: notably, an abnormal number of cellular debris with their long and irregular insertions into the ILMs—Muller cells mostly—probably a consequence of the globe's axial elongation. Furthermore, Muller cells, confirmed as the most common macroglial cells of the retina, can react to mechanical stretching (e.g. Axial elongation in myopic eye) developing a form of reactive gliosis. Immunofluorescence confirmed altered expression levels and distributions of collagen chains: in the MF eyes, collagen a3/a4 (IV) was prominently localized on the retinal side of the ILMs, whereas a5 (IV) was evenly distributed.

All these factors, together, can contribute to modify the elastic properties of the ILM, thus its biomechanics. To evaluate the intrinsic biomechanical stiffness of a material, is commonly used Young's modulus; it was measured between 0.75 and 1.5 MPa in healthy ILMs.

Young's modulus of the ILM in MF was significantly higher and its distribution pattern was irregular.

The increased ILM's rigidity in MF generates a centripetal traction and prevents ILM to follow the sclera's elongated contour assumed during—and due to—the progressive axial elongation.

Arteriolar elasticity*

Thanks again to the advent of OCT, in 2005 Ikuno Y. et al. firstly reported the presence of microfolds developed in the retina of myopic eyes after surgery. They collected post-operative OCT images of eyes with MF which underwent vitrectomy, ILM peeling, and gas tamponade. Vertical OCT scans identified horizontal microfolds, usually appearing 1 month after surgery, described as a projection of retinal vessels toward the vitreous cavity. Merging OCT images with SLO images and color fundus photographs, it was demonstrated that the location of microfolds coincided exactly with the retinal vessels, and that the vessels were always the retinal arteriole. It was proposed that microfolds formation is due to the retinal redundancy usually observed after ILM peeling. Furthermore, the exact coincidence of microfolds location with retinal arterioles led to speculate that, once ILM is surgically removed—and simultaneously its elastic traction due to her stiffness and inability to follow scleral contour—the sclerotic retinal arterioles exert an inward traction. That phenomenon should be accounted to the insufficient vascular flexibility, which becomes manifest after axial length elongation or posterior staphyloma formation (or both) in high myopic eyes. It was supposed a role, besides ILM/ERM complex and staphyloma, in the pathogenesis of MTM for this internal tractional force exerted by arterioles. Finally, they proposed another possible role for this arteriolar tractional force, together with paravascular vitreo-retinal adhesion: the formation of the so-called "paravascular break", typically small and round and resulting in retinal break formation from posterior vitreous detachment.

Later on, Sayanagi K. et al. demonstrated the presence of paravascular microfolds also in non-vitrectomized myopic eyes (even if less frequently), and near to venous vessels. Those evidences led to consider microfolds a common myopic eye condition, detectable by OCT even in non-surgically treated eyes, and accountable to the different elasticity of the vascular tree.

4.2 Staphyloma

Several studies have demonstrated important ultramicroscopic changes in scleral composition, leading to scleral tissue abnormalities and thus to biomechanical properties alterations.

In the sclera of a myopic eye, the expression of Collagen type I is reduced; furthermore, the change in the subtype ratio (III/I and V/I) alters the collagen accumulation, degradation and synthesis. The collagen fibrils are smaller with a wider variability range of diameters (from 60 to 70 nm), the fiber bundles are thinner; abnormal star-shaped fibrils are more common and the fibers arrangement is predominantly lamellar. Other studies emphasized the role of collagen crosslinking as a determinant in the refractive development of a mammalian eye: the reduction of the crosslinking seemed to be responsible for the scleral weakness, thus for the elongation and expansion of the globe.

Experimental models of induced myopia in tree shrews (mammals related to primates) have shown a significant reduction in scleral glycosaminoglycans (GAG) especially in the posterior pole (hydroxyproline and sulfated glycosaminoglycans). The reduction in collagen accumulation and proteoglycan content weakens scleral structure, allowing axial elongation.

Anomalies can be also found in the cellular population of sclera's tissue: Wu et al. highlighted the role of scleral hypoxia in the trans-differentiation of fibroblasts into myofibroblasts. In a myopic eye, several factors concur to promote a hypoxic environment; the scleral hypoxia determines a cascade of signaling mediators that finally promote the trans-differentiation of fibroblasts into myofibroblasts. Since fibroblasts are the main source of collagen type I, while myofibroblasts are contractile cells, the trans-differentiation from the former into the latter not only accounts the change in the cellular type, but also lead to a decrease in Type I collagen production.

All these changes and alterations in the scleral tissue induce an ectasia of the sclera, called staphyloma.

The presence of the staphyloma is an important anatomic predisposing factor for MTM development, as is its shape: it has to be small in diameter and deep, and—less importantly—with an irregular shape. In the presence of a deep and small-radius staphyloma, ILM and arteriolar wall can't follow the scleral profile and generate a vertical retinal stretching.

4.3 *Vitreoretinal Adhesion*

It can be an independent cause of traction or an additional factor in cases of schisis-like MTM.

The surgical experience teaches that the vitreous is "the great pretender" in high myopia. Vitreous undergoes some changes in myopic eyes, which can affect its relationship with the retinal surface. Firstly, high myopia is associated with vitreous liquefaction; it's observed an earlier onset of posterior vitreous detachment (PVD) than in non-myopic eyes. Furthermore, it was observed a faster enlargement of the posterior precortical vitreous pocket (PPVP) in myopic eyes, which is a "boat-shaped" vitreous lacuna in front of the posterior pole. The earlier vitreous liquefaction in high myopia leads to a larger PPVPs, which in turn may cause earlier partial and complete PVDs.

In 2003 Kobayashi H. et al. analyzed the effect of vitreous surgery in myopic eyes with retinoschisis. In their study, the preoperative OCT showed a foveal retinal detachment and foveal retinoschisis in all the nine eyes studied. They performed vitreous surgery (core vitrectomy with removal of the premacular vitreous cortex and internal limiting membrane in the posterior staphyloma, 30% SF6 gas tamponade) and in 8 out of 9 eyes a resolution of the retinal detachment or retinoschisis was observed.

Thus, they assumed that the tangential contraction of pre-macular vitreous might cause foveal retinal detachment and retinoschisis and subsequent development of a full-thickness macular hole.

Their data were coherent with those presented by Benhamou N. et al. and clearly suggested that highly myopic eyes with foveal detachment and/or retinoschisis are at high risk for macular hole development. Furthermore, Benhamou N. et al. reported the OCT findings of a partially detached posterior hyaloid above foveal area, with traction on the fovea. They pointed out that in high myopic eyes, the posterior hyaloid might remain attached to the retina despite apparently complete vitreous detachment.

In 2007 Panozzo e Mercanti surgically observed that multiple sheets of posterior vitreous cortex are still adherent to the retina and bridging the borders of the staphyloma, both in the presence of false PVD (large liquefied lacunae or posterior precortical vitreous pocket) or in cases of true PVD (hyaloid splitting). Those sheets of tissue are often invisible to OCT, since the depth of the staphyloma.

The vitreous cortex and its interaction with inner retinal surface, thus, plays a role in different scenarios: producing well-detectable VR-adhesion, so an anteroposterior vitreomacular traction associated with stage 1 PVD; generating tangential traction on macular surface, with a resultant force normal to the macular plane (leading to both, tractions and MH); providing a proliferation field for glial and fibroblast cells coming from the ILM.

5 Myopic Traction maculopathy (MTM): Natural History and Classifications

5.1 Natural History

Different scenarios can be counted under the MTM conditions: vitreomacular traction (VMT), retinal thickening (leading to schisis-like appearance in macular area), lamellar macular holes (LMH) and full-thickness macular holes (FTMH), and retinal/foveal detachment (RD/FD).

As already mentioned, the traction mechanisms causing the myopic traction maculopathy are diverse. The anatomic and functional success rate of a surgical repair is the higher, the more complete is the removal of the major traction mechanism; thus, the progression or the resolution of a myopic traction maculopathy is related to the presence or the release of retinal tractions.

In 2013 Shimada N. et al. conducted an extensive retrospective study following the evolution of 207 eyes with MTM for 2 years.

In order to standardize the staging criteria on which to base the follow-up of these eyes with MTM, they defined 5 stages according to the location and the extent of the "schisis":

- no macular retinoschisis (S0);
- extra-foveal macular retinoschisis (S1);
- fovea-only macular retinoschisis (S2);
- foveal but not entire macular area macular retinoschisis (S3);
- entire macular area macular retinoschisis (S4).

(They considered the size of the outer schisis only; the size of the inner schisis was not considered).

An improvement/resolution of MTM was defined as a reduction in the height or extent of the macular retinoschisis (as well, no development of an inner lamellar MH, foveal RD or full-thickness MH).

A progression of the MTM was defined as an increase in the height or extent of the retinoschisis or the development of an inner lamellar MH, foveal RD, or full-thickness MH.

The remainder eyes were classified as stable.

Under these conditions, they described the natural course of the MTM during the observation period, as largely stable: in the milder stages, the progression rate was lower than 8%, while S4 showed a 42.9% of progression. Interestingly, the more advanced stage (S4) was not necessarily the worst, but simply the more unstable, having a higher rate of progression and resolution as well. The eyes in S4 stage can experience a worsening due to multiple factors: axial elongation, macular chorioretinal atrophy, vitreomacular traction resulting from a perifoveal PVD, and intrinsic noncompliance of the ILM. The resolution is due to the completion of a spontaneous incomplete PVD (mostly in younger patients), or to the disruption of the ILM (just one case reported in the study); those results further confirmed the role of traction forces in the pathogenesis of MTM. The particular unstable behavior of S4 should also influence management options. Overall, emerged a stable behavior of the pathology, with a slow progression profile; few cases showed improvement (3.9%), slightly few (11.6%) showed worsening (most of them belonging to the S4 stage, that corresponds to the larger macular involvement).

Those conclusions—interestingly—were coherent with those of Gaucher D. et al.; in 2006 they published the results of long-term follow ups of 29 eyes with MTM, trying to figure out an evolution's model for this condition and to identify prognostic factors. They analyzed the changes in visual acuity, biomicroscopy, fundoscopy and OCT images during a period of at least two years. Firstly, they noticed that changes in visual acuity are not strictly correlated to the macular thickness (a parameter used to quantify the effect of the schisis-like damage); more then 30% of the eyes showed no worsening on the OCT scans during 2 years follow-up, revealing a quite stable over-the-time behavior of MTM. The presence of pre-macular structures (defined as hyperreflective line on OCT scans: a partially detached epimacular membrane, a partially detached and condensed posterior hyaloid, or a posterior hyaloid lined with fibrous membranous proliferations) or foveal detachment were identified as major factors for poor prognosis. A remarkable point was also highlighted: the inner boundary of the "splitted" retina appears hyperreflective on OCT scans, separated from the underlying retinal tissue but linked to them through column-like structures. These aspects give the appearance of a "retinoschisis"; furthermore, it was observed that the curve of the inner retinal surface followed the general curve of the staphyloma, but was flatter than the outer retinal tissues which follow the scleral contour. They accounted the different rigidity of the ILM as responsible for this behavior: the consequence is that an intraretinal cleavage occurs before the photoreceptors become detached from the retinal pigment.

Although the complexity of the pathogenesis and the interaction of different forces on the field, the hypothesis made by Gaucher was consistent with the surgical observation made by Khun some years earlier (Fig. 3): structured as a multi-layered tissue with different intrinsic elastic properties, the retinal sheet lies between an elongated sclera (with an irregular contour due to the different curvature radius inside staphyloma), and the pre-retinal structures (ILM, sheets of vitreous cortex variously arranged on retinal surface, and vasculature).

Trying to simplifying all the biomechanical properties, the geometric rule named Gauss law can help to understand the forces on the field and to predict the natural course of MTM: a stretched non elastic tissue forced to follow an irregular concave contour will assume a regular concave shape.

Appling this law to a retina lying on an irregular scleral contour, we may predict that usually MTM will demonstrate no progression in a dome-shaped macula or in a focal staphyloma, as shown in our clinical experience; whereas progression is more frequent among eyes with irregular, small-radius and asymmetric staphylomas.

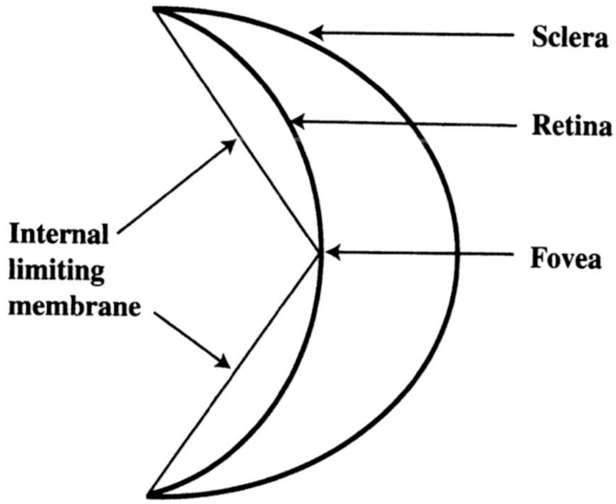

Fig. 3 Schematic representation of the eye's posterior pole before removal of the partially elevated internal limiting membrane. From Kuhn F. "Internal limiting membrane removal for macular detachment in highly myopic eyes." Am J Ophthalmol. 2003

5.2 *Classification Systems for MTM*

In the first part of this capitol different classifications of MM were analyzed. In the field of tractional-MM (MTM), several manifestations can be found; Shimada N. et al. focused on the "schisis" aspect of the pathology (as previously discussed), creating a classification based on the location and the extent of the schisis. Though the effort of summarize the spectrum of all the MTM manifestations, that classification covers only the schisis aspect of the MTM; furthermore, only the outer schisis was considered, such as the "opening" of the retina in its outer layers.

In 2020 Parolini B. et al. proposed a wider classification of the MTMs, the "Myopic Traction Maculopathy Staging System" (MSS). They tried to describe all the manifestations of the MTM as different stages of one evolving disease. Four stages describe the "retinal patters" (the location of the retinal layers involved and the eventual RD; from 1 to 4), while three stages describe the evolution of the "foveal patterns" (from splitting to MH; from a to c). Different stages were identified as a "continuous spectrum" of manifestations, all dependent on the different tractional forces acting on the field; the clinical course of the condition is the consequence of the predominant force. The progression of the retinal patterns depends on centrifugal forces perpendicular to the retina, while the progression of the foveal patters depends on centrifugal forces tangential to the retina. The co-action of both, determines all the possible combinations of retinal damage and, consequently, OCT findings.

Basing on the literature evidences of the main different physio-pathologic mechanisms characterizing an eye with a MTM condition, the clinical behavior of the pathology, the OCT findings and surgical experiences, we have elaborated a new clinicopathological classification of MTM.

Its purpose is to be useful not only for descriptions of different OCT findings, but primarily for prognosis and surgical approaches.

Considering the tractional forces and their extension, the prognosis and the timing of surgical intervention, the MTM is divided in three forms (Fig. 14):

- Type 1: intraretinal tractions
- Type 2: vitreoretinal traction
- Type 3: the mixed forms.

- The MTM Type 1—Focal traction

The MTM type 1 in *dome shaped macula* is usually stable; this behavior is due to the regular scleral contour (in accordance to the Gauss Law) (Fig. 4); long-term follow-up can show stability over the time (Fig. 5).

In some cases, it's possible to obtain a spontaneous regression. Not a clear cause can be identified in those spontaneous resolutions, but probably the release of some OCT-invisible tractions can be accounted as responsible for those events.

Surgery in these cases is not a priority; longer observation is needed to better define the possible progression pattern.

The MTM type 1 in *asymmetrical staphyloma* shows a similar stable over the time behavior (Fig. 6); in some cases, longer observation period allows to detect a slight but clear improvement, whose origin mostly remains unknown. It's a very slow process, not related to ILM modification, but apparently accountable to a "shortening" of the staphyloma.

- The MTM Type 1—Diffuse tractions

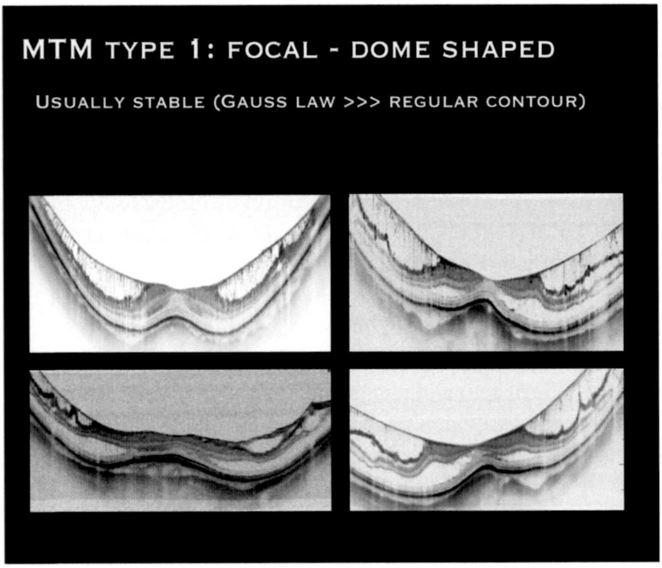

Fig. 4 MTM-1: dome shaped, Gauss law. Archive of Panozzo G.

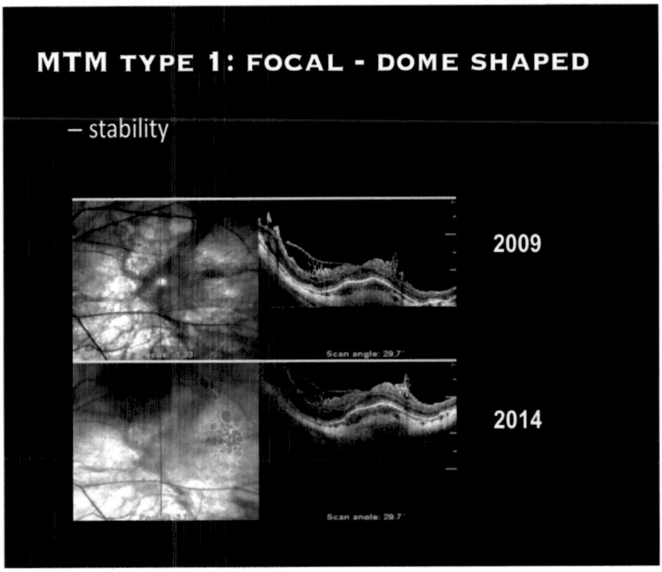

Fig. 5 MTM-1: long term stability shown by OCT. Archive of Panozzo G.

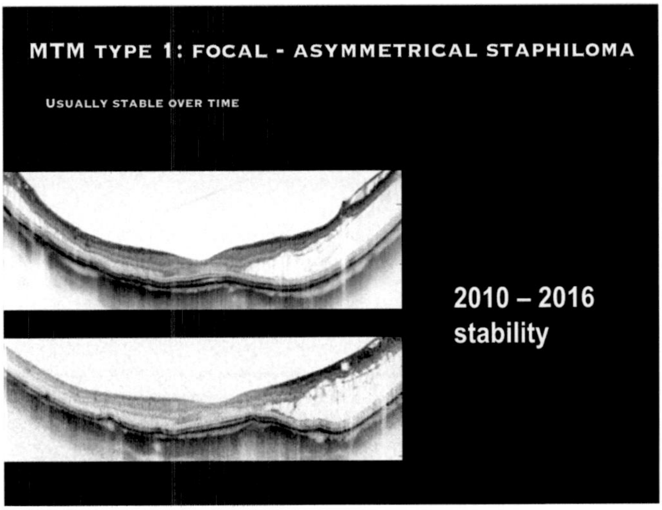

Fig. 6 MTM-1, stable behavior even in asymmetrical staphyloma. Archive of Panozzo G.

The diffuse intraretinal tractions are mostly related to the ILM tractional activity. Those cases can develop the typical "schisis-like" thickening, till reach the foveal detachment. According to the literature, this form is mostly stable, but 11% of cases worsen over the time; 4% of cases spontaneously improves. The progression rate is very slow and usually takes years (Figs. 7 and 8).

In that cases, visual acuity is not the best way to evaluate the progressive retinal damage. Microperimetry is a much more sensible test: even with a stable OCT picture it can demonstrate a progressive retinal deterioration that may suggest a surgical resolution.

Though quite unusual and very slow, the progression (Fig. 9) till the development of foveal detachment is a dangerous alert that requires prompt intervention.

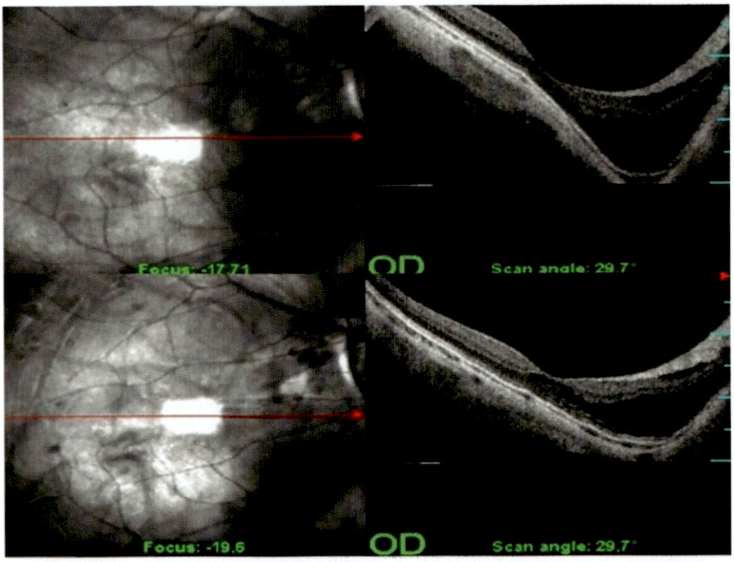

Fig. 7 OCT follow-up shows possible "shortening" of the staphyloma: the same OCT scan taken 7 years later seems to evidence a dramatic decrease of focal staphiloma . Archive of Panozzo G.

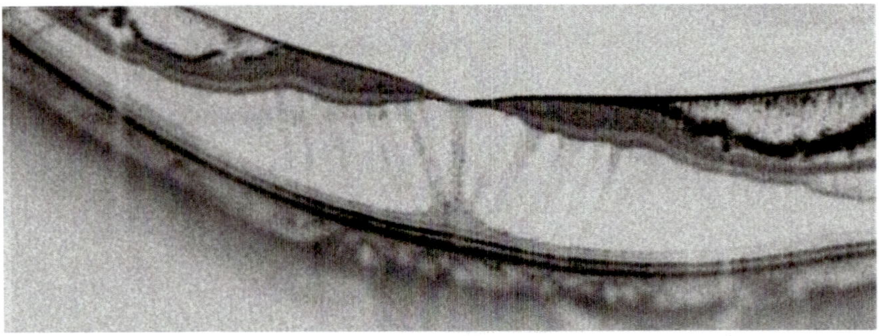

Fig. 8 MTM-1: vertical elevation of outer plexiform layer (schisis-like maculopathy) generated by tangental traction from the non-elastic due ILM, also stretched from inner retinal surface. Archive of Panozzo G.

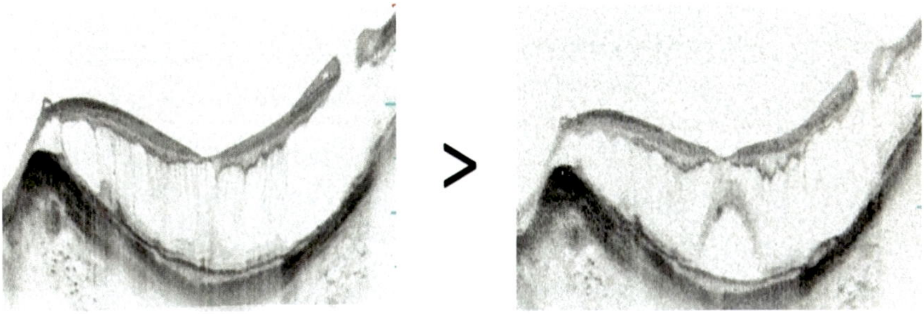

Fig. 9 Development of foveal detachment, an alert of prompt intervention. Archive of Panozzo G.

The development of a foveal detachment must be considered and treated as a myopic impending macular hole. In the presence of a deep staphyloma, the progression to a full thickness hole may happen in few days; the worst final-stage scenario is the complete posterior macular detachment. Immediate surgery, even with a stable visual acuity, must be recommended.

In Fig. 10 is shown the fast evolution of a foveal detachment to a macular hole with a complete posterior detachment in just two weeks.

In the presence of a wide foveal detachment (Fig. 11), or of a steep staphyloma, the release of all retinal tractions leads to its flattening; but this flattening may create

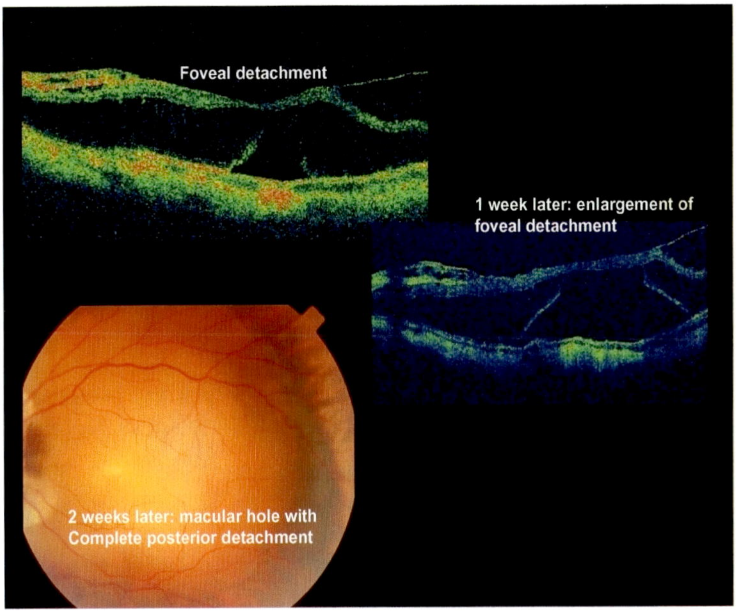

Fig. 10 Rapid evolution of a foveal detachment towards a complete posterior retinal detachment. Archive of Panozzo G.

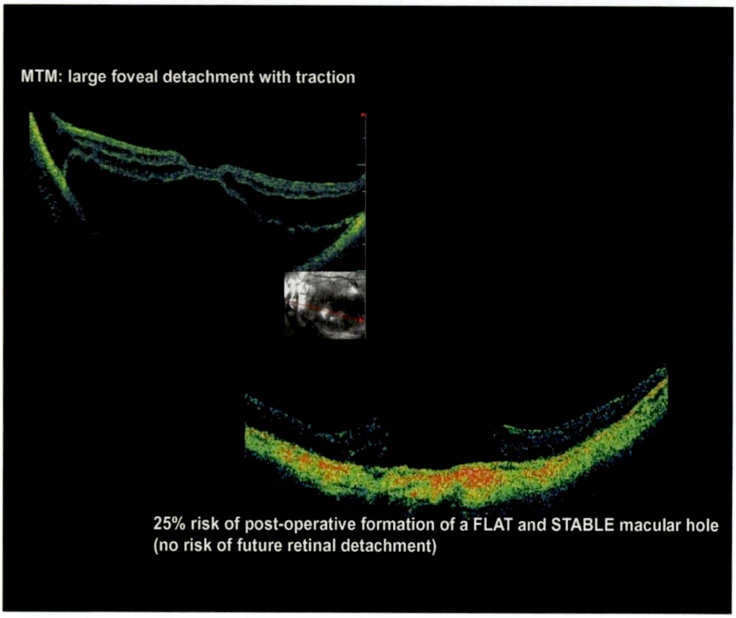

Fig. 11 Development of flat and stable full thickness macular hole aftervitrectomy and surgical release of tractions in a foveal detachment case. Archive of Panozzo G.

a full thickness macular hole. In those cases, there is no risk of future detachment, as in the non-myopic holes, because there is no more traction, but the incidence of macular hole formation in these cases is about 25%.

- MTM Type 2

MTM showing vitreoretinal traction is defined as Type 2.

As previously described, tractions exerted by the vitreoretinal interface can act in different directions: tangential to the retinal surface and perpendicular to the retinal surface. The former can be further categorized into mild and severe forms; the latter, basing to their attachment to the retinal surface, in foveal and extrafoveal.

In Fig. 12 some cases of advanced tangential form of MTM-2 are shown.

In Fig. 13 are depicted the more dangerous cases: foveal antero-posterior traction determining an impending hole or full thickness holes. Prompt surgery is required for these cases.

- MTM Type 3

Finally, there are some forms showing both kind of tractional mechanisms. They are classified as Type 3 MTM.

As a purpose of this classification, stages identify also the typical clinical behavior. In Fig. 14, forms appearing in green usually are stable and can be simply followed;

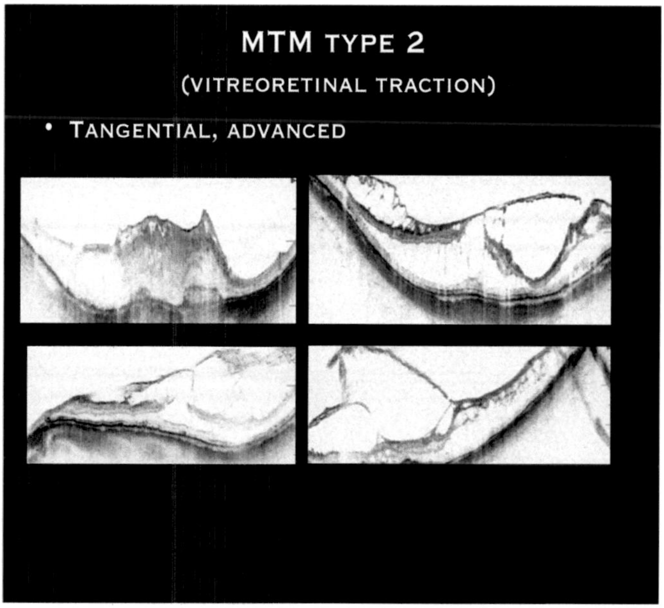

Fig. 12 MTM-2 advanced tangential tractions. Archive of Panozzo G.

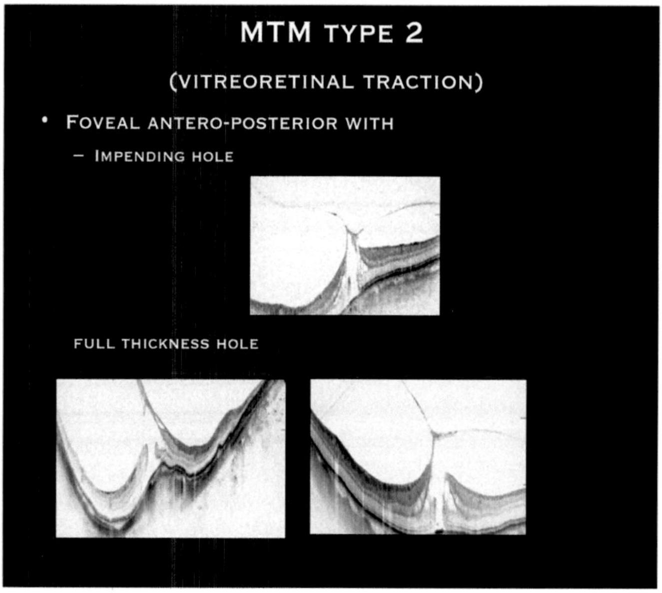

Fig. 13 MTM-2 with the development of FTMH. Archive of Panozzo G.

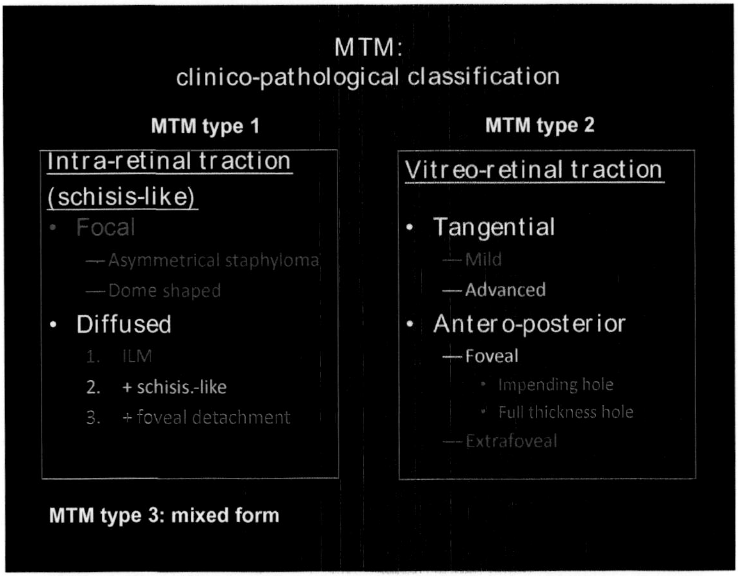

Fig. 14 Clinical classification of MTM (G. Panozzo). Three different types of traction are described and require different approaches. The color indicates the most appropriate management for each stage. Green: stability, follow up. Yellow: long follow-up, may require surgery. Red: prompt surgery

in yellow, forms that may progress and need surgery; in red, forms that need prompt surgery.

6 Myopic Traction Maculopathy (MTM): Treatment Options

6.1 Indications

A. Visual symptoms. In most of cases, MTM is not the only pathologic feature and potential cause of visual impairment in highly myopic eyes. Mild or severe amblyopic anisometropia may be a cause of low vision, making difficult to judge the functional impact of any anatomical event. Macular area may also be patchy or diffusely atrophic or Fuch's scar may chronically reduce VA. Even an active but subclinical choroidal neovascularization may be evaluated. Very often the clinical situation is also complicated by pseudophakia with barely opaque posterior capsule or dense and diffuse vitreous opacities. Unless in the presence of a dangerous and rapidly progressive form (see Fig. 14) indicating prompt surgery, it is therefore advisable to indicate surgery only in the presence of a reduction of visual function not attributable to other causes. Most of the time, in case of bilateral low vision, patients may be very precise indicating even a subtle decrease in vision or new features in their chronic and stable metamorphopsia, and their report is often the only reason that guides to surgery, considered as the only way to clean all media opacities and remove any factor possibly limiting vision, including MTM.

B. MTM stage or progression jeopardizing visual function. As described in Fig. 14, in most of the cases MTM is a stable disease that does not or minimally affect visual function. When MTM is focal and is limited to an asymmetrical staphyloma (Fig. 15) or to the declivous parts of a dome shaped macula (Type 1: intraretinal traction with schisis-like shape, Fig. 16), most of the cases it remains stable and does not progress to the fovea, without affecting visual function.

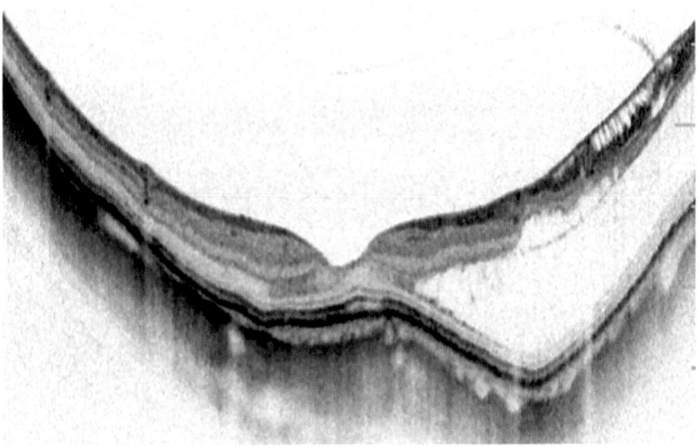

Fig. 15 Asymmetrical staphyloma with MTM. Archive of Panozzo G.

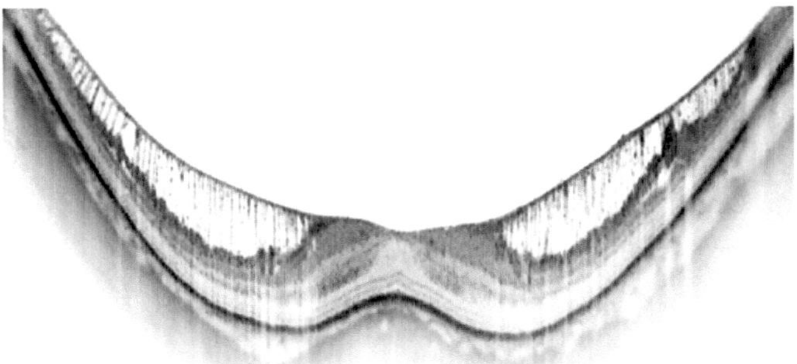

Fig. 16 Dome shaped macula with MTM. Archive of Panozzo G.

Central and diffuse schisis-like is also usually stable (Fig. 17) or may even regress, but in about 3% of cases it slowly progresses in many months or even years with visual decrease, and in this case, when this progression is clearly documented (Fig. 18) surgery may be scheduled.

On the contrary, prompt surgery is mandatory when schisis-like becomes associated with foveal neurosensory detachment (Fig. 19). This feature, that may be seen at the first examination or developing during follow up, must be considered as an impending myopic macular hole, in most of cases suddenly leading

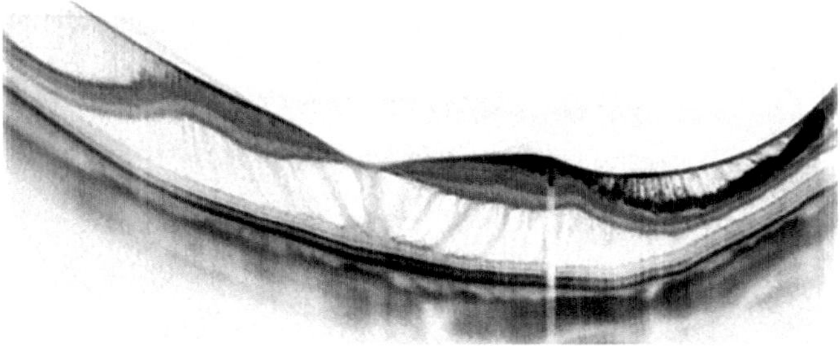

Fig. 17 Central and diffuse MTM. Archive of Panozzo G.

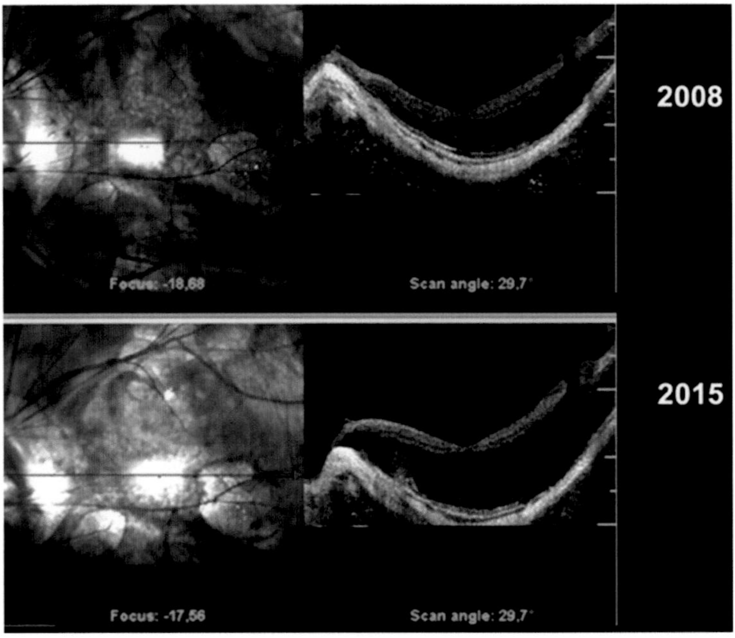

Fig. 18 Progression of an MTM. Archive of Panozzo G.

to a full thickness hole with macular detachment, and therefore requesting an immediate surgical resolution.

In cases of vitreo-retinal traction (MTM type 2) with impending or full thickness macular hole (Fig. 20) surgery is obviously indicated, while in the presence of even advanced but stable vitreo-macular adhesions the decision for a surgical approach must be based on the balance of functional benefits and intra/postoperative risks present in that specific clinical situation.

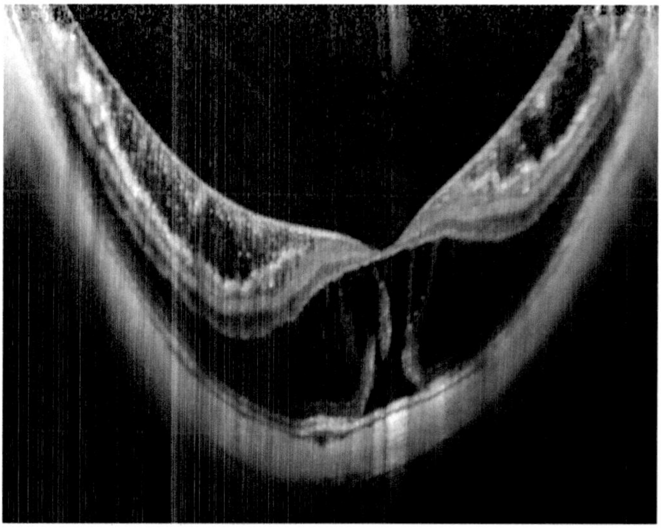

Fig. 19 MTM complicated by foveal neurosensory detachment. Archive of Panozzo G.

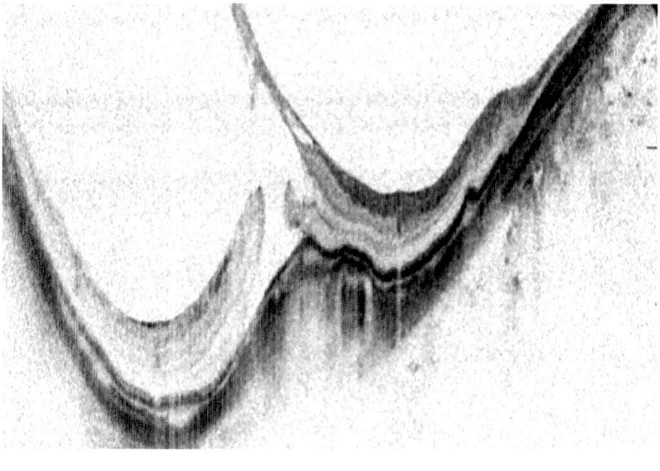

Fig. 20 MTM-2 complicated by FTMH. Archive of Panozzo G.

6.2 *Vitrectomy*

A. Traction release. The surgical target to resolve MTM is releasing all tractions inside the staphyloma forcing the macula to stretch. As previously described, there may be two types of traction present in each case and both must be resolved: the first one may be determined by vitreous cortex (partial and anomalous vitreous detachment) or its fragments and epiretinal membranes, generating a tangential/diffuse or vertical/focal traction (Figs. 21 and 22); the second type is determined by a tight and stretched ILM (Fig. 23).

These two elements are often combined in the same eye (Fig. 24). The third traction force involved in MTM, generated by stretched arteriolar walls (Fig. 25)

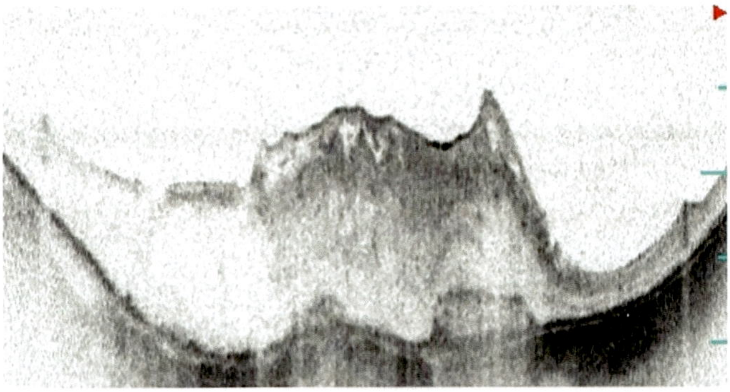

Fig. 21 An example of diffuse tangential traction on the retina. Archive of Panozzo G.

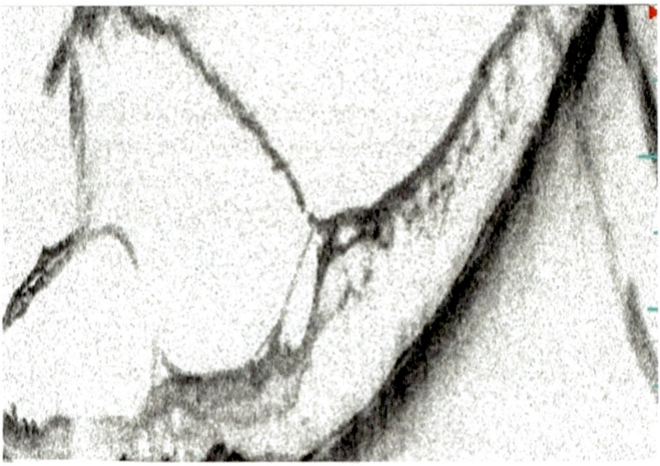

Fig. 22 An example of vertical focal traction on the retina. Archive of Panozzo G.

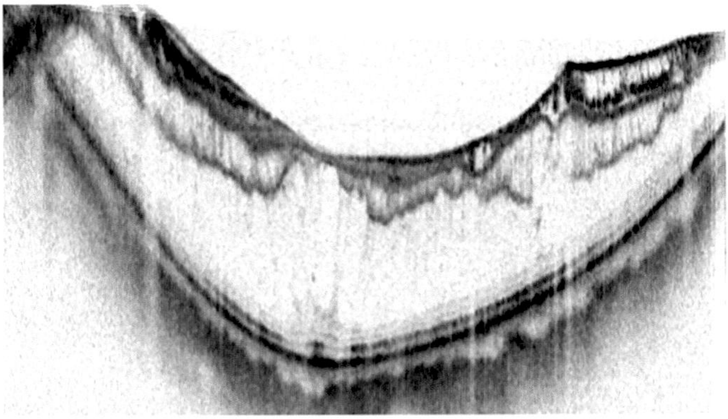

Fig. 23 An example of traction exerted by the ILM on the retina. Archive of Panozzo G.

cannot be resolved, but these focal points of stable traction usually don't impede a global retinal flattening after surgery.

B. Core or complete PPV. Surgery for MTM is focused to posterior staphyloma, and it is a form of macular vitrectomy. There may be therefore two different approaches: a core vitrectomy, leaving most of the peripheral vitreous body untouched, or a complete vitrectomy with shaving of vitreous base. Both approaches have pros and cons in high myopia: due to firm and anomalous vitreoretinal adhesions at the borders of the staphyloma and more peripherally often present in these eyes, persistence in trying to elevate a firmly attached cortical vitreous may create a iatrogenic hole very difficult to resolve in these hypopigmented eyes, while a partial vitrectomy may itself lead to postoperative breaks and retinal detachment. If the surgeon choice is a final fluid/gas exchange,

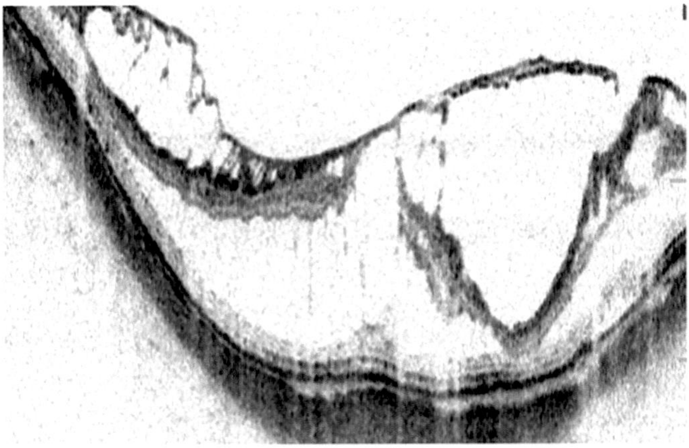

Fig. 24 An example of a combined tractional mechanism on the retina. Archive of Panozzo G.

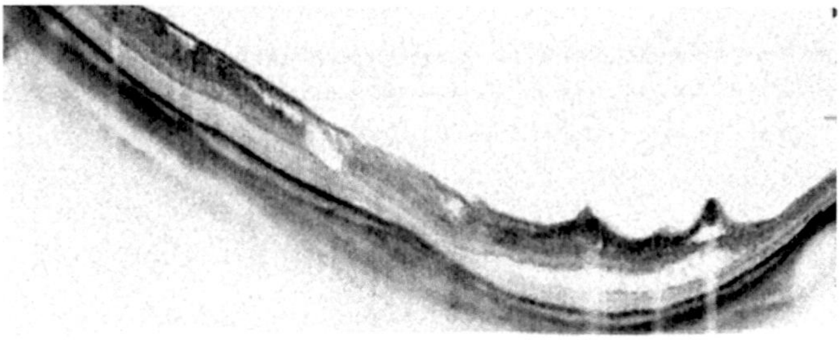

Fig. 25 Stretched arteriolar wall exerting traction on the retina. Archive of Panozzo G.

a complete vitrectomy is preferable, but we personally favor a core vitrectomy without gas exchange, having no postoperative complications.

C. Dyes and creation of complete PVD. Vitrectomy and peeling in high myopic eyes may be very challenging, and all Authors describe the use of dyes in both phases of surgery. During core and/or peripheral vitrectomy, triamcinolone may be very helpful in highlighting multiple sheets of vitreous cortex usually found in these eyes, and to be sure to create a complete vitreoretinal separation, in case of core vitrectomy at least until the borders of staphyloma, while an intense ILM staining is mandatory during peeling, and among various options most Authors agree that indocyanine green gives the best visualization in these hypo and patchy-pigmented eyes.
D. ILM peeling and tamponade. Although some case series described positive results even without ILM peeling, according to the review and metanalysis of Meng B. et al., ILM peeling leads to better and more stable surgical outcomes. ILM peeling should be enlarged as much close to the border of the staphyloma as possible, without obviously jeopardizing the integrity of the retina and absolutely try to avoid any iatrogenic posterior retinal break. When shallow neuroretinal detachment is present and only a very thin layer of inner tissue is visible at preoperative OCT examination (Fig. 19), a foveal-sparing ILM peeling may be the right choice to avoid the high risk of creating a full thickness macular hole, without decreasing the anatomic results. The same review by Meng B. et al. also describes how gas tamponade doesn't lead to better or more rapid postoperative retinal flattening. As described in our case series, we always peel ILM unless this maneuver jeopardizes the integrity of the retina, because we consider this membrane a main cause of MTM formation, and never use gas tamponade to improve or accelerate retinal flattening as this method is never used at the end of ERM peeling in non-myopic eyes.
E. Time for retinal flattening. After vitrectomy and ILM peeling the retina slowly flattens to the scleral bed. This process may take many months (Fig. 26), is independent from the use of gas tamponade and remains stable over time, as a sign that MTM is a tractional disease. In cases of irregular shape of the staphyloma a shallow neuro-retinal detachment may persist in the deepest areas, while the

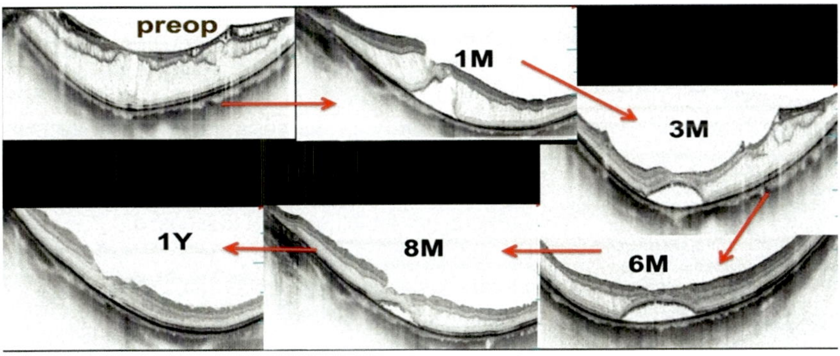

Fig. 26 The slow process of retinal flattening after surgery. Archive of Panozzo G.

peaks of tangential retinal traction generated by the small arteries remain stable over time without preventing the general retinal flattening.

6.3 Macular Buckle

While this technique is preferred by many authors in case of full thickness macular hole with posterior retinal detachment, giving in most cases stable anatomical results, its role in case of MTM is controversial, and comparative studies are not available. An exhaustive postoperative OCT examination combined with RMI study of the shape and deepness of the staphyloma may guide the surgeon to the better choice. As suggested by Parolini B. et al. as well as by other Authors, it seems reasonable that when MTM is determined by vitreoretinal adhesion or by an evident ILM stiffness and tangential traction (Figs. 23 and 24), vitrectomy could be the method of choice. On the contrary, when the amplitude of retinal stretching is particularly elevated due to the presence of a very deep staphyloma that may obstacle a complete retinal flattening, in this case macular buckle, isolated or in combination with vitrectomy may be preferable.

A. Technical features. Many types of buckles are available, with different shapes and positioning techniques.

   An interesting option in our opinion is offered by the Ando's plombe due to its versatility, modified by Mateo with an illuminated light pipe for precise localization, and also a new 3-D printing-assisted buckle that guarantees a perfect personalized shape.

B. Effect on posterior circulation. Many reports describe alterations of choroidal circulation after episcleral surgery with encircling or radial buckle. The compressive effect that a macular buckle exerts on the choroidal vessels generates a temporary thickening of the choroid, but due to the already poor choroidal blood flow typical of staphylomas this chronic compression could contribute to the progressive chorioretinal atrophic evolution typical of these eyes.

6.4 Scleral Shortening

In these very last years, few studies were published on the efficacy of scleral shortening combined with vitrectomy in eyes with macular hole and retinal detachment, but even as an isolated procedure to treat MTM. This shortening may be obtained by a scleral temporal flap parallel to the corneal limbus or by suturing an allogenic patch. According to these series, the shortening of the bulb seems long lasting, generating a progressive resolution of MTM without the risks induced by a complex procedure such as vitrectomy or macular buckle. More studies with longer follow ups are anyway necessary to validate this interesting procedure.

6.5 Functional Results

As previously mentioned, many contemporary factors contribute to visual function in high myopic eyes, and independently from the surgical procedure the effects of retinal flattening on final visual acuity are difficult to analyze and are greatly affected by the functional and anatomical preoperative conditions of the single eye. Surgery usually stops the progressive visual impairment and most series report anyway a significant range of improvement (1–5 lines).

7 Conclusion

A high myopic eye is a different world: different anatomy, structural differences, different forces on the field. The pathologies that affect these eyes are the same, but their manifestation and natural course may change consistently in this particular environment. Understanding and keeping in mind these differences is fundamental for a correct approach to the myopic eye.

Myopic Traction Maculopathy is the best example of this difference: a fascinating disorder generating striking OCT images and deserving knowledge to be understood, patience during follow-ups, and also a firm hand and apnea skills during surgery.

Bibliography

1. Feldkaemper M, Schaeffel F. An updated view on the role of dopamine in myopia. Exp Eye Res. 2013;114:106–19. https://doi.org/10.1016/j.exer.2013.02.007. Epub 2013 Feb 19. PMID: 23434455.
2. Norton TT, Siegwart JT Jr. Light levels, refractive development, and myopia—a speculative review. Exp Eye Res. 2013;114:48–57. https://doi.org/10.1016/j.exer.2013.05.004. Epub 2013 May 13. PMID: 23680160; PMCID: PMC3742693.

3. Morgan I, Rose K. How genetic is school myopia? Prog Retin Eye Res. 2005;24(1):1–38. https://doi.org/10.1016/j.preteyeres.2004.06.004. PMID: 15555525.
4. Watson PG, Young RD. Scleral structure, organisation and disease. A review. Exp Eye Res. 2004;78(3):609–23. https://doi.org/10.1016/s0014-4835(03)00212-4. PMID: 15106941.
5. Matthijs Blankesteijn W. Has the search for a marker of activated fibroblasts finally come to an end? J Mol Cell Cardiol. 2015;88:120–3. https://doi.org/10.1016/j.yjmcc.2015.10.005. Epub 2015 Oct 22. PMID: 26454160.
6. Trier K, Olsen EB, Ammitzboll T. Regional glycosaminoglycans composition of the human sclera. Acta Ophthalmol. 1990;68(3):304–6.
7. Spaide RF. Staphyloma: part 1. In: Spaide RF, Ohno-Matsui K, Yannuzzi LA, editors. Pathologic myopia. New York: Springer; 2014. p. 167–76. https://doi.org/10.1007/978-1-4614-8338-0_12
8. Frisina R, Gius I, Palmieri M, Finzi A, Tozzi L, Parolini B. Myopic traction maculopathy: diagnostic and management strategies. Clin Ophthalmol. 2020;14:3699–708. https://doi.org/10.2147/OPTH.S237483. PMID: 33173268; PMCID: PMC7646438.
9. Curtin BJ. The posterior staphyloma of pathologic myopia. Trans Am Ophthalmol Soc. 1977;75:67–86. PMID: 613534; PMCID: PMC1311542.
10. Ohno-Matsui K. Proposed classification of posterior staphylomas based on analyses of eye shape by three-dimensional magnetic resonance imaging and wide-field fundus imaging. Ophthalmology. 2014;121(9):1798–809. https://doi.org/10.1016/j.ophtha.2014.03.035. Epub 2014 May 9. PMID: 24813630.
11. Ohno-Matsui K, Jonas JB, Spaide RF. Macular Bruch membrane holes in highly myopic patchy chorioretinal atrophy. Am J Ophthalmol. 2016;166:22–8. https://doi.org/10.1016/j.ajo.2016.03.019. Epub 2016 Mar 24. PMID: 27018232
12. Ruiz-Moreno JM, Arias L, Montero JA, Carneiro A, Silva R. Intravitreal anti-VEGF therapy for choroidal neovascularisation secondary to pathological myopia: 4-year outcome. Br J Ophthalmol. 2013;97(11):1447–50. https://doi.org/10.1136/bjophthalmol-2012-302973. Epub 2013 Sept 11. PMID: 24026146.
13. Ikuno Y, Fujimoto S, Jo Y, Asai T, Nishida K. Choroidal thinning in high myopia measured by optical coherence tomography. Clin Ophthalmol. 2013;7:889–93. https://doi.org/10.2147/OPTH.S44138. Epub 2013 May 15. PMID: 23696696; PMCID: PMC3658536.
14. Ohno-Matsui K, Kawasaki R, Jonas JB, Cheung CM, Saw SM, Verhoeven VJ, Klaver CC, Moriyama M, Shinohara K, Kawasaki Y, Yamazaki M, Meuer S, Ishibashi T, Yasuda M, Yamashita H, Sugano A, Wang JJ, Mitchell P, Wong TY. META-analysis for Pathologic Myopia (META-PM) Study Group. International photographic classification and grading system for myopic maculopathy. Am J Ophthalmol. 2015;159(5):877–83.e7. https://doi.org/10.1016/j.ajo.2015.01.022. Epub 2015 Jan 26. PMID: 25634530.
15. Curtin BJ, Karlin DB. Axial length measurements and fundus changes of the myopic eye. Am J Ophthalmol. 1971;71(1 Pt 1):42–53. https://doi.org/10.1016/0002-9394(71)91092-0. PMID: 5099937.
16. Avila MP, Weiter JJ, Jalkh AE, Trempe CL, Pruett RC, Schepens CL. Natural history of choroidal neovascularization in degenerative myopia. Ophthalmology. 1984;91(12):1573–81. https://doi.org/10.1016/s0161-6420(84)34116-1. PMID: 6084222.
17. Hayashi K, Ohno-Matsui K, Shimada N, Moriyama M, Kojima A, Hayashi W, Yasuzumi K, Nagaoka N, Saka N, Yoshida T, Tokoro T, Mochizuki M. Long-term pattern of progression of myopic maculopathy: a natural history study. Ophthalmology. 2010;117(8):1595–611, 1611.e1–4. https://doi.org/10.1016/j.ophtha.2009.11.003. Epub 2010 Mar 5. PMID: 20207005.
18. Fang Y, Du R, Nagaoka N, Yokoi T, Shinohara K, Xu X, Takahashi H, Onishi Y, Yoshida T, Ohno-Matsui K. OCT-based diagnostic criteria for different stages of myopic maculopathy. Ophthalmology. 2019;126(7):1018–32. https://doi.org/10.1016/j.ophtha.2019.01.012. Epub 2019 Jan 29. PMID: 30703442.
19. Ruiz-Medrano J, Montero JA, Flores-Moreno I, Arias L, García-Layana A, Ruiz-Moreno JM. Myopic maculopathy: current status and proposal for a new classification and grading system (ATN). Prog Retin Eye Res. 2019;69:80–115. https://doi.org/10.1016/j.preteyeres.2018.10.005. Epub 2018 Nov 1. PMID: 30391362.

20. Ip M, Garza-Karren C, Duker JS, Reichel E, Swartz JC, Amirikia A, Puliafito CA. Differentiation of degenerative retinoschisis from retinal detachment using optical coherence tomography. Ophthalmology. 1999;106(3):600–5. https://doi.org/10.1016/S0161-6420(99)90123-9. PMID: 10080221.
21. Morita H, Ideta H, Ito K, Yonemoto J, Sasaki K, Tanaka S. Causative factors of retinal detachment in macular holes. Retina. 1991;11(3):281–4. https://doi.org/10.1097/00006982-199111030-00002. PMID: 1961986.
22. Phillips CI, Dobbie JG. Posterior staphyloma and retinal detachment. Am J Ophthalmol. 1963;55:332–5.
23. Abdel-Latif S. Macular hole with central retinal detachment in high myopia with posterior staphyloma. Br J Ophthalmol. 1969;53:62–3.
24. Cree IA. Ophthalmic pathology—an atlas and textbook. J Clin Pathol. 1998;51(1):85. PMCID: PMC500453.
25. Rochon-Duvigneaud M. Déformation et lésions de l'œil myope: in Mawas J, introduction à l'étude de la myopie et des chorio-retinites myopiques. Bulletin de la Societé d'Ophtalmologie de Paris. 1938;1:1–10.
26. Takano M, Kishi S. Foveal retinoschisis and retinal detachment in severely myopic eyes with posterior staphyloma. Am J Ophthalmol. 1999;128(4):472–6. https://doi.org/10.1016/s0002-9394(99)00186-5. PMID: 10577588.
27. Panozzo G, Mercanti A. Optical coherence tomography findings in myopic traction maculopathy. Arch Ophthalmol. 2004;122(10):1455–60. https://doi.org/10.1001/archopht.122.10.1455. PMID: 15477456.
28. Gallemore RP, Jumper JM, McCuen BW 2nd, Jaffe GJ, Postel EA, Toth CA. Diagnosis of vitreoretinal adhesions in macular disease with optical coherence tomography. Retina. 2000;20(2):115–20. PMID: 10783942.
29. Henaine-Berra A, Zand-Hadas IM, Fromow-Guerra J, García-Aguirre G. Prevalence of macular anatomic abnormalities in high myopia. Ophthalmic Surg Lasers Imaging Retina. 2013;44(2):140–4. https://doi.org/10.3928/23258160-20130219-01. Epub 2013 Feb 25. PMID: 23438042.
30. Kuhn F. Internal limiting membrane removal for macular detachment in highly myopic eyes. Am J Ophthalmol. 2003;135(4):547–9. https://doi.org/10.1016/s0002-9394(02)02057-3. PMID: 12654379.
31. Johnson MW. Posterior vitreous detachment: evolution and complications of its early stages. Am J Ophthalmol. 2010;149(3):371–82.e1. https://doi.org/10.1016/j.ajo.2009.11.022. PMID: 20172065.
32. Kampik A, Kenyon KR, Michels RG, Green WR, de la Cruz ZC. Epiretinal and vitreous membranes. Comparative study of 56 cases. Arch Ophthalmol. 1981;99(8):1445–54. https://doi.org/10.1001/archopht.1981.03930020319025. PMID: 7020665.
33. Smiddy WE, Green WR, Michels RG, de la Cruz Z. Ultrastructural studies of vitreomacular traction syndrome. Am J Ophthalmol. 1989;107(2):177–85. https://doi.org/10.1016/0002-9394(89)90219-5. PMID: 2913812.
34. Smiddy WE, Maguire AM, Green WR, Michels RG, de la Cruz Z, Enger C, Jaeger M, Rice TA. Idiopathic epiretinal membranes. Ultrastructural characteristics and clinicopathologic correlation. Ophthalmology. 1989;96(6):811–20; discussion 821. https://doi.org/10.1016/s0161-6420(89)32811-9. PMID: 2740079.
35. Ishida S, Yamazaki K, Shinoda K, Kawashima S, Oguchi Y. Macular hole retinal detachment in highly myopic eyes: ultrastructure of surgically removed epiretinal membrane and clinicopathologic correlation. Retina. 2000;20(2):176–83. PMID: 10783951.
36. Bando H, Ikuno Y, Choi JS, Tano Y, Yamanaka I, Ishibashi T. Ultrastructure of internal limiting membrane in myopic foveoschisis. Am J Ophthalmol. 2005;139(1):197–9. https://doi.org/10.1016/j.ajo.2004.07.027. PMID: 15652854.
37. Yokota R, Hirakata A, Hayashi N, Hirota K, Rii T, Itoh Y, Orihara T, Inoue M. Ultrastructural analyses of internal limiting membrane excised from highly myopic eyes with myopic traction maculopathy. Jpn J Ophthalmol. 2018;62(1):84–91. https://doi.org/10.1007/s10384-017-0542-9. Epub 2017 Oct 25. PMID: 29071469

38. Chen L, Wei Y, Zhou X, Zhang Z, Chi W, Gong L, Jiang X, Zhang S. Morphologic, biomechanical, and compositional features of the internal limiting membrane in pathologic myopic foveoschisis. Invest Ophthalmol Vis Sci. 2018;59(13):5569–78. https://doi.org/10.1167/iovs.18-24676. PMID: 30480705.
39. Flores-Moreno I, Lugo F, Duker JS, Ruiz-Moreno JM. The relationship between axial length and choroidal thickness in eyes with high myopia. Am J Ophthalmol. 2013;155(2):314–19.e1. https://doi.org/10.1016/j.ajo.2012.07.015. Epub 2012 Oct 1. PMID: 23036569.
40. Shen L, You QS, Xu X, Gao F, Zhang Z, Li B, Jonas JB. Scleral and choroidal thickness in secondary high axial myopia. Retina. 2016;36(8):1579–85. https://doi.org/10.1097/IAE.0000000000000947. PMID: 26735565.
41. Ikuno Y, Gomi F, Tano Y. Potent retinal arteriolar traction as a possible cause of myopic foveoschisis. Am J Ophthalmol. 2005;139(3):462–7. https://doi.org/10.1016/j.ajo.2004.09.078. PMID: 15767054.
42. Sayanagi K, Ikuno Y, Gomi F, Tano Y. Retinal vascular microfolds in highly myopic eyes. Am J Ophthalmol. 2005;139(4):658–63. https://doi.org/10.1016/j.ajo.2004.11.025. PMID: 15808161.
43. Curtin BJ, Iwamoto T, Renaldo DP. Normal and staphylomatous sclera of high myopia. An electron microscopic study. Arch Ophthalmol. 1979;97(5):912–5. https://doi.org/10.1001/archopht.1979.01020010470017. PMID: 444126.
44. McBrien NA, Gentle A. Role of the sclera in the development and pathological complications of myopia. Prog Retin Eye Res. 2003;22(3):307–38. https://doi.org/10.1016/s1350-9462(02)00063-0. PMID: 12852489.
45. McBrien NA, Norton TT. Prevention of collagen crosslinking increases form-deprivation myopia in tree shrew. Exp Eye Res. 1994;59(4):475–86. https://doi.org/10.1006/exer.1994.1133. PMID: 7859823.
46. Wu H, Chen W, Zhao F, Zhou Q, Reinach PS, Deng L, Ma L, Luo S, Srinivasalu N, Pan M, Hu Y, Pei X, Sun J, Ren R, Xiong Y, Zhou Z, Zhang S, Tian G, Fang J, Zhang L, Lang J, Wu D, Zeng C, Qu J, Zhou X. Scleral hypoxia is a target for myopia control. Proc Natl Acad Sci U S A. 2018;115(30):E7091–100. https://doi.org/10.1073/pnas.1721443115. Epub 2018 July 9. PMID: 29987045; PMCID: PMC6064999.
47. Itakura H, Kishi S, Li D, Nitta K, Akiyama H. Vitreous changes in high myopia observed by swept-source optical coherence tomography. Invest Ophthalmol Vis Sci. 2014;55(3):1447–52. https://doi.org/10.1167/iovs.13-13496. PMID: 24508787.
48. Kobayashi H, Kishi S. Vitreous surgery for highly myopic eyes with foveal detachment and retinoschisis. Ophthalmology. 2003;110(9):1702–7. https://doi.org/10.1016/S0161-6420(03)00714-0. PMID: 13129865.
49. Benhamou N, Massin P, Haouchine B, Erginay A, Gaudric A. Macular retinoschisis in highly myopic eyes. Am J Ophthalmol. 2002;133(6):794–800. https://doi.org/10.1016/s0002-9394(02)01394-6. PMID: 12036671.
50. Panozzo G, Mercanti A. Vitrectomy for myopic traction maculopathy. Arch Ophthalmol. 2007;125(6):767–72. https://doi.org/10.1001/archopht.125.6.767. PMID: 17562987.
51. Shimada N, Tanaka Y, Tokoro T, Ohno-Matsui K. Natural course of myopic traction maculopathy and factors associated with progression or resolution. Am J Ophthalmol. 2013;156(5):948–57.e1. https://doi.org/10.1016/j.ajo.2013.06.031. Epub 2013 Aug 20. PMID: 23972301.
52. Gaucher D, Haouchine B, Tadayoni R, Massin P, Erginay A, Benhamou N, Gaudric A. Long-term follow-up of high myopic foveoschisis: natural course and surgical outcome. Am J Ophthalmol. 2007;143(3):455–62. https://doi.org/10.1016/j.ajo.2006.10.053. Epub 2006 Dec 8. PMID: 17222382.
53. Parolini B, Palmieri M, Finzi A, Besozzi G, Lucente A, Nava U, Pinackatt S, Adelman R, Frisina R. The new myopic traction maculopathy staging system. Eur J Ophthalmol. 2021;31(3):1299–312. https://doi.org/10.1177/1120672120930590. Epub 2020 June 8. PMID: 32506945.
54. Ikuno Y, Sayanagi K, Ohji M, Kamei M, Gomi F, Harino S, Fujikado T, Tano Y. Vitrectomy and internal limiting membrane peeling for myopic foveoschisis. Am J Ophthalmol. 2004;137(4):719–24. https://doi.org/10.1016/j.ajo.2003.10.019. PMID: 15059711.

55. Gohil R, Sivaprasad S, Han LT, Mathew R, Kiousis G, Yang Y. Myopic foveoschisis: a clinical review. Eye (Lond). 2015;29(5):593–601. https://doi.org/10.1038/eye.2014.311. Epub 2015 Mar 6. PMID: 25744445; PMCID: PMC4429265.
56. Meng B, Zhao L, Yin Y, Li H, Wang X, Yang X, You R, Wang J, Zhang Y, Wang H, Du R, Wang N, Zhan S, Wang Y. Internal limiting membrane peeling and gas tamponade for myopic foveoschisis: a systematic review and meta-analysis. BMC Ophthalmol. 2017;17(1):166. https://doi.org/10.1186/s12886-017-0562-8. PMID: 28886700; PMCID: PMC5591565.
57. Shimada N, Sugamoto Y, Ogawa M, Takase H, Ohno-Matsui K. Fovea-sparing internal limiting membrane peeling for myopic traction maculopathy. Am J Ophthalmol. 2012;154(4):693–701. https://doi.org/10.1016/j.ajo.2012.04.013. Epub 2012 July 25. PMID: 22835515.
58. Elwan MM, Abd Elghafar AE, Hagras SM, Abou Samra WA, Saleh SM. Long-term outcome of internal limiting membrane peeling with and without foveal sparing in myopic foveoschisis. Eur J Ophthalmol. 2019;29(1):69–74. https://doi.org/10.1177/1120672117750059. Epub 2018 Mar 22. PMID: 29565695.
59. Parolini B, Frisina R, Pinackatt S, Gasparotti R, Gatti E, Baldi A, Penzani R, Lucente A, Semeraro F. Indications and results of a new l-shaped macular buckle to support a posterior staphyloma in high myopia. Retina. 2015;35(12):2469–82. https://doi.org/10.1097/IAE.0000000000000613. PMID: 26079474.
60. Mateo C, Dutra Medeiros M, Alkabes M, Burés-Jelstrup A, Postorino M, Corcóstegui B. Illuminated Ando plombe for optimal positioning in highly myopic eyes with vitreoretinal diseases secondary to posterior staphyloma. JAMA Ophthalmol. 2013;131(10):1359–62. https://doi.org/10.1001/jamaophthalmol.2013.4558. PMID: 23949132.
61. Zou J, Tan W, Li F, Zhou G, Li L, Xiong S, Wang X, Xu H. Outcomes of a new 3-D printing-assisted personalized macular buckle combined with para plana vitrectomy for myopic foveoschisis. Acta Ophthalmol. 2021;99(6):688–94. https://doi.org/10.1111/aos.14711. Epub 2020 Dec 16. PMID: 33326163.
62. Sugawara R, Nagaoka T, Kitaya N, Fujio N, Takahashi J, Takahashi A, Yokota H, Yoshida A. Choroidal blood flow in the foveal region in eyes with rhegmatogenous retinal detachment and scleral buckling procedures. Br J Ophthalmol. 2006;90(11):1363–5. https://doi.org/10.1136/bjo.2006.097485. Epub 2006 Aug 16. PMID: 16914476; PMCID: PMC1857488.
63. Tang N, Zhao X, Chen J, Liu B, Lu L. Changes in the choroidal thickness after macular buckling in highly myopic eyes. Retina. 2021;41(9):1858–66. https://doi.org/10.1097/IAE.0000000000003125. PMID: 33492079.
64. Zhang P, Ye CX, Hou LX, Hao YH, Wang K, Shang QL. A pilot study on vitrectomy combined with scleral shortening for eyes with myopic macular retinoschisis-2y follow-up results. Int J Ophthalmol. 2021;14(2):263–8. https://doi.org/10.18240/ijo.2021.02.13. PMID: 33614456; PMCID: PMC7840361.
65. Ye J, Pan AP, Zhu S, Zheng L, Lu F, Xue AQ. Posterior scleral contraction to treat myopic foveoschisis in highly myopic eyes. Retina. 2021;41(5):1047–56. https://doi.org/10.1097/IAE.0000000000002997. PMID: 33079788.

Macular Surgery in Highly Myopic Eyes

Mª Cristina Bohórquez, Anniken Burés-Jelstrup, Luis Miguel Salazar, and Carlos Mateo

Abstract This chapter provides a comprehensive overview of macular surgery in highly myopic eyes, focusing on anatomical features and surgical management techniques. Anatomical considerations include posterior staphyloma, vitreous gel characteristics, and the internal limiting membrane in highly myopic eyes. Surgical management covers various conditions such as myopic traction maculopathy, including retinoschisis and lamellar macular hole, as well as full-thickness macular hole with and without retinoschisis. Additionally, it discusses surgical techniques for retinal detachment secondary to full-thickness macular hole, including pars plana vitrectomy and macular buckling. The chapter delves into important points to consider and surgical techniques specific to each condition, highlighting the nuances and challenges associated with macular surgery in highly myopic eyes.

Keywords Macular traction maculopathy · High myopia · Macular retinoschisis · Posterior staphyloma · Macular hole · Macular hole retinal detachment

Abbreviations

PS	Posterior staphyloma
CNV	Choroidal neovascularisaton
MRI	Magnetic resonance imaging
BCVA	Best corrected visual acuity
MTM	Myopic traction maculopathy
PVD	Posterior vitreous
OCT	Optical coherence tomography
PPVP	Posterior precortical vitreous pocket

Supplementary Information The online version contains supplementary material available at https://doi.org/10.1007/978-3-031-63508-3_13.

M. C. Bohórquez · A. Burés-Jelstrup · L. M. Salazar · C. Mateo (✉)
Instituto de Microcirugía Ocular. Miranza-Veonet, Barcelona, Spain
e-mail: carlosmateo@me.com

F. Patelli et al. (eds.), *Macular Surgery*, https://doi.org/10.1007/978-3-031-63508-3_13

ILM	Internal limiting membrane
RS	Retinoshisis
RPE	Retinal pigment epithelium
FS	Foveoschisis
IS/OS	Photoreceptor inner segment/outer segment
PPV	Pars plana vitrectomy
BSS	Balanced saline solution
C3F8	Octafluoropropane
LMH	Lamellar macular hole
FTMH	Full thickness macular hole
MHRD	Macular hole with retinal detachment
LHEP	Lamellar hole-associated epiretinal proliferation
ERM	Epiretinal membrane
MH	Macular hole
a-PRP	Autologous platelet-rich plasma
APC	Autologous platelet concentrate
RD	Retinal detachment
SF6	Sulfur hexafluoride
PFCL	Perfluorocarbon liquid

When considering macular surgery in highly myopic eyes, it's important to describe the particular anatomic and physiologic reasons why a highly myope patient implies a major surgical challenge. The definition of pathological myopia has been recently updated and is currently defined as eyes with characteristic myopic fundus findings and a refractive error of ≥ 8 negative diopters [1].

1 Anatomic Features of the Macular Area in Highly Myopic Eyes

1.1 Posterior Staphyloma

Posterior staphyloma (PS) is the hallmark of pathologic myopia and plays an important role in the etiology and physiopathology of different fundus alterations in the myopic eye, such as choroidal neovascularization (CNV), choroidal atrophy and myopic traction maculopathy [2–4].

As described by Spaide R, a PS is an outpouching of a circumscribed posterior fundus region and has a curvature radius that is smaller than the curvature radius of the adjacent eye wall [5]. It is present in approximately 50% of patients with pathologic myopia [6].

In 1977 Curtin sorted these lesions into 10 types. Although this classification is still quoted widely, recent technologies, like three-dimensional magnetic resonance imaging (MRI) and wide field optical coherence tomography, have made it possible to understand more about these lesions and to come out with a simpler classification, presented by Ohno Matsui in 2014 [7, 8].

PS is considered a sequel of axial elongation which leads to morphological changes in the posterior pole, characterized by a relatively abrupt scleral thinning starting at its edge, with a pronounced derangement of the scleral collagen fibrils and a marked choroidal thinning, of unclear etiology [9]. It is believed that the main risk factors for PS development include elongated axial length and older age. With increasing age, the incidence and size of the staphyloma increases.

In highly myopic eyes with PS, as compared to highly myopic eyes without PS, best corrected visual acuity (BCVA) was significantly worse and myopic macular complications were significantly more common. Johnson M. et al. described some pathogenic mechanisms of myopic traction maculopathy (MTM) and expressed that this entity virtually always occurs within a PS, as a result of outward forces acting within the eye wall [10].

1.2 Vitreous Gel

Highly myopic eyes show vitreous liquefaction and posterior vitreous detachment (PVD) at an earlier age than non-myopic eyes. The higher the degree of myopia, the younger the age at which PVD begins [11]. This liquefaction and the ensuing PVD, partial or complete, in which the cortical vitreous pulls on and then away from the retinal surface, are the key factors to develop several retinal complications, including a retinal tear, retinal detachment and vitreomacular traction syndrome. In myopic patients, this finding is associated with the development of MTM, epiretinal membrane formation and macular hole[12]. Anomalous or incomplete PVD is defined as a partial vitreous detachment with persistent attachment in the macular region featuring an anomalous strength of adhesion to one or more structures in the posterior pole, resulting in tractional deformation of retinal tissue and favoring traction, which may lead to schisis development.

A complete PVD is rare in eyes with MTM and there is no actual explanation for this finding [13].

Some of the most frequent vitreous interface findings in theUltra-Wide field optical coherence tomography (OCT) exam of a highly myopic patient are:

(1) PVD asymmetrical to the fovea
(2) Location of these asymmetrical PVDs usually correspond to the sites where the sclera is displaced more posteriorly
(3) Multiple PVD images
(4) Posterior pre-cortical vitreous pocket (PPVP) with characteristic features
(5) Vitreoretinal adhesion to the retinal vessels.

The posterior pre-cortical vitreous pocket (PPVP), a "lacuna" in front of the posterior pole, formed between the vitreous cortex (in contact with the internal limiting membrane), and the vitreous cavity, expresses a different behavior of the vitreous in highly myopic patients in contrast tonon-myopic eyes. The PPVP reflects earlier vitreous liquefaction with further stimulation ofan earlier posterior vitreous detachment (PVD), which in turn plays an important role in the development of various vitreoretinal disorders in high myopia [14, 15].

Wide-Field OCTs shows a more extensive length of the vitreous surface (a region of up to 23 × 20 mm and a depth of 5 mm), allowing the clinician to have a better understanding of the vitreous detachment process and the changes at the PPVP area in these patients [16].

Finally, highly myopic eyes may have a residual vitreous cortex that adhere and remain attached to the surface of the retina. Itakura and Kishi showed in their study how the vitreous cortex frequently remains attached to the retina in highly myopic eyes despite the presence of a Weiss ring [14].

Nowadays we know there is a splitting of the vitreous cortex because of its lamellar structure, creating a phenomenon called vitreoschisis [17]. This special feature makes the surgical procedure more challenging and explains the undesired results seen in some specific cases.

Vitreoschisis is not only present in high myopic patients but has also been observed in eyes with macular holes and macular pucker, as well as in a variety of retinovascular disorders such as diabetic retinopathy and Eales disease, suggesting that the vitreous histopathology may play an important role in the development of these entities as well.

1.3 Internal Limiting Membrane in the High Myopic Eye

The internal limiting membrane (ILM) represents a part of the vitreoretinal interface, and its particular location entails some important functions. It has been demonstrated that the ILM contributes significantly to the biomechanical strength of the central retina. Wollensak and collaborators reported in 2006 their results on the study of the biomechanical significance of human ILM, demonstrating that after ILM removal, the mean force of the central retina was reduced significantly by 53,6% and the ultimate elongation by 27,3%, compared to controls, demonstrating a remarkably increased fragility of the retina after its removal [18].

In the myopic patient, the ILM plays an important role when a PS is present. It has been believed for decades that the ILM in these patients has an abnormal configuration which makes it more rigid [19, 20]. It is possible to observe an intrinsic noncompliance effect, which represents one of the major traction mechanisms involved in the development of MTM. This mechanism confers a relative tautness on the inner retina over a PS. The outer retina conforms to the concavity of the PS, but the inner retina is unable to do so, thus, the retina stretches apart gradually over time, generating a macular retinoschisis (RS). When the surgeon relaxes the inner retina by peeling the ILM this problem resolves [10].

Yokota et al., published in 2018, their results from a retrospective case series study, which included 7 patients with macular RS who underwent pars plana vitrectomy. The ultrastructural analysis of the ILM revealed the presence of cellular proliferation and abnormal production of collagen, in addition to basement membranes produced by the glial and retinal pigment epithelium (RPE)-like cells merging within the ILM of these patients. They believed this newly synthesized collagen in addition to glial and RPE-like cell proliferation could create tangential traction in eyes with MTM [13].

In 2005, Bando and Ikuno had already reported their results of a similar study including 15 specimens from 15 patients. In this study they compared two groups of patients, ones with high myopia and RS and the others with idiopathic macular holes. They also found newly synthesized collagen on ILMs from highly myopic patients, and no cells from emmetropic patients with idiopathic macular holes [19]. These findings suggest that active collagen synthesis occurs within the ILM in highly myopic eyes, probably synthetized by fibroblast-like cells and fibrous glial cells with an important associated tractional component.

2 Myopic Traction Maculopathy (MTM)

Named as myopic traction maculopathy (MTM) by Pannozo and Mercanti, it is nowadays considered a spectrum of pathological conditions [21].

Traction mechanisms causing MTM are diverse, and a great proportion of patients require surgical management to relieve the associated mechanism [22].

Sayanagi and collaborators also added the effect of arteriolar traction as a possible cause of RS and MTM [23]. In summary, these are the principal factors associated to traction and inner retinal noncompliance in MTM etiology:

1. Vitreomacular traction (from perifoveal PVD)
2. Remnant cortical vitreous layer (after PVD)—vitreoschisis
3. Epiretinal membrane
4. Intrinsic noncompliance of the ILM (ultrastructural changes within the ILM in some myopic patients)
5. Retinal arteriolar stiffness.

2.1 *Retinoschisis (RS)/Foveoschisis (FS)*

The prevalence of retinoschisis (RS) in the general population is about 0.8% and its prevalence among high myopes rises to 6.5–32.9%.

RS is considered the most prevalent feature found in patients with MTM (with a prevalence of around 80%), followed by lamellar macular hole (25%) as well as the earliest retinal alteration occurring in the progression of the anomaly [21]. RS as a possible cause of retinal detachment was first described by Calbert Phillips [24]. In his paper he wanted to depict the common finding of a retinal detachment localized to, "or apparently originating from" the macular area in myopic patients with the presence of a PS in some cases, without the evidence of a hole. However, the first investigators to describe RS as we now know it by means of OCT were Takano and Kishi in 1999 [25].

RS is described as a progressive separation of the retinal layers (internal, external or both), which remain connected by Henle's fibers and stretched in multiple columnar structures. OCT findings have enabled the clinician to improve the characterization of the anomalies encountered in these patients and at the same time appreciate the different features converging in the same anomaly [8]. Its pathogenesis remains debatable, being the most common hypothesis an antero-posterior traction due to a PS and the presence of tangential traction caused by stretched retinal vessels and an abnormally rigid ILM [26]. Anomalous or incomplete PVD as well as contraction of an attached cortical vitreous are important associated factors as well [27].

The term englobes a wide range of different anatomic alterations within the same pathology, as we can see inthe classification chapter above, staged according to its severity and its treatment alternatives. Based on these findings we can characterize each patient and define a specific treatment. The natural history of this condition is usually progressive, and its appearance may represent the prior stage of what could come next, being the final stage a macular hole with an associated retinal detachment [28].

There are, however, exceptions: Shimada et al. published a series of 207 eyes with RS in MTM, where they observed improvement by OCT in 3.9% of patients. Most of the patients showing this regression, developed a PVD and in one case, a spontaneous disruption of the ILM occurred [22].

In general terms we could divide our patients with RS into two categories: those who only require observation and those who require a surgical approach. Each one of these two broad categories include different clinical approaches.

Observation

Along with patients' complaints and progression of visual acuity compared with previous visits, OCT findings are crucial when deciding the optimal treatment approach.

Treating a highly myope patient usually requires an observational period that needs to be long enough to ensure there are actual changes in their OCT. In the clinical practice it is usual to have an annual visit where the specialist reports OCT findings, BCVA and presence or absence of metamorphopsia and other macula-related clinical symptoms. If there are no clinical symptoms, and visual acuity is stable, it is quite probable that the OCT remains unchanged. These patients will receive general recommendations and will be asked to come back earlier if some new symptoms appear.

There could be, though, some mild OCT changes inan asymptomatic patient. These changes are considered mild and establish the beginning of RS. As long as the patient remains asymptomatic and the visual acuity stable (or shows only a mild reduction), the patient can be observed. With our current knowledge, we know these findings can remain stable for years or show a very low progression. It's important to consider though, that the younger the patient the more probable the progression within a certain period of time.

Surgical Management

During follow-up, surgery would be suggested in patients who have suffered a drop in visual acuity, associated with progression of the foveal structural changes controlled by OCT, such as worsening of the RS and the onset of a foveal detachment. Regarding visual acuity, metamorphopsia may be an associated symptom, but it is necessary to rule out the presence of CNV or an early onset macular hole without RS. The presence of a foveal detachment and/or disruption within the ellipsoid layer (photoreceptor inner segment/outer segment—IS/OS) and the external limiting membrane, suggest the need of surgery in the near future. The presence of a full thickness macular hole or the presence of a retinal detachment with or without a macular hole are findings that make surgery necessary.

The surgical technique is still controversial. There have been several attempts to control the pathology, avoiding the progressive loss of visual acuity and the risks associated with the intervention.

Gas Injection

In order to avoid higher risks, in 2019, I-Hsin Ma and collaborators published their long-term results of gas tamponade without vitrectomy in RS with foveal detachment. The rate of foveal reattachment after one session of intravitreal gas injection was 70%, at 3 months follow-up. However, during subsequent follow-up, some of the cases experienced recurrence, and underwent a new gas injection, obtaining reattachment of the retina in approximately 65% of cases avoiding the onset of a macular hole [29].

Pars plana vitrectomy alone, macular buckling or a combination of these procedures, have been reported in the literature with different rates of success and complications.

Pars Plana Vitrectomy (PPV): General Concepts

PPV is the most common technique used to treat progressive RS. One of the challenges of high myopic eyes is the increased axial length, which is too long for the conventional instruments used in surgery. These instruments limit the access to the posterior pole, and when trying to reach this area, the surgeon may deform the corneal surface and thus, diminish visualization.

There are several alternatives which may help overcome this issue:

A. Extending the Limbus to Cannula distance to 6.0 mm. Remember there are some anatomic differences between myopic and emmetropic eyes, one of these involves the insertion of the ora serrata which is located posteriorly in myopic eyes, meaning that the entrance of the instruments for the dominant hand could be placed 5 or even 6mm from the limbus [30].
B. One way to identify the ora serrata insertion consists in performing transillumination with the intraocular light held by the non-dominant hand, being able to localize the entrance area and to insert the cannula without touching the retina.
C. Another option to gain some extra length is to remove the cannula while working in the macular area.
D. Some authors have described the use of a temporary macular buckle to shorten the axial length during surgery [31].

As we have described above, the vitreous in highly myopic patients represents a major challenge during PPV. One tip to overcome this issue and facilitate its complete removal, is to stain it with triamcinolone, which will enhance its visualization making sure it is removed completely, althoughit is not always an easy task to accomplish despite the enhanced visualization. Some other dyes have also been used, offering no better results than triamcinolone [32].

Due to the presence of a strong attachment from the cortical vitreous to the retinal vessels, RPE or peripheral lattice degenerations, PPV could induce iatrogenic tears that may cause a retinal detachment, if left untreated. In some cases, we can find spindle-like inner retinal defects next to stretched retinal vessels. These are considered cleavage lesions among the internal layers, and not full thickness retinal defects and in general, they don´t need to be treated [33–35] (Video 1).

It is generally accepted that PPV in a high myope patient counteracts tangential forces due to vitreous traction and ILM rigidity (or intrinsic non-compliance), but it has no effect on the arteriolar stiffness or the perpendicular traction created by the PS.

Another thingto acknowledge is the development of a macular hole after PPV in high myopes, reported in 20–27% of cases in some of the published series [36–38]. These published reports have led to look for a different surgical option, the macular buckle alone or in combination with PPV [8, 28, 39]. These published series have shown good clinical results based on correcting the perpendicular traction exerted by the PS.

Internal Limiting Membrane (ILM) Peeling

ILM peeling has remained a controversial technique ever since the beginning, with some series showing good visual outcomes in surgeries without peeling and diminishing the risk of developinga macular hole [40, 41].

Though ILM peeling canbe performed without dyeing, the use of some dyes (indocyaninegreen and Brilliant Blue G) might increase visualization of the ILM and enhance its rigidity, making it easier to peel and obtaining large pieces of the ILM, which would help avoid multiple pinching procedures [42, 43].

Dyes

Different dyes have been used to stain the ILM, such as Brilliant Blue G, Tripan Blue and a low concentration of indocyaninegreen with a short exposure time, in order to minimize its toxicity. Even after dyeing, visualization of the ILM might be difficult because of the presence of vitreoschisis and, in some cases, remnants of the vitreous cortex still attached to the inner retina.To deal with this situation we suggest the use of a flexible loop to gently brush over the retinal surface to remove all these remnants, and then, using a dye to have the best possible exposure.

Sparing the Fovea Technique (Fig. 1)

The risk of developing a macular hole after PPV seems to increase in patients with a previous IS/OS defect in the OCT [44]. Nowadays the preferred technique among surgeons is to perform the ILM peeling sparing the fovea, which consists in doing an ILM peeling following a circled pattern without crossing the foveal area, leaving a fragment of ILM around this area of approximately 1 disc diameter (1DD), and the remnants of ILM around this area are then trimmed with the vitreous cutter or micro scissors [45–47] (Video 2).

In the literature we can find different techniques to protect the macular area and prevent the appearance of a macular hole, with the foveal sparing technique. In 2016, Jin et al., described the "parafoveal multiple curvilinear peeling" which consists in creating ILM circled parafoveal peeling, preserving 500 microns of the perifoveal ILM. Xie et al. also reported a "continuous arc-shaped fold-back peel of the ILM" consisting in applying shearing forces to create arc-shaped tears of the ILM, preserving around 1/3 of the optic disc diameter [48, 49]. Some other series do not show any increased risk of macular hole formation with complete ILM peeling [50, 51].

In patients with a deep central PS, extra care is recommended during the ILM peeling, especially while working with a contact lens with high magnification. It is important to be aware of the presence of this anatomic defect and avoid touching the temporal wall of it, to prevent the formation of retinal tears, subretinal hemorrhages and in some cases, choroidal hemorrhages (Fig. 2).

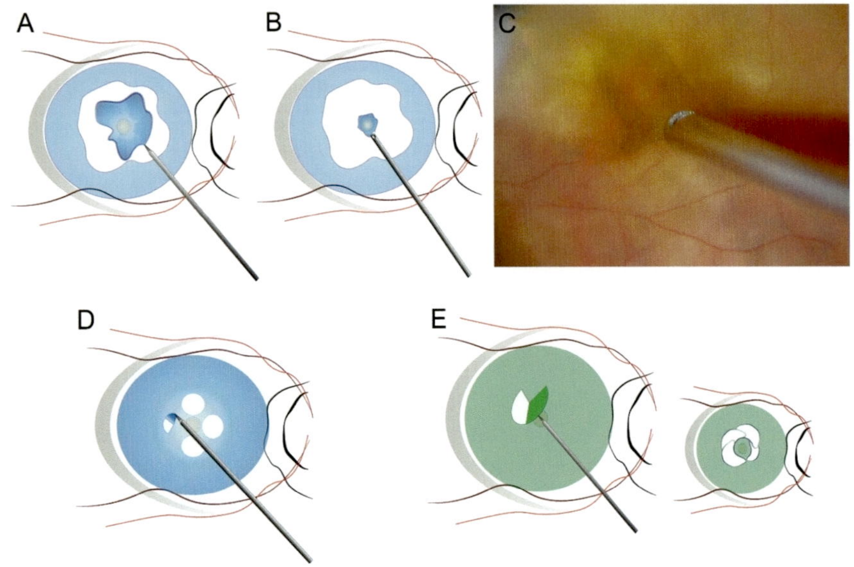

Fig. 1 (A) ILM peeling in a circular way from the periphery to the centre of the macula, sparing the fovea. (B) Elevated ILM is trimmed towards the foveal centre with the vitreous probe [45]. (C) Intraoperative view of figure (B). (D) Rounded ILM peeling around the fovea leaving 500 μ around the foveal area [48]. (E) Multiple arc shaped ILM peeling, leaving approximately 1/3-disc diameter of unpeeled ILM around the fovea [49]

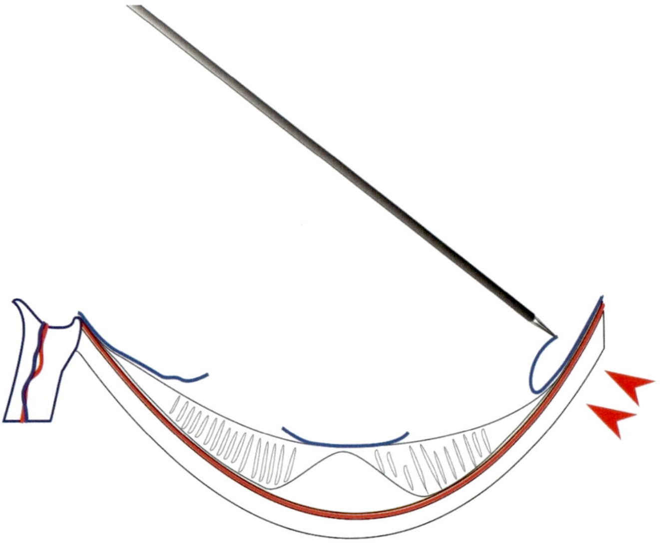

Fig. 2 Under high magnification, extreme caution must be taken to avoid touching the temporal wall of the staphyloma

Tamponade

A tamponade substance is used in those cases (mostly retinal tears) where there is a need to create an interface to avoid the entrance of fluid from the vitreous cavity into the subretinal space, using the superficial and interfacial tension of the element chosen as a tamponade. With this concept in mind, the typical progressive macular RS does not have a retinal tear in its pathogenesis, so the use of a tamponade at the end of the vitrectomy is expected to have a different effect. Some authors suggest its use might resolve the RS during a short period of time, partly due to its buoyancy force. There are different opinions among the medical community regarding the use or not of any tamponade element after PPV in highly myopic patients. Hirakata et al., showed in his retrospective 14 cases series, the formation of a macular hole in 2 patients after using gas as a tamponade at the end of surgery. His hypothesis was that the gas bubble may push the subretinal fluid present inside the macular detachment towards the weak and thin central fovea, causing the development of a macular hole[41]. Meng et al. in 2017 reported that PPV with gas tamponade was associated with more complications than non-tamponade and that the use of tamponade did not influence BCVA or anatomic response [27].

On the other hand, Zheng et al. showed, in a retrospective series of 18 patients, that the injection of octafluoropropane (C3F8) at the end of the procedure, resulted in a more rapid anatomical resolution and greater improvement of BCVA, than when left with balanced saline solution (BSS) at the end of surgery. In his series there was no randomization, and the criteria to leave C3F8 or BSS at the end of surgery was based on the surgeon's preference [52]. In 2022 Zhang et al. showed his results with the use of air as a tamponade in contrast to C3F8. Although this was not a randomized study, they concluded that the use of air could lead to better outcomes than eyes treated with C3F8, reporting 2 cases of post-operative macular hole in the C3F8 group [53].

Predictive Factors of surgical outcomes for RS

RS is the entity associated with best visual prognosis after surgery within the MTM spectrum, compared to the other disorders englobed in this pathology such as lamellar macular hole, full thickness macular hole and macular hole retinal detachment. Patients with RS alone achieved anatomical recovery in the shortest time and have the best postoperative BCVA [54]. In general terms, a good baseline BCVA and absence of foveal detachment on preoperative OCT examination are predictive of a good postoperative visual outcome, according to different studies [55]. Linn et al. published a retrospective case series, where they concluded that patients with RS with preoperative IS/OS disruption and thinner central foveal thickness tend to have poorer visual outcomes [56]. Fujimoto et al. suggested that retinal thickness changes and recovery of photoreceptors cells are important OCT findings related to final BCVA [57].

Within this entity there is a group of patients exhibiting a variety of findings at the OCT in the macular area. Besides from the macular thickness and presence or absence of subretinal fluid, there is another feature to consider when talking

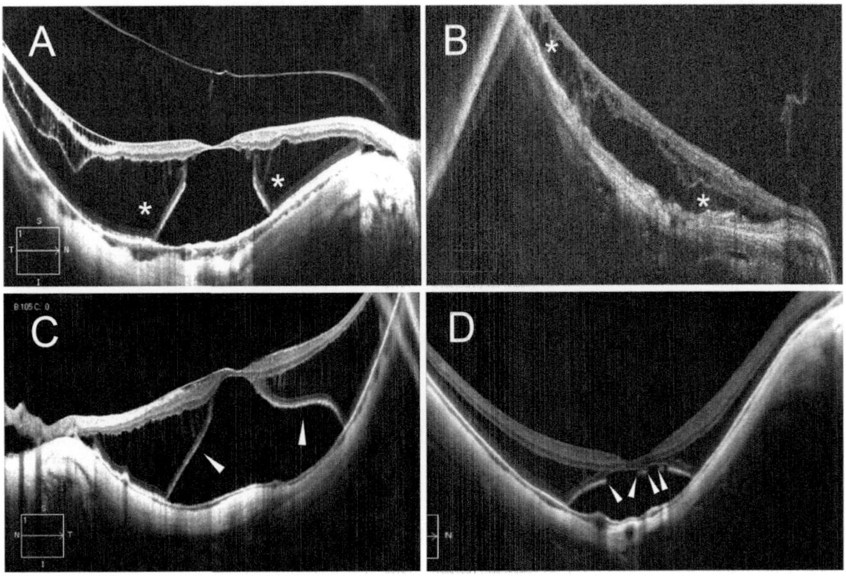

Fig. 3 (A) OCT image of RS with foveal detachment. High density of tissular columns (Henle´s layer fibres and Müller cells) in the outer retina (asterisk). These findings predict a better prognosis than those in image (B). (B) OCT image shows less density of tissular columns and disorganization of the outer retina (asterisk). These findings are correlated with a worse visual prognosis. (C) OCT showing preservation of the distal ends of the photoreceptors (arrowheads). This finding is related to better outcomes than those in image (D), where large areas of absence of distal ends of the photoreceptors are seen (arrowheads)

about prognosis, which is the presence or absence of Henle's layer fibers. In our experience, a diminished number of Henle´s fibers or its absence in the OCT, is a strong indicatorof poor visual prognosis. In most of these cases we prefer not to perform surgery to avoid possible complications, knowing thatvisual prognosis will be poor even though we accomplish a good anatomical outcome [58].

It is widely accepted then, that the better preoperative vision, the better postoperative visual acuity. Additional clues we can see on OCT and that can limit visual prognosis are: (Fig. 3).

A. Presence of a foveal detachment
B. Less density of Henle's layer fibers and Müller cells in the outer retina
C. Absence of areas of terminal ends of photoreceptors.

2.2 *Lamellar Macular Hole (LMH)*

LMH is considered, by definition, as a macular lesion with partial-thickness loss of foveal tissue [59] and is a common macular structural abnormality in patients with high myopia (4.8–20.7%). Its clinical course may differ from that in idiopathic LMH, related to the adherent vitreous cortex and epiretinal membrane exerting a complex anteroposterior and tangential traction and because the ILM could be more rigid, and a PS is often present. In non-myopic eyes, LMH has a stable clinical course, and rarely progresses to a full thickness macular hole (FTMH) (1–4%) [60].

In high myopic eyes, MTM induces traction and the LMH manifests different structural related changes. Some of these may remain stable or show minimal progression for a long period of time and others may progress to a FTMH or macular hole with retinal detachment (MHRD), causing severe vision loss [60].

LMH was described by Witkins in 2006 as a macular lesion with an irregular foveal contour, a break in the inner fovea, intraretinal splitting and an intact foveal photoreceptor layer [61]. Nowadays its diagnosis is made based on the updated criteria proposed by the International Vitreomacular Traction Study (IVTS) Group, including the following characteristics:

(1) irregular foveal contour
(2) defect in the inner fovea (with or without actual loss of tissue)
(3) separation between the inner and outer retinal layers in the fovea
(4) absence of full-thickness foveal defect [60].

An epiretinal proliferation over the ILM, named lamellar hole-associated epiretinal proliferation (LHEP), has been described in some of these patients (30%) (Fig. 4). This LHEP has no hyporeflective spaces between the two anatomical structures and no contractile properties [62]. LHEP is not an exclusive feature of LMH, as it can be found in other pathologies, but it is a common finding to consider during surgery because its behavior differs to the one of the ILM or the epiretinal membrane (ERM) and therefore could affect surgical outcomes. LHEP is often more difficult to start peeling than typical ERMs, since this tissue is more elastic and typically yellow, possibly from xanthophyll pigment (unpublished data, Richard Spaide, 2013). There has also been described a relatively firm adhesion between this tissue and the edges of the hole [63].

On SD-OCT imaging, LHEP appears as a homogenous material with medium reflectivity and variations in thickness. Lying on the epiretinal surface, LHEP assumes a mound configuration that, either partially or completely, surrounds the lamellar hole, molding the inner retinal anatomy. In his study, Spaide et al. hypothesized that this epiretinal proliferative material possesses similar traits to that of the middle retinal layers, suggesting this tissue could possibly originate from a proliferation of Müller cells, in an attempt of the eye to restabilize the retinal structure [62]. In general, eyes with LHEP are associated with poorer visual acuity, larger LMH diameters, thinner retinal thickness, and higher incidence of IS/OS disruption compared with eyes without it [59].

In 2017, Yang et al. published his results about surgical outcomes of LMH or FTMH associated with epiretinal proliferation in high myopic patients. First, he reported a higher prevalence of LHEP in highly myopic eyes (66.2%) than in previous studies (22.9–30%). Little is known about the clinical and surgical features of LHEP in highly myopic eyes, but in his observations, he described that LHEP in eyes

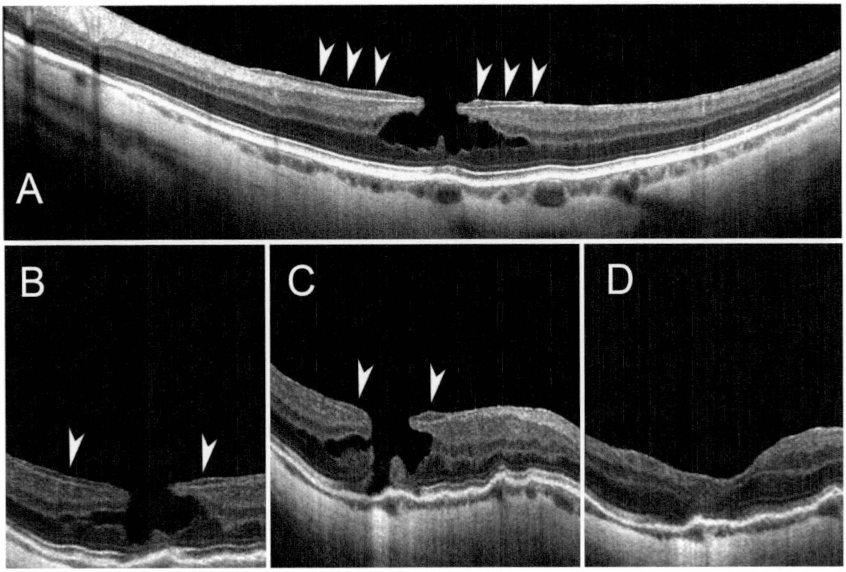

Fig. 4 (A, B) OCT images showing the presence of a LMH with a hyporeflective tissue over the ILM, surrounded by a hyperreflective line (LHEP) (white arrow heads). This epiretinal proliferation hinders a correct visualization of the ILM after dye injection. (B, C) Progress from a LMH to a FTMH. (C) Postoperative restoration of the foveal area, with absence of the epiretinal proliferation

with high myopia tended to have a broader extension, LHEP and posterior hyaloid adhesion occurred more often and, lastly, subjects with LHEP and high myopia were younger than those non-myopic with LHEP. Unfortunately, this study is a retrospective one with a small sample size, but the results obtained suggested that the presence of LHEP could help seal the macular hole[63].

Being described as a progressive feature, highly myope patients with a LMH with or without epiretinal proliferation need to be observed for a long time to describe changes, subjective ones noted by the patient (symptoms related to macular disruption) and objective ones noted by the specialist (decrease in visual acuity or OCT changes).

As well as in RS, the decision to treat a patient would rely on changes described by the patient or the specialist, both comprising visual acuity changes. The treatment is surgical and involves PPV with peeling of the epiretinal proliferation and/or the ERM and the ILM, usually sparing the fovea to avoid formation of a FTMH, and the technique is the same as the one described for RS.

2.3 Full Thickness Macular Hole (FTMH) Without Retinoschisis (RS)

According to the literature, development of a macular hole (MH) in highly myopic eyes involves complex traction forces from various directions, including vitreous antero-posterior traction, oblique or tangential traction from partially detached or undetached posterior hyaloid, traction from ERM, ILM induced tangential traction, posterior outward traction fromthe PS, and retinal vessel traction [64].

All these factors, whether alone or in combination, may induce MH formation through mechanisms different from those underlying idiopathic MH, explaining its different behavior and prognosis.

Importants Points to Consider in FTMH Without RS

1. FTMH tends to appear at a younger age in highly myopes, compared to emmetropic or non-myopic patients. Kobayashi et al. demonstrated that age at onset showed a significant decrease in relation to axial length and myopic refraction, with a mean age of 52.1 years in eyes with severe myopia versus 69.8 years in eyes with emmetropia and hyperopia [65].
2. High myopia represents the most frequent cause of MH in the population under 55 years, and OCT is mandatory in these cases to confirm the diagnosis, even in asymptomatic cases [66].
3. Two types of MH might be seen in the highly myopic patient, based on the presence or absence of macular RS. In the absence of RS, Kobayashi showed no significant statistical difference between area, volume, and depth of the MH in a highly myopic patient, versus an emmetropic one using a confocal scanning diode laser (670 nm) retinal tomograph [65]. Nevertheless, Tamer Mahmoud recently published an article showing that transversal OCT measurements might underestimate the real size of a myopic MH and suggested adding the axial length into the OCT device itself, to obtain a more accurate value [67]. This finding is relevant, considering that eyes with an axial length greater than 30 mm are considered at a greater risk of anatomical failure during surgery [68].

The presence of a MH without RS can also be seen during or after PPV for MTM [69]. The success rate in cases of MH without RS is better than that in cases of MH with RS [70].

FTMH Without RS—Surgical Technique

Basic Steps:

A. Check the patient's previous OCT before surgery. In high myopes you can see the presence of a hyporeflective tissue surrounded by a hyperreflective area, which will limit the dyeing process of the ILM. This tissue is difficult to manipulate and peel because of its composition.It has a yellowish color, and its appearance is completely different from that of the ILM or a common ERM. We recommend using a flexible loop (Finesse® Flex Loop, Alcon Lab.) to grasp it, and then re-dye, to obtain a good visualization of the ILM.

B. Dye injection: The most frequent dyes used to stain the ILM are Brilliant Blue G, and indocyanine green used at a low concentration and with a limited time of exposure to avoid toxicity. Repeated dyeing is often needed to warrant a complete ILM dissection.
C. ILM dissection and inverted flap: The ILM is peeled around the foveal area, obtaining a flap which will lay inverted over the MH, while keeping it attached to one of its margins. After the inverted macular flap technique was described as an alternative to treat large MH in emmetropic eyes, several authors have described their results using the same or similar techniques to pursue anatomic success in highly myopic eyes (Video 3).

Michalewska showed, in a series of 19 eyes with a mean axial length of 29.4 mm, a MH closure rate of 100% without any recurrences [71]. Mete et al. showed, in his series of 34 eyes with a mean axial length of 29.6 mm, a closure rate of 91% and a significant statistical difference between preoperative and postoperative BCVA [72].

Oleñik et al. described a series of 33 eyes with a mean axial length of 32.48 mm and a 100% rate of primary closure with just 2 recurrences. Although preoperative BCVA was different and unrelated in these 3 series, BCVA in postoperative patients reached almost 20/50 [73]. Rizzo also demonstrated better results with the inverted flap technique rather than the conventional technique to treat MH in highly myopic eyes. In his series he showed an 88.4% closure rate versus 38.9% in those cases with the standard technique [74].

Different approaches to the inverted flap: Inverted flap technique has evolved since it was first described, according to the surgeons' preferences. Direction of the flap might change (superior to inferior, temporal to nasal), stuffing the ILM inside the hole or just laying it on top of the foveal area (envelope or flower-petal technique) [75–77] (Fig. 5).

This variety of options just facilitates the procedure, giving each and every surgeon the most comfortable technique according to their needs and expectations.

Another technique described by Mahmoud and Finn is the "retracting door" technique where the nasal side of the ILM is peeled crossing the foveal area and including a small portion of the temporal zone, forming a temporal "hinge". The once-taut ILM relaxes and retracts as it is draped, a more nasal portion of ILM covers and helps closing the hole [78].

D. Other options: recently, some authors have used autologous platelet-rich plasma (a-PRP) or autologous platelet concentrate (APC), as hole closure inductors because of its high concentration of growth factors that promote wound healing. This specific technique has become an alternative to treat large MH, recurrent MH, and MH in highly myopic patients. Kim and collaborators described their results comparing 2 groups of patients, one group treated with the mainstay

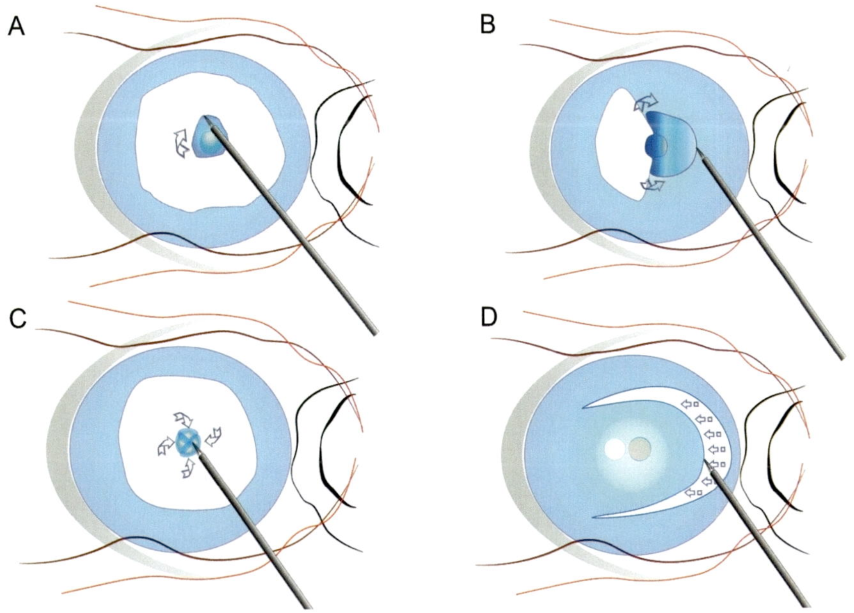

Fig. 5 (A) Superior to inferior inverted flap. (B) Temporal to nasal inverted flap leaving the nasal quadrant untouched [76]. (C) "all in" or "flower-petal" technique [75]. (D) "Retracting door" technique [78]

technique, which is PPV, posterior hyaloid detachment, in this specific case, peeling of the ILM around the MH by a minimum of one-disc diameter (1DD), fluid/air exchange and gas injection; versus the same technique with the injection of the APC/aPRP before gas injection. Unfortunately, the use of an inverted flap during the procedure was at the surgeon's discretion using it in either one of the groups, probably being the reason why there were no significant differences, with no additional benefit of APC injection in these patients [79]. In contrast, Figueroa published her results of a prospective, single center, nonrandomized study, where all the patients achieved closure of the MH using APC with the same technique used by Kim. They both concluded that this technique is an easier procedure and may guarantee similar surgical outcomes as other techniques described [80]. Buzzi and collaborators discuss the use of a-PRP as an adjuvant to revisional PPV for refractory FTMH, obtaining similar results to the ones reported by Figueroa, and also adding functional results with a significant improvement in BCVA from baseline to final visits, correlating with restoration of the neuroepithelial external layers in many of the cases [81].

It is important to keep in mind that PPV in eyes with MTM might induce central RPE atrophy, which will increase progressively in time. In MH patients, these findings might reach 13% of cases [82] (Fig. 6).

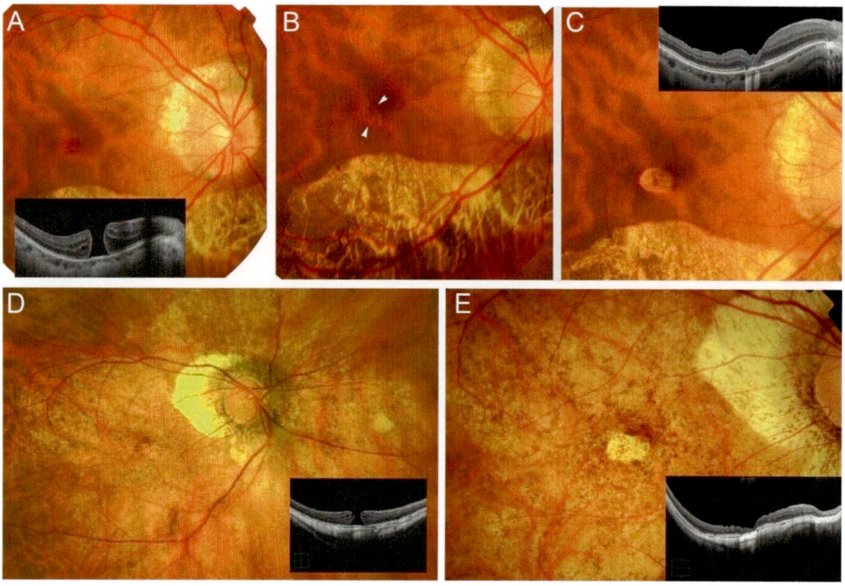

Fig. 6 (A) OCT image of a FTMH in an eye with an axial length of 29.7 mm. (B) Two months after surgery, the MH is closed but some mild RPE disturbances are observed (arrowheads) (C) 10 months after surgery, RPE atrophy is now evident. (D) OCT image of a FTMH in an eye with an axial length of 31 mm. (E) 3 years after surgery, image shows central atrophy of the RPE. OCT image shows the dimples of the inner surface of the retina, representing the area of ILM removal

2.4 *Full-Thickness Macular Hole (FTMH) with Retinoschisis (RS)*

There are not many studies differentiating MH with RS as a different entity from MH in high myopic eyes without RS. Probably many of these patients end up included in a big reported series of MH in high myopia without any differentiation.

In 2006 Ikuno and Tano described a MH associated with RS. They published their study including 8 eyes who underwent ILM peeling, previously stained with indocyanine green, obtaining MH closure in 1 case and 1 more after a re-intervention using intravitreal gas injection. The rest of the cases remained open after re-interventions [83].

After this article was published, many others came out showing similar results, highlighting the difficulty to obtain a complete MH closure in the presence of macular RS with the standard ILM peeling technique [68, 84]. Jo and collaborators stated that RS negatively impacts PPV for highly myopic MH [85].

It's from these results that the macular buckle reappears in the horizon as a technique aimed to counteract the pulling effect from the PS in order to obtain better anatomical and functional results. In 2014, a retrospective study by Burés-Jelstrup et al. analyzed 16 eyes that underwent PPV and macular buckling in highly myopic patients with MH associated with macular RS, obtaining an anatomic hole closure of 100% and a functional acuity improvement of 81% [86].

In 2016, a prospective study published by Cacciamani et al., treated 15 eyes with macular buckling for FTMH with RS and reported the closure of the MH with RS in 100% of the cases and a functional visual acuity improvement in 86% of the cases [87].

The macular buckling technique has a steep learning curve and potential complications may arise. This, and the addition of new techniques developed to treat the macular area in myopic eyes, has led to a new approximation to treat these patients.

Recently, a retrospective series, including 12 eyes, has reported a 91% success rate in MH closure using the ILM inverted flap technique (superior or inferior) reaching a functional recovery in about 75% of the cases [88] (Video 4).

2.5 *Retinal Detachment Secondary to FTMH (MHRD)*

Retinal Detachment (RD) originated from a MH has been considered a very complex entity for decades. While the exact pathogenesis for RD in these patients remains unknown, many hypotheses have been suggested as its possible etiology. As we mentioned above, the pathophysiology associated with MTM along with factors linked to pathological traction, (vitreomacular traction, intrinsic non-compliance of the ILM, presence of a deep PS, among others) show the natural progress of the disease, ending in some cases with the development of a MHRD if left untreated [10]. Some other authors also link the etiology to the presence of large areas of chorioretinal atrophy leading to a weak adhesion between the retina and the underlying RPE [1].

MH associated with RS and a deep PS are the ones more frequently associated with RD [89]. It is important to keep in mind that the RS will disappear in most cases once the attachment of the photoreceptors to the RPE disappears during the detachment, due to the retina's intrinsic elasticity.

A FTMH is not the only factor associated with a RD involving the macular area in highly myopic patients. If a FTMH has been ruled out with the help of an OCT, there are some other places in the macular area where we may look for full thickness ruptures explaining the presence of a RD, and its location is not always easy to find. The most common places for these other ruptures are:

1. Next to the stretched retinal vessels. It is frequent to observe spindle-like inner retinal defects around major temporal vessels not associated with a RD, but keep in mind that sometimes a full retinal tear may be present.
2. Areas of RPE atrophy in the PS. During the slit-lamp examination it is difficult to determine the presence or absence of lesions in this area so, with the help of an OCT it is possible to find these small full thickness ruptures (in some cases there is more than one rupture associated). It is also frequent to find atrophic outer retinal layers attached to the RPE, with no bridges connecting with the inner retina, showing chronicity and poor visual prognosis within these areas.

3. Around the optic disc. It is very common to observe atrophic areas around the optic disc. The use of an OCT, carefully assessing the peripapillary area, might help us find possible breaks.

If the decision for macular buckling has already been made to treat a special case, consider that the MH might not be at the center of the PS dome, but next to its nasal margins on the slope, making it closer to the optic disc, and therefore making the procedure more complicated.

Surgical Treatment for MHRD

Ever since it was first described, MHRD has been known as a pathology with a limited visual prognosis. In pre-PPV era, the macular buckling technique appeared as an option to counteract the pulling effect of the PS, with no clear conclusions about its usefulness so, in mostcases, this entity was treated with diathermy and cryotherapy to close the MH and avoid a recurrent RD, which always left a postoperative central scotoma [90–98].

With the appearance of PPV and its improvements over the 90s and early 2000s, the macular buckling technique was put aside, and just small, isolated groups showed apparently good results [99–101]. But more recently this technique has reappeared and has showed competing results to PPV (Fig. 7).

PPV for MHRD

Initial results with PPV and ILM peeling using indocyanine green to stain the ILM were also poor in some published series, accounting for the complexity of the procedure due to all the associated factors related to high myopia, already described. Ikuno et al. showed, in 2003, a closure rate of about 44%, corroborated by OCT. These results marked the end of the era where it was impossible to be certain about the actual MH closure, thus a tendency to overestimate these results was quite probable. In his study, Ikuno showed retinal reattachment in 100% of cases, with a tendency to improve visual acuity in 86% of cases when the MH was closed and 33% when the MH remained open [102].

In 2011, Nishimura showed a retrospective study where he reported a 55% MH closure rate and 92% of retinal reattachment, using silicone oil as a tamponade for a period of 6 months, although with high intraocular pressure levels reported after its removal. There were no statistical differences in BCVA between open and closed holes after surgery [103]. Closure of the MH after PPV with peeling of ILM and silicone oil has been described among 11% and 86% of the cases, with a reattachment rate between 75 and 95% of cases. In series including patients with longer axial lengths, the results tend to be worse [104–107].

Choosing the perfect tamponade at the end of surgery remains a controversial matter. A multicenter study, with an initial reattachment rate of 69%, showing worse

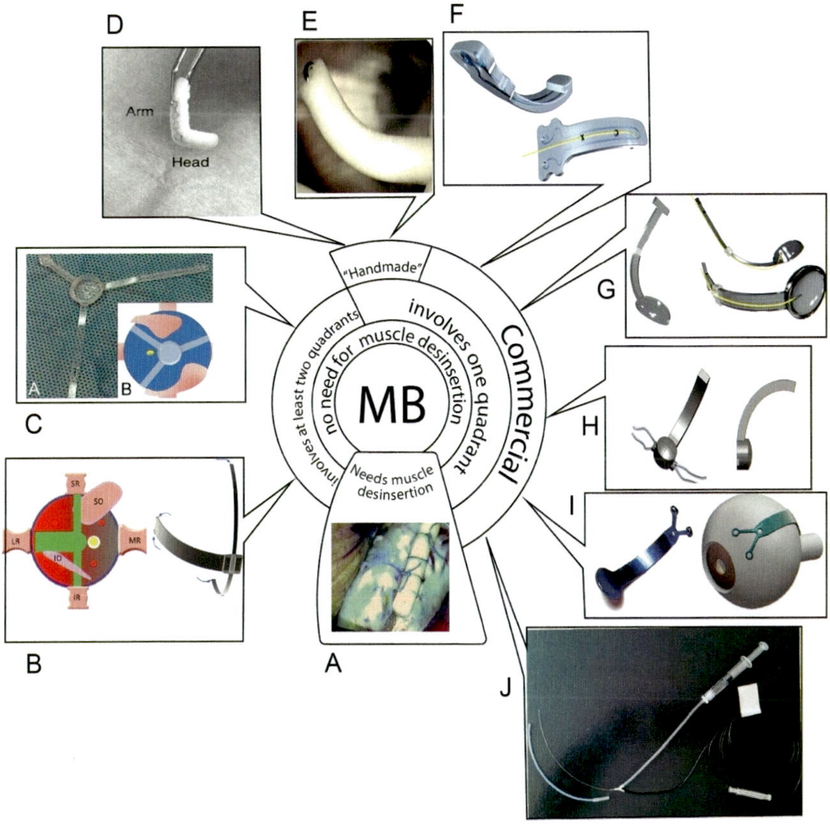
D
Arm
Head
E
F
G
H
I
J
C
A
B
B
SR
SO
LR
IO
MR
IR
A
"Handmade"
Commercial
involves one quadrant
no need for muscle desinsertion
involves at least two quadrants
MB
Needs muscle desinsertion

◀**Fig. 7** Some of the macular buckles used and described in the literature: (A) From Siam et al.: a 2 mm diameter silastic sponge rod, radially placed. It requires exposure of all 4 recti muscles and disinsertion of the superior oblique tendon to place the posterior sutures [119]. A vertical 7.5 × 5.5 mm sponge has also been used along the vertical axis [97, 101]. (B) T-shape macular buckle described by Devin F. in 2011 (FCI, Carl Zeiss Meditec) [117]; it consists in a three arm device where a 2 mm band is threaded through a 7 mm solid silicone with a convex ending platform to induce macular indentation. There is no need for posterior sutures or muscle disinsertion but the conjunctiva has to be open in all quadrants. Main complications associated with this technique are the risks of inducing a choroidal detachment or compressing the inferotemporal vorticose vein when placing the buckle. Another potential risk is crossing through the ending fibers of the inferior oblique muscle [117, 125]. (C) Similar to (B) but with a central silicone capsule (8 mm diameter) that is filled with saline solution through a closed channel in the short arm [124]. (D) A titanium stent is inserted into a 7 mm large, 5 mm thick and 3 mm long oval silicone sponge. Once the titanium is inside, the sponge is bent to create a 90-degree angle and is then inserted in the superotemporal quadrant to obtain the buckling effect in the macular area [123, 128]. (E) Similar to (D), a 0.5 mm orthodontic steel is inserted into a 7 mm sponge and bent to obtain the desired macular buckling effect [120]. (F) Ando Plombe (Ondeko Corporation. Japan): semi-transparent hard silicone rod with titanium wires inside that can be bent. Two sizes are available to be selected depending on the axial length (25 and 27 mm long) The distal end has a 5 × 5 mm flat and square indenting platform [100, 115]. An optic fiber may be inserted into the indenting platform to facilitate a correct placement [130]. (G) AJL Macular Buckle (AJL Ophthalmic. Spain). Customizable in relation to the axial length. Rigid and made of silicone coated PMMA with a rounded and convex 8 mm diameter indenting platform. A groove in the center of the indenting platform allows for insertion of an optic fiber to facilitate correct centering. (H) The AMB (Micromed. Italy) is made of silicone rubber with a stalk and a convex 5 mm diameter terminal plate. The dimensions of the quadrangular stalk to handle the device are 2 × 2 × 10 mm. Two lateral winglets in the indenting plate allow sutures to be placed to fix the device to the anterior sclera [87, 118]. (I) Akduman Macular Buckle is made of titanium and has two holes in the anterior arms to place the sutures. The indenting platform is flat and concave towards the sclera [126]. (J) El Rayes Flextip Suprachoroidal Buckling; a 450 μm catheter (MedOne Surgical. USA) is advanced through the suprachoroidal space to the macular area, where a long lasting Hyaluronic acid (Perlane; D-med, Sweden) is injected, obtaining a customized indenting effect [122]

prognosis with longer axial lengths, did not find any differences between Sulfur hexafluoride (SF6) or C3F8 as tamponade between successful and failed initial reattachments [108]. In contrast, Uemoto et al. showed a better reattachment rate when using C3F8 due to its long-lasting effect, in contrast to SF6 [109]. In 2013 a retrospective series compared silicone oil and C3F8 reattachment rates, obtaining a 94% rate in the C3F8 group versus 54% in the silicone oil group [110]. Some other factors also need to be taken under consideration, such as the contralateral eye, need for airplane transportation or pre-existing glaucoma.

Inverted ILM flap technique has clearly improved the prognosis for both outcomes (MH closure and retinal reattachment) in highly myopic eyes with MHRD [111–114]. The results of different studies clearly show this trend, although BCVA has not improved as it was expected. In 2016 Chen and collaborators published their results comparing standard ILM peeling technique with inverted flap technique, obtaining a MH closure rate of 100% in cases with the inverted flap technique versus 35% of closure with the standard technique. Final retinal reattachment was obtained with 100% of cases [111].

Macular buckling re-appeared around the year 2010, with different groups of surgeons looking for more promising alternatives to treat these patients, doing it as an isolated technique or in combination with PPV [28, 39, 115–126].

To our knowledge, there is only one randomized study reported by Ma J and collaborators in 2017, including patients with an axial length superior to 30 mm, where there is a direct comparison between surgery with the standard technique, including PPV and peeling of the ILM, versus PPV and peeling of the ILM, plus a macular buckling procedure. Both macular reattachment and MH closure rates were clearly superior in the combined group in the 12-month follow-up. Additionally, they reported a BCVA improvement in this group of patients, ever since the 6th post-op month [127]. In 2015, Parolini et al. published her results comparing macular buckle alone, versus macular buckle with PPV in cases with MHRD, in both groups they obtained a reattachment rate of 100% and MH closure in 60% of cases, with improved BCVA in every case [128].

Key points in PPV for MHRD:

Two types of MHRD have been described:

1. Retinal detachment comprising the periphery

There is usually more movement within the retina, compromising the detachment of the posterior hyaloid, especially in the mid periphery. Take into account that there is usually a tight adherence between the posterior hyaloid and the retina within the areas of lattice and other areas where accumulation of pigment might be seen. Avoid creating iatrogenic ruptures around these areas.

- How to aspirate the subretinal fluid: In general, if the retinal detachment affects the periphery, it is possible to displace the fluid in that direction using perfluorocarbon liquid (PFCL) and perform a small superior retinotomy to aspirate it. Another alternative would be to aspirate the fluid through the MH, doing a previous air exchange and using a small gauge cannula. This technique is, though, complex, and there are many things to consider such as the low magnification and a worse visualization of the retina when working under air.
- Points to have in mind:
  - Try to avoid direct contact with the RPE underneath the MH and avoid touching its margins to prevent enlarging it.
  - Even the contact of the viscous subretinal fluid through the MH might enlarge it.

2. Macular detachment in the staphyloma.
   - In cases where the RD does not affect the periphery, one option may be to use PFCL, but keeping in mind that it may block the MH, making it impossible for the subretinal fluid to go out. Using high magnification and a 41-gauge cannula (under fluid), it is possible to aspirate the subretinal fluid, reattaching the MH, and then stain the ILM to perform an inverted flap technique [129] (Fig. 8) (Video 5).

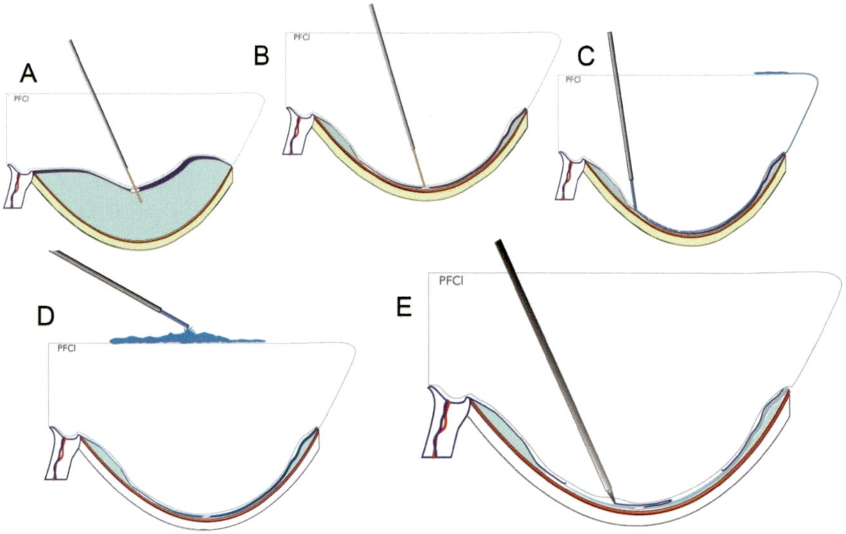

Fig. 8 (A) While PFCL is over the macular area, the MH will stay blocked, avoiding fluid from leaking beneath the retina. The rest of the vitreous cavity is filled with BSS to improve visualization, which facilitates the use of a 41G cannula to slowly aspirate the subretinal fluid through the MH, sealing the MH over the RPE (B). (C) Slowly proceed to inject the dye into the retina/PFCL interface, which will cause an immediate staining of the ILM, while the excess of dye will move to the top of the PFCL bubble, where it can then be aspirated (D). (E) Once the retina is stabilized, ILM peeling with the inverted flap technique is easily performed [129]

- Another option consists in performing a small retinotomy at the edge of the staphyloma through which the subretinal fluid can be aspirated after having injected PFCL. This retinotomy should be placed far from the foveal area, since RPE atrophy secondary to the photocoagulation of the retinotomy could, later, affect the fovea.

Macular Buckling for MHRD (Ando Plombe and AJL Macular Buckle) (Video 6)

Surgical steps of combined macular buckle + PPV (Fig. 9).

1. Conjunctival incision at approximately 1 mm from the superotemporal limbus exposing superior and lateral recti muscles.
2. Superior and temporal recti muscles are braided with 4/0 silk sutures to expose the superotemporal quadrant.
3. With a two-armed 5/0 nylon, a mattress suture is placed pointing to the theoretical center of the macula between the insertion of both superior and inferior oblique muscles. This suture will serve as the pivoting axis for the final placement of the macular buckle.

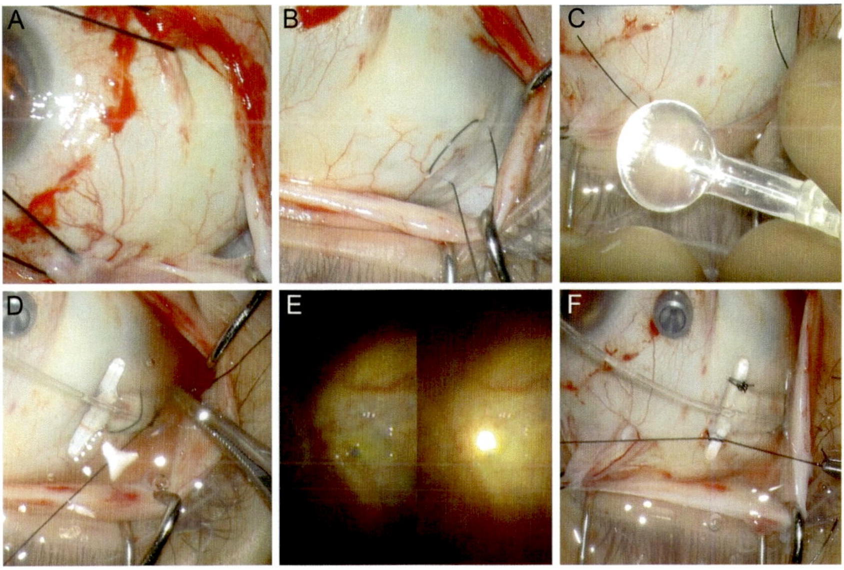

Fig. 9 (A) After a 120 ° superotemporal peritomy, superior and temporal muscles are braided with 4/0 silk sutures to expose the superotemporal quadrant. (B) A 5/0 nylon mattress suture is placed pointing towards the macular area, between the insertion of both oblique muscles. The more posterior the buckle is placed, the more indenting effect is achieved and contrary, the more anterior, the less buckling effect. (C) An optic fibre is inserted into the groove to the centre of the indenting platform and the light is then turned off (remember that the light can induce phototoxicity and thus, should be turned on only when strictly necessary). (D) After PPV, the AJL macular buckle (or the Ando Plombe) is inserted into the mattress suture that is knotted. (E) Under wide field visualization, the light of the optic fibre is then turned on and the transillumination helps localizing the centre of the indenting platform. (F) Once the indenting platform is in the correct place, additional sutures in the anterior arm of the macular buckle are added and the optic fibre is pulled out

It is preferable to perform these maneuvers before performing PPV because the eye has a better tone.

4. PPV and the maneuvers previously described. An additional advantage is the fact that the blue or green color of the inverted flap over the macular hole will help a correct visualization and centering of the macular buckle.
5. Insertion of the macular buckle into the mattress suture will help stabilize the buckle in its position
6. Under wide-field visualization, the light of the optic fiber is turned on to confirm the position of the indenting device [130]. If the indenting illuminated device is too nasal to the MH, move its anterior end towards the nasal side and this will move thedevice temporarily. On the contrary, if the illuminated device is located to the temporal side, move the anterior end temporarily. If the device is located in the superior arcade, push the macular buckle through the mattress suture in order for it to be more posterior. On the contrary, if the buckling effect is seen in the inferior arcade, pull the macular buckle anteriorly. These maneuvers to achieve

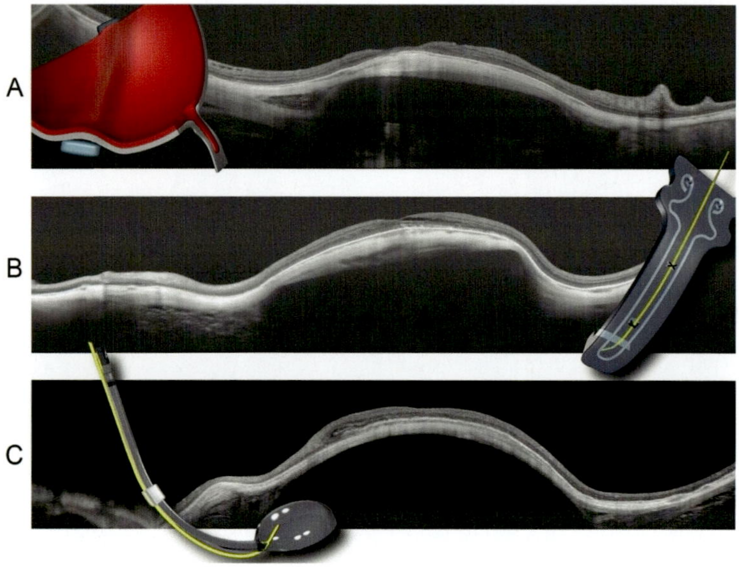

Fig. 10 Proportional OCT images of different macular buckles inducing different macular profiles. (A) 4 mm wide hard silicone tire from inferonasal to superonasal quadrants, crossing the macular area. (B) Ando Plombe: pay attention to the square angled edges of the 5 × 5 mm indenting platform. (C) AJL Macular Buckle with a rounded indenting platform. Optic fibre from (B) and (C) are withdrawn at the end of surgery, after correct position is achieved

appropriate location of the device are greatly facilitated with the initial mattress suture. Remember to leave the light on as less as possible to avoid potential phototoxicity.

7. Remove the PFCL
8. Inject the selected tamponade.

Different macular buckles may result in different postoperative OCT profiles (Fig. 10).

Complications after macular buckling (Fig. 11):

1. Progressive RPE disturbance and atrophy of the central macula that may compromise final visual acuity in some cases (Fig. 11A, B).
2. Choroidal hemorrhage: More frequent in nasal-to-nasal buckles where there is a risk for choroidal compression.
3. Serous foveal detachment mimicking "Dome Shape macula" that shortly disappears after removal of the macular buckle[131] (Fig. 11C–G)
4. Incorrect positioning of the macular buckle (Fig. 1H, I)
5. Hyperopic shift that may be an issue in pseudophakic eyes.

Key points in MTM

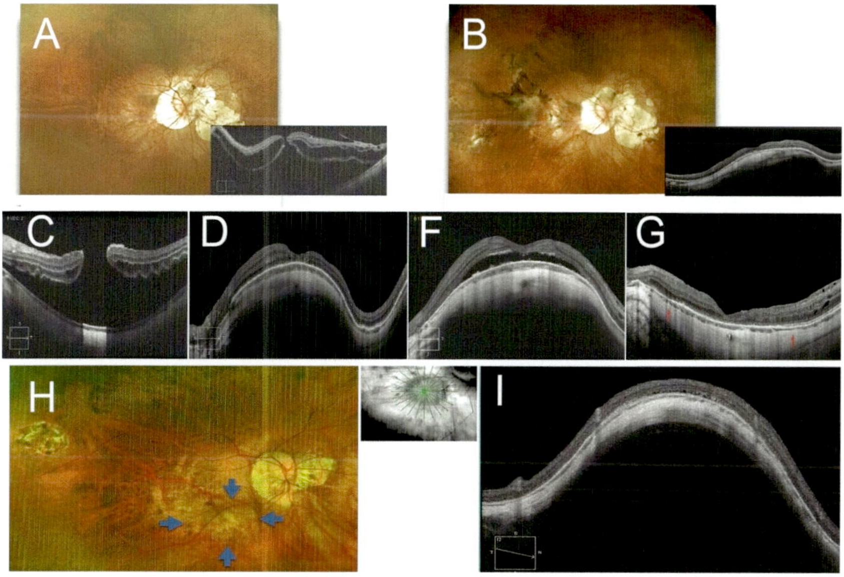

Fig. 11 (A) MHRD in an eye with PS. (B) One year after combined PPV and macular buckling, important RPE disturbances are observed. RPE atrophy is especially evident along the margins of the macular buckle. In the OCT image, MH is closed and no subfoveal RPE atrophy is observed. (B) Non-proportional OCT image of a recurrent MHRD. (D) After combined PPV and macular buckle, MH is closed, and the retina is reattached (non-proportional OCT image). (F) 3 years postoperatively, the patient noticed a decrease in visual acuity. OCT shows an increased choroidal thickness and presence of subretinal fluid. (G) Few days after removal of the macular buckle, OCT showed a decrease in choroidal thickness and absence of subretinal fluid [131]. (H–I) Incorrect positioning of the indenting platform, which is located in the inferotemporal arcade

- MTM tends to show progression in the long term, especially when the central macula is involved. Consider performing periodic OCTs in patients with deep staphylomas.
- Outer retinal defects or breaks in the outer retina may be signs of progression in eyes with retinoschisis.
- Review all the OCT cuts in the macula, not only one cut (macula is a three-dimensional structure not a two-dimensional OCT cut).
- FTMH may be asymptomatic in the beginning and difficult to see by biomicroscopy.
- A longer axial length and presence of retinoschisis may be signs of poor prognosis in FTMH in patients with high myopia.

References

1. Laviers H, Li JPO, Grabowska A, Charles SJ, Charteris D, Haynes RJ, et al. The management of macular hole retinal detachment and macular retinoschisis in pathological myopia; a UK collaborative study. Eye Lond Engl. 2018;32(11):1743–51.
2. Hayashi K, Ohno-Matsui K, Shimada N, Moriyama M, Kojima A, Hayashi W, et al. Long-term pattern of progression of myopic maculopathy: a natural history study. Ophthalmology. 2010;117(8):1595–611, 1611.e1–4.
3. Hsiang HW, Ohno-Matsui K, Shimada N, Hayashi K, Moriyama M, Yoshida T, et al. Clinical characteristics of posterior staphyloma in eyes with pathologic myopia. Am J Ophthalmol. 2008;146(1):102–10.
4. Ohno-Matsui K, Kawasaki R, Jonas JB, Cheung CMG, Saw SM, Verhoeven VJM, et al. International photographic classification and grading system for myopic maculopathy. Am J Ophthalmol. 2015;159(5):877-883.e7.
5. Spaide RF, Ohno-Matsui K, Yannuzzi LA, editors. Pathologic myopia. 2nd ed. Cham: Springer; 2021.
6. Ohno-Matsui K, Wu PC, Yamashiro K, Vutipongsatorn K, Fang Y, Cheung CMG, et al. IMI pathologic myopia. Invest Ophthalmol Vis Sci. 2021;62(5):5.
7. Ohno-Matsui K. Proposed classification of posterior staphylomas based on analyses of eye shape by three-dimensional magnetic resonance imaging and wide-field fundus imaging. Ophthalmology. 2014;121(9):1798–809.
8. Frisina R, Gius I, Palmieri M, Finzi A, Tozzi L, Parolini B. Myopic traction maculopathy: diagnostic and management strategies. Clin Ophthalmol Auckl NZ. 2020;14:3699–708.
9. Ohno-Matsui K, Jonas JB. Posterior staphyloma in pathologic myopia. Prog Retin Eye Res. 2019;70:99–109.
10. Johnson MW. Myopic traction maculopathy: pathogenic mechanisms and surgical treatment. Retina Phila Pa. 2012;32(Suppl 2):S205-210.
11. Yonemoto J, Ideta H, Sasaki K, Tanaka S, Hirose A, Oka C. The age of onset of posterior vitreous detachment. Graefes Arch Clin Exp Ophthalmol Albrecht Von Graefes Arch Klin Exp Ophthalmol. 1994;232(2):67–70.
12. Holekamp NM. The vitreous gel: more than meets the eye. Am J Ophthalmol. 2010;149(1):32–6.
13. Yokota R, Hirakata A, Hayashi N, Hirota K, Rii T, Itoh Y, et al. Ultrastructural analyses of internal limiting membrane excised from highly myopic eyes with myopic traction maculopathy. Jpn J Ophthalmol. 2018;62(1):84–91.
14. Itakura H, Kishi S, Li D, Nitta K, Akiyama H. Vitreous changes in high myopia observed by swept-source optical coherence tomography. Invest Ophthalmol Vis Sci. 2014;55(3):1447–52.
15. She X, Ye X, Chen R, Pan D, Shen L. Characteristics of posterior precortical vitreous pockets and cloquet's canal in patients with myopia by optical coherence tomography. Invest Ophthalmol Vis Sci. 2019;60(14):4882–8.
16. Shinohara K, Shimada N, Moriyama M, Yoshida T, Jonas JB, Yoshimura N, et al. Posterior staphylomas in pathologic myopia imaged by widefield optical coherence tomography. Invest Ophthalmol Vis Sci. 2017;58(9):3750–8.
17. Gupta P, Yee KMP, Garcia P, Rosen RB, Parikh J, Hageman GS, et al. Vitreoschisis in macular diseases. Br J Ophthalmol. 2011;95(3):376–80.
18. Wollensak G, Spoerl E, Grosse G, Wirbelauer C. Biomechanical significance of the human internal limiting lamina. Retina. 2006;26(8):965–8.
19. Bando H, Ikuno Y, Choi JS, Tano Y, Yamanaka I, Ishibashi T. Ultrastructure of internal limiting membrane in myopic foveoschisis. Am J Ophthalmol. 2005;139(1):197–9.
20. Sayanagi K, Ikuno Y, Tano Y. Tractional internal limiting membrane detachment in highly myopic eyes. Am J Ophthalmol. 2006;142(5):850–2.
21. Panozzo G, Mercanti A. Optical coherence tomography findings in myopic traction maculopathy. Arch Ophthalmol. 2004;122(10):1455–60.

22. Shimada N, Tanaka Y, Tokoro T, Ohno-Matsui K. Natural course of myopic traction maculopathy and factors associated with progression or resolution. Am J Ophthalmol. 2013;156(5):948-957.e1.
23. Sayanagi K, Ikuno Y, Gomi F, Tano Y. Retinal vascular microfolds in highly myopic eyes. Am J Ophthalmol. 2005;139(4):658–63.
24. Phillips CI. Retinal detachment at the posterior pole. Br J Ophthalmol. 1958;42(12):749–53.
25. Takano M, Kishi S. Foveal retinoschisis and retinal detachment in severely myopic eyes with posterior staphyloma. Am J Ophthalmol. 1999;128(4):472–6.
26. Mateo C, Gómez-Resa MV, Burés-Jelstrup A, Alkabes M. Surgical outcomes of macular buckling techniques for macular retinoschisis in highly myopic eyes. Saudi J Ophthalmol Off J Saudi Ophthalmol Soc. 2013;27(4):235–9.
27. Meng B, Zhao L, Yin Y, Li H, Wang X, Yang X, et al. Internal limiting membrane peeling and gas tamponade for myopic foveoschisis: a systematic review and meta-analysis. BMC Ophthalmol. 2017;17(1):166.
28. Alkabes M, Mateo C. Macular buckle technique in myopic traction maculopathy: a 16-year review of the literature and a comparison with vitreous surgery. Graefes Arch Clin Exp Ophthalmol Albrecht Von Graefes Arch Klin Exp Ophthalmol. 2018;256(5):863–77.
29. Ma IH, Hsieh YT, Yeh PT, Yang CH, Yang CM. Long-term results and risk factors influencing outcome of gas tamponade for myopic foveoschisis with foveal detachment. Eye Lond Engl. 2020;34(2):392–9.
30. Iwama Y, Ikeda T, Nakashima H, Matsumoto E, Inoue R, Emi K. Extending the limbus-to-cannula distance to 6.0 mm during pars plana vitrectomy in highly myopic eyes. Retina Phila Pa. 2022;42(6):1199–202.
31. Al Sabti K, Raizada S. Posterior scleral indentation in long axial length eyes (axial length more than 34 mm) to assist in pars plana vitrectomy and internal limiting membrane peeling in full-thickness macular holes. Retina Phila Pa. 2023;43(4):705–10.
32. Guo S, Tutela AC, Wagner R, Caputo AR. A comparison of the effectiveness of four biostains in enhancing visualization of the vitreous. J Pediatr Ophthalmol Strabismus. 2006;43(5):281–4.
33. Chihara E, Chihara K. Apparent cleavage of the retinal nerve fiber layer in asymptomatic eyes with high myopia. Graefes Arch Clin Exp Ophthalmol Albrecht Von Graefes Arch Klin Exp Ophthalmol. 1992;230(5):416–20.
34. Komeima K, Kikuchi M, Ito Y, Terasaki H, Miyake Y. Paravascular inner retinal cleavage in a highly myopic eye. Arch Ophthalmol. 2005;123(10):1449–50.
35. Muraoka Y, Tsujikawa A, Hata M, Yamashiro K, Ellabban AA, Takahashi A, et al. Paravascular inner retinal defect associated with high myopia or epiretinal membrane. JAMA Ophthalmol. 2015;133(4):413.
36. Uchida A, Shinoda H, Koto T, Mochimaru H, Nagai N, Tsubota K, et al. Vitrectomy for myopic foveoschisis with internal limiting membrane peeling and no gas tamponade. Retina. 2014;34(3):455–60.
37. Panozzo G. Vitrectomy for myopic traction maculopathy. Arch Ophthalmol. 2007;125(6):767.
38. Gaucher D, Haouchine B, Tadayoni R, Massin P, Erginay A, Benhamou N, et al. Long-term follow-up of high myopic foveoschisis: natural course and surgical outcome. Am J Ophthalmol. 2007;143(3):455-462.e1.
39. Susvar P, Sood G. Current concepts of macular buckle in myopic traction maculopathy. Indian J Ophthalmol. 2018;66(12):1772.
40. Kwok AKH. Vitrectomy and gas tamponade without internal limiting membrane peeling for myopic foveoschisis. Br J Ophthalmol. 2005;89(9):1180–3.
41. Hirakata A, Hida T. Vitrectomy for myopic posterior retinoschisis or foveal detachment. Jpn J Ophthalmol. 2006;50(1):53–61.
42. Wollensak G, Spoerl E, Wirbelauer C, Pham DT. Influence of indocyanine green staining on the biomechanical strength of porcine internal limiting membrane. Ophthalmologica. 2004;218(4):278–82.

43. Haritoglou C, Mauell S, Benoit M, Schumann RG, Henrich PB, Wolf A, et al. Vital dyes increase the rigidity of the internal limiting membrane. Eye. 2013;27(11):1308–15.
44. Gao X, Ikuno Y, Fujimoto S, Nishida K. Risk factors for development of full-thickness macular holes after pars plana vitrectomy for myopic foveoschisis. Am J Ophthalmol. 2013;155(6):1021-1027.e1.
45. Shimada N, Sugamoto Y, Ogawa M, Takase H, Ohno-Matsui K. Fovea-sparing internal limiting membrane peeling for myopic traction maculopathy. Am J Ophthalmol. 2012;154(4):693–701.
46. Ho TC, Yang CM, Huang JS, Yang CH, Yeh PT, Chen TC, et al. Long-term outcome of foveolar internal limiting membrane nonpeeling for myopic traction maculopathy. Retina Phila Pa. 2014;34(9):1833–40.
47. Seppey C, Wolfensberger T. Vitrectomy with fovea-sparing internal limiting membrane peeling for myopic foveoschisis. Klin Monatsblätter Für Augenheilkd. 2017;234(04):497–500.
48. Jin H, Zhang Q, Zhao P. Fovea sparing internal limiting membrane peeling using multiple parafoveal curvilinear peels for myopic foveoschisis: technique and outcome. BMC Ophthalmol. 2016;16(1):180.
49. Xie ZG, He QY, Zhu J, Du W, Tong J, Chen F. A modified surgical technique of fovea-sparing internal limiting membrane peeling: continuous arc-shaped foldback peeling. J Ophthalmol. 2020;23(2020):1–6.
50. Al-Badawi AH, Abdelhakim MASE, Macky TA, Mortada HA. Efficacy of non-fovea-sparing ILM peeling for symptomatic myopic foveoschisis with and without macular hole. Br J Ophthalmol. 2019;103(2):257–63.
51. Elwan MM, Abd Elghafar AE, Hagras SM, Abou Samra WA, Saleh SM. Long-term outcome of internal limiting membrane peeling with and without foveal sparing in myopic foveoschisis. Eur J Ophthalmol. 2019;29(1):69–74.
52. Zheng B, Chen Y, Chen Y, Zhao Z, Zhang Z, Zheng J, et al. Vitrectomy and internal limiting membrane peeling with perfluoropropane tamponade or balanced saline solution for myopic foveoschisis. Retina. 2011;31(4):692–701.
53. Zhang J, Yu Y, Dai D, Liu W. Vitrectomy with internal limiting membrane peeling and gas tamponade for myopic foveoschisis. BMC Ophthalmol. 2022;22(1):214.
54. Duan TQ, Tan W, Yang J, Li FL, Xiong SQ, Wang XG, et al. Morphological characteristics predict postoperative outcomes after vitrectomy in myopic traction maculopathy patients. Ophthalmic Surg Lasers Imaging Retina. 2020;51(10):574–82.
55. Lee DH, Moon I, Kang HG, Choi EY, Kim SS, Byeon SH, et al. Surgical outcome and prognostic factors influencing visual acuity in myopic foveoschisis patients. Eye Lond Engl. 2019;33(10):1642–8.
56. Lim LS, Ng WY, Wong D, Wong E, Yeo I, Ang CL, et al. Prognostic factor analysis of vitrectomy for myopic foveoschisis. Br J Ophthalmol. 2015;99(12):1639–43.
57. Fujimoto S, Ikuno Y, Nishida K. Postoperative optical coherence tomographic appearance and relation to visual acuity after vitrectomy for myopic foveoschisis. Am J Ophthalmol. 2013;156(5):968-973.e1.
58. García-Ben A, Baquero-Aranda I, García-Basterra I, García-Campos JM. Relationship between integrity of henle fibers and visual acuity in myopic foveoschisis. Retina. 2022;42(4):689–96.
59. Pang CE, Spaide RF, Freund KB. Comparing functional and morphologic characteristics of lamellar macular holes with and without lamellar hole-associated epiretinal proliferation. Retina Phila Pa. 2015;35(4):720–6.
60. Hsia Y, Ho TC, Yang CH, Hsieh YT, Lai TT, Yang CM. Clinical characteristics and long-term evolution of lamellar macular hole in high myopia. PLoS ONE. 2020;15(5):e0232852.
61. Witkin AJ, Ko TH, Fujimoto JG, Schuman JS, Baumal CR, Rogers AH, et al. Redefining lamellar holes and the vitreomacular interface: an ultrahigh-resolution optical coherence tomography study. Ophthalmology. 2006;113(3):388–97.

62. Pang CE, Spaide RF, Freund KB. Epiretinal proliferation seen in association with lamellar macular holes: a distinct clinical entity. Retina Phila Pa. 2014;34(8):1513–23.
63. Lai TT, Yang CM. Lamellar hole-associated epiretinal proliferation in lamellar macular hole and full-thickness macular hole in high myopia. Retina Phila Pa. 2018;38(7):1316–23.
64. Lin CW, Ho TC, Yang CM. The development and evolution of full thickness macular hole in highly myopic eyes. Eye Lond Engl. 2015;29(3):388–96.
65. Kobayashi H, Kobayashi K, Okinami S. Macular hole and myopic refraction. Br J Ophthalmol. 2002;86(11):1269–73.
66. Coppé AM, Ripandelli G, Parisi V, Varano M, Stirpe M. Prevalence of asymptomatic macular holes in highly myopic eyes. Ophthalmology. 2005;112(12):2103–9.
67. Scoles D, Mahmoud TH. Inaccurate measurements confound the study of myopic macular hole. Ophthalmol Retina. 2022;6(2):95–6.
68. Suda K, Hangai M, Yoshimura N. Axial length and outcomes of macular hole surgery assessed by spectral-domain optical coherence tomography. Am J Ophthalmol. 2011;151(1):118-127.e1.
69. Ohno-Matsui K. Pathologic myopia. Asia-Pac J Ophthalmol Phila Pa. 2016;5(6):415–23.
70. Kuriyama S, Hayashi H, Jingami Y, Kuramoto N, Akita J, Matsumoto M. Efficacy of inverted internal limiting membrane flap technique for the treatment of macular hole in high myopia. Am J Ophthalmol. 2013;156(1):125-131.e1.
71. Michalewska Z, Michalewski J, Dulczewska-Cichecka K, Nawrocki J. Inverted internal limiting membrane flap technique for surgical repair of myopic macular holes. Retina Phila Pa. 2014;34(4):664–9.
72. Mete M, Alfano A, Guerriero M, Prigione G, Sartore M, Polito A, et al. Inverted internal limiting membrane flap technique versus complete internal limiting membrane removal in myopic macular hole surgery: a comparative study. Retina Phila Pa. 2017;37(10):1923–30.
73. Oleñik A, Rios J, Mateo C. Inverted internal limiting membrane flap technique for macular holes in high myopia with axial length ≥30 mm. Retina Phila Pa. 2016;36(9):1688–93.
74. Rizzo S, Tartaro R, Barca F, Caporossi T, Bacherini D, Giansanti F. Internal limiting membrane peeling versus inverted flap technique for treatment of full-thickness macular holes: a comparative study in a large series of patients. Retina Phila Pa. 2018;38(Suppl 1):S73–8.
75. Habib AM, Mansour A, Fouad YA. Flower-petal inverted flap for internal limiting membrane in myopic eyes with macular hole and rhegmatogenous retinal detachment. Indian J Ophthalmol. 2022;70(2):667–9.
76. Avci R, Mavi Yildiz A, Yilmaz S. Conventional internal limiting membrane peeling versus temporal inverted internal limiting membrane flap for large macular holes. Eur J Ophthalmol. 2021;31(2):679–87.
77. Avci R, Mavi Yildiz A, Yilmaz S. Evaluation of inner retinal dimples and internal limiting membrane flap configuration after temporal inverted ILM flap technique. Eur J Ophthalmol. 2021;31(2):649–55.
78. Finn AP, Mahmoud TH. Internal limiting membrane retracting door for myopic macular holes. Retina Phila Pa. 2019;39(Suppl 1):S92–4.
79. Kim M, Won JY, Choi SY, Kim M, Ra H, Jee D, et al. Therapeutic efficacy of autologous platelet concentrate injection on macular holes with high myopia, large macular holes, or recurrent macular holes: a multicenter randomized controlled trial. J Clin Med. 2021;10(12):2727.
80. Figueroa MS, Govetto A, de Arriba-Palomero P. Short-term results of platelet-rich plasma as adjuvant to 23-G vitrectomy in the treatment of high myopic macular holes. Eur J Ophthalmol. 2016;26(5):491–6.
81. Buzzi M, Parisi G, Marolo P, Gelormini F, Ferrara M, Raimondi R, et al. The short-term results of autologous platelet-rich plasma as an adjuvant to re-intervention in the treatment of refractory full-thickness macular holes. J Clin Med. 2023;12(5):2050.
82. Fang Y, Yokoi T, Shimada N, Du R, Shinohara K, Takahashi H, et al. Development of macular atrophy after pars plana vitrectomy for myopic traction maculopathy and macular hole retinal detachment in pathologic myopia. Retina Phila Pa. 2020;40(10):1881–93.

83. Ikuno Y, Tano Y. Vitrectomy for macular holes associated with myopic foveoschisis. Am J Ophthalmol. 2006;141(4):774–6.
84. Ikuno Y, Sayanagi K, Soga K, Oshima Y, Ohji M, Tano Y. Foveal anatomical status and surgical results in vitrectomy for myopic foveoschisis. Jpn J Ophthalmol. 2008;52(4):269–76.
85. Jo Y, Ikuno Y, Nishida K. Retinoschisis: a predictive factor in vitrectomy for macular holes without retinal detachment in highly myopic eyes. Br J Ophthalmol. 2012;96(2):197–200.
86. Burés-Jelstrup A, Alkabes M, Gómez-Resa M, Rios J, Corcóstegui B, Mateo C. Visual and anatomical outcome after macular buckling for macular hole with associated foveoschisis in highly myopic eyes. Br J Ophthalmol. 2014;98(1):104–9.
87. Cacciamani A, Lazzeri S, Rossi T, Scarinci F, Parravano M, Ripandelli G, et al. Adjustable macular buckling for full-thickness macular hole with foveoschisis in highly myopic eyes: long-term anatomical and functional results. Retina Phila Pa. 2016;36(4):709–16.
88. Rodriguez-Vargas G, Ortiz-Coto F, Burés-Jelstrup A, Mateo C. Vitrectomy for macular hole with macular foveoschisis in myopic tractional maculopathy PPV for MH-MFS. J Ophthalmol Vis Sci. 2023;8(1):1–5.
89. Ohsugi H, Ikuno Y, Matsuba S, Ohsugi E, Nagasato D, Shoujou T, et al. Morphologic characteristics of macular hole and macular hole retinal detachment associated with extreme myopia. Retina Phila Pa. 2019;39(7):1312–8.
90. Schepens CL, Okamura ID, Brockhurst RJ. The scleral buckling procedures. I. Surgical techniques and management. AMA Arch Ophthalmol. 1957;58(6):797–811.
91. Adams ST. Retinal detachment due to macular and small posterior holes. Arch Ophthalmol. 1961;66:528–33.
92. Rosengren B. The silver plomb method in macular holes. Trans Ophthalmol Soc UK. 1966;86:49–53.
93. Howard GM, Campbell CJ. Surgical repair of retinal detachments caused by macular holes. Arch Ophthalmol. 1969;81(3):317–21.
94. Siam A. Macular hole with central retinal detachment in high myopia with posterior staphyloma. Br J Ophthalmol. 1969;53(1):62–3.
95. Klöti R. Silver clip for central retinal detachments with macular hole. Mod Probl Ophthalmol. 1974;12:330–6.
96. Margherio RR, Schepens CL. Macular breaks. 2. Management. Am J Ophthalmol. 1972;74(2):233–40.
97. Theodossiadis GP. A simplified technique for the surgical treatment of retinal detachments resulting from macula holes (author's transl). Klin Monatsbl Augenheilkd. 1973;162(6):719–28.
98. Feman SS, Hepler RS, Straatsma BR. Rhegmatogenous retinal detachment due to macular hole. Management with cryotherapy and a Y-shaped sling. Arch Ophthalmol. 1974;91(5):371–2.
99. Landolfo V, Albini L, Romano A. Macular hole-induced retinal detachment: treatment with an "armed-silicone" implant. Ophthalmic Surg. 1986;17(12):810–2.
100. Sasoh M, Yoshida S, Ito Y, Matsui K, Osawa S, Uji Y. Macular buckling for retinal detachment due to macular hole in highly myopic eyes with posterior staphyloma. Retina Phila Pa. 2000;20(5):445–9.
101. Theodossiadis GP, Theodossiadis PG. The macular buckling procedure in the treatment of retinal detachment in highly myopic eyes with macular hole and posterior staphyloma: mean follow-up of 15 years. Retina Phila Pa. 2005;25(3):285–9.
102. Ikuno Y, Sayanagi K, Oshima T, Gomi F, Kusaka S, Kamei M, et al. Optical coherence tomographic findings of macular holes and retinal detachment after vitrectomy in highly myopic eyes. Am J Ophthalmol. 2003;136(3):477–81.
103. Nishimura A, Kimura M, Saito Y, Sugiyama K. Efficacy of primary silicone oil tamponade for the treatment of retinal detachment caused by macular hole in high myopia. Am J Ophthalmol. 2011;151(1):148–55.
104. Nadal J, Verdaguer P, Canut MI. Treatment of retinal detachment secondary to macular hole in high myopia: vitrectomy with dissection of the inner limiting membrane to the edge of the staphyloma and long-term tamponade. Retina Phila Pa. 2012;32(8):1525–30.

105. Xie A, Lei J. Pars plana vitrectomy and silicone oil tamponade as a primary treatment for retinal detachment caused by macular holes in highly myopic eyes: a risk-factor analysis. Curr Eye Res. 2013;38(1):108–13.
106. Meng L, Wei W, Li Y, Han X, Shi X, Yang M. Treatment of retinal detachment secondary to macular hole in highly myopic eyes: pars plana vitrectomy with internal limiting membrane peel and silicone oil tamponade. Retina Phila Pa. 2014;34(3):470–6.
107. Arias L, Caminal JM, Rubio MJ, Cobos E, Garcia-Bru P, Filloy A, et al. Autofluorescence and axial length as prognostic factors for outcomes of macular hole retinal detachment surgery in high myopia. Retina Phila Pa. 2015;35(3):423–8.
108. Nakanishi H, Kuriyama S, Saito I, Okada M, Kita M, Kurimoto Y, et al. Prognostic factor analysis in pars plana vitrectomy for retinal detachment attributable to macular hole in high myopia: a multicenter study. Am J Ophthalmol. 2008;146(2):198–204.
109. Uemoto R, Saito Y, Sato S, Imaizumi A, Tanaka M, Nakae K. Better success of retinal reattachment with long-standing gas tamponade in highly myopic eyes. Graefes Arch Clin Exp Ophthalmol Albrecht Von Graefes Arch Klin Exp Ophthalmol. 2003;241(10):792–6.
110. Mancino R, Ciuffoletti E, Martucci A, Aiello F, Cedrone C, Cerulli L, et al. Anatomical and functional results of macular hole retinal detachment surgery in patients with high myopia and posterior staphyloma treated with perfluoropropane gas or silicone oil. Retina Phila Pa. 2013;33(3):586–92.
111. Chen SN, Yang CM. Inverted internal limiting membrane insertion for macular hole-associated retinal detachment in high myopia. Am J Ophthalmol. 2016;162:99-106.e1.
112. Matsumura T, Takamura Y, Tomomatsu T, Arimura S, Gozawa M, Kobori A, et al. Comparison of the inverted internal limiting membrane flap technique and the internal limiting membrane peeling for macular hole with retinal detachment. PLoS ONE. 2016;11(10):e0165068.
113. Baba R, Wakabayashi Y, Umazume K, Ishikawa T, Yagi H, Muramatsu D, et al. Efficacy of the inverted internal limiting membrane flap technique with vitrectomy for retinal detachment associated with myopic macular holes. Retina Phila Pa. 2017;37(3):466–71.
114. Yuan J, Zhang LL, Lu YJ, Han MY, Yu AH, Cai XJ. Vitrectomy with internal limiting membrane peeling versus inverted internal limiting membrane flap technique for macular hole-induced retinal detachment: a systematic review of literature and meta-analysis. BMC Ophthalmol. 2017;17(1):219.
115. Tanaka T, Ando F, Usui M. Episcleral macular buckling by semirigid shaped-rod exoplant for recurrent retinal detachment with macular hole in highly myopic eyes. Retina Phila Pa. 2005;25(2):147–51.
116. Ando F, Ohba N, Touura K, Hirose H. Anatomical and visual outcomes after episcleral macular buckling compared with those after pars plana vitrectomy for retinal detachment caused by macular hole in highly myopic eyes. Retina Phila Pa. 2007;27(1):37–44.
117. Devin F, Tsui I, Morin B, Duprat JP, Hubschman JP. T-shaped scleral buckle for macular detachments in high myopes. Retina Phila Pa. 2011;31(1):177–80.
118. Stirpe M, Ripandelli G, Rossi T, Cacciamani A, Orciuolo M. A new adjustable macular buckle designed for highly myopic eyes. Retina Phila Pa. 2012;32(7):1424–7.
119. Siam ALH, El Maamoun TA, Ali MH. Macular buckling for myopic macular hole retinal detachment: a new approach. Retina Phila Pa. 2012;32(4):748–53.
120. Mortada HA. A novel episcleral macular buckling: wire-strengthened sponge exoplant for recurrent macular hole and retinal detachment in high myopic eyes. Med Hypothesis Discov Innov Ophthalmol J. 2013;2(1):14–9.
121. Alkabes M, Burés-Jelstrup A, Salinas C, Medeiros MD, Rios J, Corcostegui B, et al. Macular buckling for previously untreated and recurrent retinal detachment due to high myopic macular hole: a 12-month comparative study. Graefes Arch Clin Exp Ophthalmol Albrecht Von Graefes Arch Klin Exp Ophthalmol. 2014;252(4):571–81.
122. El Rayes EN. Supra choroidal buckling in managing myopic vitreoretinal interface disorders: 1-year data. Retina Phila Pa. 2014;34(1):129–35.
123. Parolini B, Frisina R, Pinackatt S, Gasparotti R, Gatti E, Baldi A, et al. Indications and results of a new l-shaped macular buckle to support a posterior staphyloma in high myopia. Retina Phila Pa. 2015;35(12):2469–82.

124. Liu B, Ma W, Li Y, Luo Y, Jin C, Liang X, et al. Macular buckling using a three-armed silicone capsule for foveoschisis associated with high myopia. Retina Phila Pa. 2016;36(10):1919–26.
125. Mura M, Iannetta D, Buschini E, de Smet MD. T-shaped macular buckling combined with 25G pars plana vitrectomy for macular hole, macular schisis, and macular detachment in highly myopic eyes. Br J Ophthalmol. 2017;101(3):383–8.
126. Akduman L. A titanium macular buckle implant designed for an easy placement in myopic macular holes. Retin Cases Brief Rep. 2022.
127. Ma J, Li H, Ding X, Tanumiharjo S, Lu L. Effectiveness of combined macular buckle under direct vision and vitrectomy with ILM peeling in refractory macular hole retinal detachment with extreme high axial myopia: a 24-month comparative study. Br J Ophthalmol. 2017;101(10):1386–94.
128. Parolini B, Frisina R, Pinackatt S, Mete M. A new L-shaped design of macular buckle to support a posterior staphyloma in high myopia. Retina Phila Pa. 2013;33(7):1466–70.
129. La Mantia A, Mateo C. Modified perfluorocarbon liquid/internal limiting membrane interface staining in myopic macular hole retinal detachment. Eur J Ophthalmol. 2023;33(1):602–6.
130. Mateo C, Dutra Medeiros M, Alkabes M, Burés-Jelstrup A, Postorino M, Corcóstegui B. Illuminated Ando plombe for optimal positioning in highly myopic eyes with vitreoretinal diseases secondary to posterior staphyloma. JAMA Ophthalmol. 2013;131(10):1359–62.
131. Mateo C, Burés-Jelstrup A. Macular buckling with ando plombe may increase choroidal thickness and mimic serous retinal detachment seen in the tilted disk syndrome. Retin Cases Brief Rep. 2016;10(4):327–30.

Macular Surgery for Diabetic Macular Edema

Ricarda Gisela Schumann, Armin Wolf, and Denise Vogt

Abstract Diabetic macular edema (DME) is a leading cause of vision loss in individuals with diabetes. While pharmacological therapies have been the primary approach to managing DME, surgical interventions have gained attention as an alternative or adjunctive treatment option. Given the advanced understanding of the key factors in the development and progression of DME, the rationale for vitrectomy and peeling of the inner limiting membrane seems well circumscribed. Vitreous cells, known as hyalocytes, play an important role in synthesizing the extracellular matrix and regulating the intraocular immune response, thereby modulating inflammation and the release of pro-angiogenic factors in diabetic eyes. This chapter provides an overview of the surgical techniques and innovations in the field of macular surgery for DME, along with an analysis of their efficacy and safety based on recent research.

Keywords Diabetic macular edema · Diabetic retinopathy · Epiretinal membrane · Hyalocytes · Inner limiting membrane · Membrane peeling · Posterior vitreous detachment · Vitrectomy · Vitreous cortex

1 Introduction

Diabetic macular edema (DME) is a sight-threatening complication of diabetic retinopathy and the most common cause of vision loss in working-age adults [1, 2]. Given the increasing prevalence of diabetes worldwide, DME poses a major

R. G. Schumann (✉)
Eye Center and Vascular Medicine Schwabing, Ludwig-Maximilians-University Munich, Munich, Germany
e-mail: ricarda.schumann@med.uni-muenchen.de

A. Wolf · D. Vogt
Department of Ophthalmology, University Ulm, Ulm, Germany
e-mail: armin.wolf@uniklinik-ulm.de

D. Vogt
e-mail: denise.vogt@uniklinik-ulm.de

F. Patelli et al. (eds.), *Macular Surgery*, https://doi.org/10.1007/978-3-031-63508-3_14

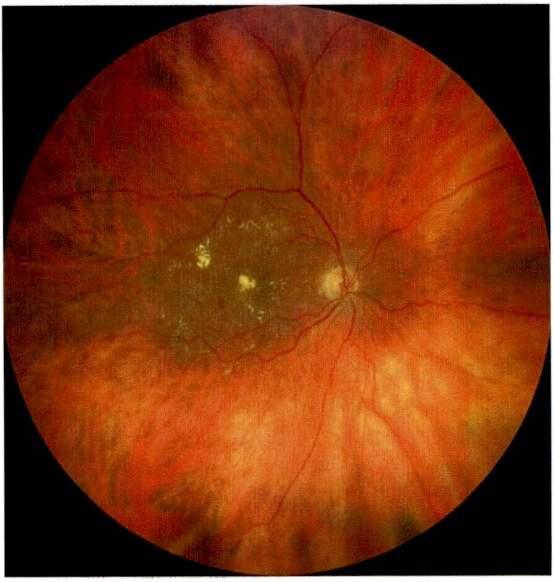

Fig. 1 Fundus photograph of diabetic macular edema with exudates and epiretinal membrane in non-proliferative diabetic retinopathy

medical and socioeconomic challenge (Fig. 1). Despite advances in the treatment of DME, therapy remains difficult in many cases.

2 Pathophysiology

The advanced stage of the disease is characterized by a poorly perfused retina causing hypoxia-induced release of pro-angiogenic growth factors [3, 4]. In fact, first-line treatment of DME consists of pharmacotherapy with intravitreal injections of anti-vascular endothelial growth factor (VEGF) and anti-angiopoietin-2 agents or steroids. Those mediators counteract two important pathogenetic factors, namely loss of the blood-retinal barrier and inflammation. Intravitreal injections of inhibitors of pro-angiogenic factors are effectively used in routine clinical practice for the treatment of DME [5].

In addition to these factors, molecular mechanisms induce direct damage to Müller cells and retinal pigment epithelial (RPE) cells, leading to a drainage dysfunction resulting in extracellular edema [6]. Subsequently, neurodegeneration is a major endpoint in DME that determines functional rehabilitation [7]. As a result, some patients respond only moderately or poorly to intravitreal injection therapy.

2.1 Vitreomacular Interface Changes

There are additional factors playing a significant role in the development and progression of DME such as vitreous and vitreomacular interface (VMI) abnormalities [8, 9]. The following pathologic changes were shown to be involved in the diabetic eye [10]:

- abnormal posterior vitreous detachment (PVD),
- abnormal collagen cross-linking and vitreous cortex thickening,
- thickening of the inner limiting membrane (ILM),
- formation of epiretinal membranes (ERM).

Extracellular matrix changes at the VMI are due to non-enzymatic glycosylation of collagen fibrils within the vitreous body and the ILM, the basement membrane of Mueller cells. Beside non-cellular irregularities specific cellular changes are involved in pathophysiology of DME. Resident cells in the vitreous cortex, known as hyalocytes, play a crucial role in this process resulting in development of contractile membranes at the vitreoretinal and vitreopapillary interface.

2.2 The Role of Hyalocytes

Hyalocytes are distributed as single cells within the vitreous cortex at an average distance of 20–50 μm from the inner surface of the retina in healthy eyes. Due to their role in extracellular matrix synthesis and regulation of intraocular inflammation, hyalocytes can change their phenotype and cell function. Thereby, hyalocytes are able to transdifferentiate into myofibroblast-like cells. Although myofibroblasts can transdifferentiate from numerous cell types, in diabetic eyes they are believed to predominantly originate from hyalocytes [11]. Pathologic fibrocellular changes at the vitreomacular interface (VMI) are present in all eyes irrespective of the presence of tractional epiretinal membranes.

Diabetes-related changes in the vitreous and the VMI are also reflected in attenuated neovascularization in eyes with PVD. However, PVD usually develops late or not at all in eyes of diabetic patients. Based on pathologic vitreous changes, secondary fibrocellular membrane formation is a common finding in DME.

Table1 explains the development and progression of diabetic macular edema [2, 3].

Table 1 Pathophysiology of DME: development and progression

Microangiopathy induced vascular changes
Diabetes-induced vitreous and VMI changes
Inflammatory changes
Ischemia induced angiogenesis
Neuronal dysfunction and retinal destruction

3 Macular Surgery

Macular surgery for DME is considered when specific clinical indications are met. While pharmacological intravitreal therapies have been the mainstay of treatment for DME, surgical interventions are reserved for cases that may fall into certain categories.

3.1 Indications

In accordance with guidelines for the management of DME, pars plana vitrectomy (PPV) is recommended as a therapeutic option in cases of tractional DME demonstrating contractive epiretinal membranes at the VMI (Fig. 2) [12]. In the absence of traction formation, there is currently no consensus on the role of PPV in the treatment algorithm for diabetic eyes.

However, patients who do not respond adequately to conventional treatments such as anti-VEGF therapy or corticosteroid injections may be candidates for macular

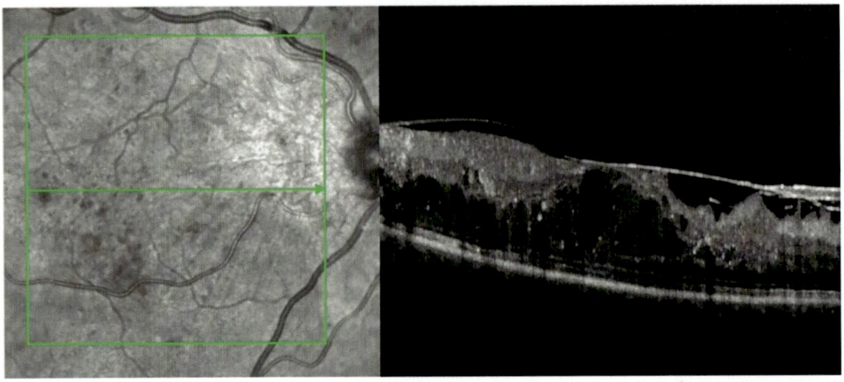

Fig. 2 High resolution optical coherence tomography in diabetic macular edema with tractional epiretinal membrane, intraretinal cystoid lesions, single hyperreflective foci, disorganization of inner retinal layers with overall intact ellipsoid zone

surgery. The indication for PPV in eyes with non-tractional DME is based on persistent or refractory DME after intensive pharmacotherapy. Especially in case of non-response to intravitreal treatment and concomitant presence of a thickened vitreous cortex without PVD, macular surgery with PPV may be considered.

Cases where DME has led to vision-threatening complications, such as tractional retinal detachment or extensive macular hemorrhage, often require surgical intervention. In these situations, surgery aims not only to alleviate edema but also to address the underlying anatomical distortions or hemorrhagic events.

Patient selection is crucial in determining the appropriateness of macular surgery. Factors considered in patient selection include vitreous cortex changes, severity of DME, visual acuity at baseline, presence of coexisting ocular conditions, and overall health status and surgical risk assessment.

The role of macular surgery as an early treatment option continues to be under debate [13–20]. While some studies reported only limited functional improvement and a short-term effect of macular thickness reduction after surgery, others showed a significant benefit for anatomical and functional results over a longer period of time in both tractional and non-tractional DME.

Taken all options into account, indication for macular surgery may be given in:

- **Tractional DME with presence of ERM**
- **Persistent or refractory DME**
- **Vitreous cortex thickening with lack of PVD**
- **Vision-threatening complications**
- **Individual patient selection criteria**

3.2 Rationale for Vitrectomy

Vitrectomy is not only potent to induce a complete vitreous detachment and to remove vitreous collagen from the retinal surface but it also has been shown to increase the rate of molecular transport by a reduction in viscosity. This effect could be beneficial in ischemic retinal disease, as it leads to a reduction in VEGF concentration and an increase in oxygen supply in ischemic areas [12, 13]. Oxygen has been shown to suppress VEGF gene expression and is therefore a potent anti-VEGF agent. Improved oxygenation of the inner retinal layers leads to an increase in vitreal diffusion coefficient and a consecutive decrease in VEGF concentration and other DME-promoting cytokines, especially in the premacular area.

Due to their role in extracellular matrix synthesis and regulation of intraocular immune responses, hyalocytes modulate inflammation in diabetic eyes and represent a source for pro-angiogenic factors such as VEGF [10]. Thus, in terms of pathogenesis, there is a strong indication for removal of hyalocytes by vitrectomy.

Table 2 explains the role of hyalocytes in diabetic macular edema [9, 10].

Table 2 Role of hyalocytes in DME

Promotion of angiogenesis
Leukocyte migration
Complement activation
Adaptive immune response
Fibrocellular ERM formation

3.3 Rationale for ILM Peeling

Clinicopathological analyses showed that pathological fibrocellular changes at the VMI are present in all eyes with DME regardless of macular edema type and severity as classified by optical coherence tomography (OCT) [11]. Multilayered fibrocellular membranes are mainly composed of hyalocytes and myofibroblasts that are embedded in masses of collagen. Multilayered ERMs consisting of hyalocytes, myofibroblasts and vitreous collagen fibrils represent the histopathologic correlate of tractive VMI changes in eyes with DME. Myofibroblasts are known for their contractile properties and their ability to produce newly formed collagen leading to thickening of collagen fibrils at the VMI leading to increased mechanical stress of retinal cells.

In order to remove all traction from the macular surface ILM peeling is needed. Without ILM peeling there is no sufficient traction relief in DME. Recent evidence on the role of the vitreous and cellular structures at the VMI in DME supports an early surgical intervention [11]. The cellular changes at the VMI in diabetic eyes explain the firm adhesions between vitreous and retinal ILM surface that can be observed during macular surgery. Nevertheless, to improve inner retinal architecture by macular surgery it is most important to remove all cellular and extra-cellular remnants from the retinal surface in these eyes.

3.4 Pros and Cons of ILM Peeling

Importantly, the decision to perform ILM peeling in the treatment of DME should be made on a case-by-case basis, taking into account the patient's specific condition, the presence of tractional forces or epiretinal membranes, the surgeon's experience, and the potential risks and benefits [25].

Pros:

Improved Macular Edema Resolution: ILM peeling can lead to better resolution of macular edema and better fluid dynamics, particularly in cases where tractional forces from the ILM contribute to the edema.

Enhanced Visual Outcomes: ILM peeling can lead to improved visual acuity, especially when accompanied by epiretinal membranes or vitreomacular traction.

Prevent Recurrence: ILM peeling can reduce the risk of recurrence of macular edema by addressing the underlying factors contributing to edema formation.
Restitution of Mueller cells: ILM peeling can release tractional stress from Mueller cells thereby increasing the cells' functionality and drainage activity with reduction in macular edema.

Cons:

Risk of Retinal Damage: ILM peeling is a delicate procedure that carries a risk of damaging the underlying neurosensory retina.
Variable Efficacy: The effectiveness of ILM peeling may vary from patient to patient and depends on the underlying pathology contributing to macular edema.
Additional Surgical Time: ILM peeling adds to the overall surgical time, which can increase the duration of the procedure and may lead to increased patient discomfort or complication rate.
Staining Complications: When vital dyes are used to stain the ILM for better visibility during peeling, there is a potential risk of complications by retinal toxicity or allergic reactions.
Need for Skilled Surgeon: ILM peeling in DME requires a high level of surgical skill and expertise. The availability of skilled surgeons may be limited in some regions.

4 Timing of Surgery

The perfect timing of macular surgery for DME may vary depending on the specific clinical scenario. Early intervention is essential in cases of acute complications, whereas surgery may be considered later in cases of chronic or persistent edema. The surgeon's experience and expertise play a crucial role in determining the optimal timing for intervention.

4.1 Preoperative Evaluation and Diagnostics

Advances in imaging techniques, including optical coherence tomography (OCT) and angiography, have enhanced the ability to assess the indications for surgery. Multimodal imaging provides valuable insights into the extent of macular edema, the presence of tractional forces, and the integrity of retinal layers. Standard imaging modalities aiding in the decision-making process include:

- **Optical coherence tomography**
- **En-face optical coherence tomography**
- **Blue light fundus autofluorescence imaging**
- **Multicolor scanning laser ophthalmoscopy**
- **Ultra wide-field color fundus photography**

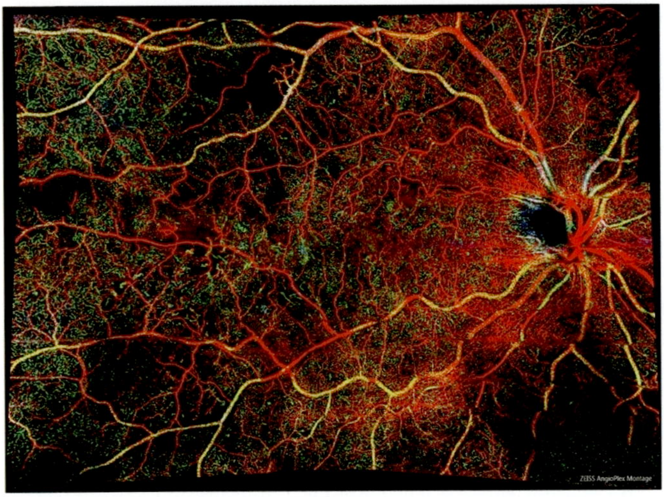

Fig. 3 Optical coherence tomography angiography montage image showing enlarged foveal avascular zone and local perfusion defects in the deep retinal plexus

- **Fluorescein angiography**
- **Optical coherence tomography angiography**
- **Ultra wide-field angiography**
- **Ultrasound examination**

It is anticipated that more advanced imaging techniques, particularly OCT angiography and wide-angle imaging (which allows imaging of up to 200° of the retina in a single image), will play a greater role in the treatment strategy of DME, taking into account factors other than ischaemia, such as inflammation and neurodegeneration (Fig. 3).

4.2 Predictive Factors for Functional Rehabilitation

There are several factors associated with final visual acuity (VA) improvement after PPV. Higher visual acuity gain is associated with lower preoperative visual acuity. Well-known biomarkers such as lack of ELM integrity, disruption of the ellipsoid zone and greater retinal thickness are associated with poorer final absolute VA [21, 22]. In addition, systemic factors also play an important role in the success of PPV in DME. For example, poorer glycemic control has been associated with poorer postoperative VA [20].

5 Surgical Techniques

Macular surgery for diabetic macular edema (DME) consists of PPV. It encompasses a range of surgical approaches such as ERM and ILM peeling aimed at addressing the underlying pathophysiology and reducing macular edema. These techniques are selected based on the specific characteristics of the DME case.

Pars plana vitrectomy (PPV)	• 23-gauge or 25-gauge self-sealing small scleral incisions • Removal of vitreous gel and cortex • Inducing posterior vitreous detachment if not present • Removal of vitreous collagen remnants from VMI
Epiretinal membrane (ERM) removal	• Removal of ERM if present to reduce tractional forces • Sequential peeling with ILM (possible)
Internal limiting membrane (ILM) peeling	• Removal of ILM • Removal of vitreous collagen remnants • Removal of cellular remnants • Using micro-forceps • Improved visualization by vital dyes (optional)
Subretinal fluid drainage	• Surgical drainage (rare)
Endotamponade	• Balanced salt solution • Gas endotamponade • Silicone oil endotamponade
Retinal endolaser therapy	• Related to retinal ischemia • Due to retinal defects or retinal detachment
Combination approaches	• Combination with cataract surgery • Combination with intravitreal agents

Each surgical technique has its unique advantages and considerations, and the choice of approach depends on the specific characteristics of the case such as presence of tractional forces, epiretinal membranes, and subretinal fluid. The selection of the most appropriate technique is made in consultation with the surgeon, taking into account the patient's condition and response to previous treatments.

It's essential to note that ILM peeling in DME is a delicate and precise surgical technique that should be performed by experienced retinal surgeons who have a thorough understanding of the specific characteristics of the patient's macular edema.

6 Innovations in Macular Surgery

Innovations in macular surgery of DME include advanced visualization techniques, drug delivery systems, and artificial intelligence applications. Advances are synergistically contributing to improved patient outcomes, increased precision, and enhanced decision-making throughout the treatment journey [23, 24].

6.1 Advanced Visualization Techniques

Advanced visualization techniques have revolutionized the way surgeons plan and perform macular surgery for DME. High-resolution OCT imaging provides detailed, real-time images of retinal structures, allowing surgeons to precisely assess the extent of edema, the integrity of retinal layers, and the presence of tractional forces. This information guides surgical decision-making and enhances the accuracy of procedures. Advances in retinal imaging such as ultra wide-field fluorescein angiography and OCT angiography aids in visualizing retinal blood vessels and detecting areas of vascular leakage, helping surgeons target specific regions for laser treatment. Advanced operating microscopes equipped with integrated imaging systems enable real-time visualization during surgery, enhancing precision and reducing the risk of complications.

6.2 Drug Delivery Systems

Innovations in drug delivery systems have expanded the armamentarium of treatments for DME and offer the potential for improved therapeutic outcomes. Sustained-release intravitreal implants, such as dexamethasone and fluocinolone acetonide implants, provide controlled and prolonged drug delivery, reducing the need for frequent injections and optimizing therapeutic efficacy. Emerging technologies include intravitreal port systems that allow for precise and customizable drug delivery. These systems enable the delivery of multiple drugs or combination therapies with minimal invasiveness. Advancements in nanotechnology are being explored to develop nano-sized drug carriers that can efficiently transport therapeutic agents to the target site within the retina, potentially reducing side effects and improving drug bioavailability.

6.3 *Artificial Intelligence Applications*

Artificial intelligence (AI) is making significant inroads into the field of macular surgery for DME, offering novel tools for diagnosis, treatment planning, and post-operative monitoring. AI algorithms can analyze OCT and angiography images to detect subtle changes in retinal morphology and vasculature associated with DME. They also assist in predicting disease progression and treatment response. AI-driven decision support systems aid surgeons in selecting the most appropriate surgical techniques, including the identification of cases that may benefit from ILM peeling, ERM removal, or other procedure. AI-powered software enables automated tracking of postoperative outcomes, including changes in macular thickness and visual acuity. This facilitates early detection of complications and the need for potential re-intervention.

In summary, macular surgery for DME is considered for cases with tractive features at the VMI, and for cases that do not respond to standard treatments, or involve vision-threatening complications, or meet specific patient selection criteria. The timing of surgery is crucial, taking into account the clinical presentation and the surgeon's judgment, generally supported by multimodal retinal imaging. Integration of advanced imaging techniques with new diagnostic devices will improve the decision making process in the future, and the development of personalized treatment for DME.

Clinical Pearls

- Macular surgery is a potent treatment option in DME based on advanced pathologic vitreous and retina changes in diabetic eyes.
- Indication for macular surgery is given in tractional DME and in persistent or refractory DME following intensive pharmacotherapy.
- Macular surgery typically includes ERM and ILM removal along with standard PPV.
- Potential risks and benefits should be individually considered before surgery.

References

1. Yau JW, Rogers SL, Kawasaki R, et al. Global prevalence and major risk factors of diabetic retinopathy. Diabetes Care. 2012;35:556–64.
2. Cheung N, Mitchell P, Wong T. Diabetic retinopathy. Lancet. 2010;376(9735):124–36.
3. Lange C, Bainbridge J. Oxygen sensing in retinal health and disease. Ophthalmologica. 2012;227(3):115–31.
4. Regula JT, Lundh von Leithner P, Foxton R, et al. Targeting key angiogenic pathways with a bispecific CrossMAb optimized for neovascular eye disease. EMBO Mol Med. 2019;11:e10666
5. El Rami H, Barham R, Sun J, et al. Evidence-based treatment of diabetic retinopathy. Semin Ophthalmol. 2017;32(1):67–74.
6. Zhang J, Zhang J, Zhang C, et al. Diabetic macular edema: current understanding, molecular mechanisms and therapeutic implications. Cells. 2022; 25:11(21):3362

7. Simó R, Stitt AW, Gardner TW. Neurodegeneration in diabetic retinopathy: does it really matter? Diabetologia. 2018;61(9):1902–12.
8. Duh EJ, Sun JK, Stitt AW. Diabetic retinopathy: current understanding, mechanisms, and treatment strategies. JCI Insight. 2017;2(14): e93751.
9. Jones Ch, Gui W, Schumann RG, et al. Hyalocytes in proliferative vitreo-retinal diseases. Expert Rev Ophthalmol. 2022;17(4):263–80.
10. Kroll P, Rodrigues E, Meyer C. Proliferative diabetic vitreo-retinopathy. In: Sebag J, editor. Vitreous—in health & disease. New York: Springer; 1984. p. 421–36.
11. Hagenau F, Vogt D, Ziada J, et al. Vitrectomy for diabetic macular edema: optical coherence tomography criteria and pathology of the vitreomacular interface. Am J Ophthalmol. 2019;200:34–46.
12. Schmidt-Erfurth U, Carcia-Arumi J, Bandello F, et al. Guidelines for the management of diabetic macular edema by the European Society of Retina Specialists (EURETINA). Ophthalmologica. 2017;237:185–222.
13. Stefaniotou M, Aspiotis M, Kalogeropoulos C, et al. Vitrectomy results for diffuse diabetic macular edema with and without inner limiting membrane removal. Eur J Ophthalmol. 2004;14:137–43.
14. Hoerauf H, Bruggemann A, Muecke M, Luke J, Muller M, Stefansson E, Hammes HP, Weiss C. Pars plana vitrectomy for diabetic macular edema. Internal limiting membrane delamination vs posterior hyaloid removal. A prospective randomized trial. Graefes Arch Clin Exp Ophthalmol. 2011; 249:997–1008
15. Bardak Y, Cekic O, Tig SU. Comparison of ICG-assisted ILM peeling and triamcinolone-assisted posterior vitreous removal in diffuse diabetic macular oedema. Eye (Lond). 2006;20:1357–9.
16. Kumagai K, Hangai M, Ogino N, Larson E. Effect of internal limiting membrane peeling on long-term visual outcomes for diabetic macular edema. Retina. 2015;35:1422–8.
17. Figueroa MS, Contreras I, Noval S. Surgical and anatomical outcomes of pars plana vitrectomy for diffuse nontractional diabetic macular edema. Retina. 2008;28:420–6.
18. Shiba T, Kamura Y, Yagi F, Sato Y. Comparison of surgical procedures for vitreous surgery in diabetic macular edema. Jpn J Ophthalmol. 2009;53:120–4.
19. Shah SP, Patel M, Thomas D, Aldington S, Laidlaw DA. Factors predicting outcome of vitrectomy for diabetic macular oedema: results of a prospective study. Br J Ophthalmol. 2006;90:33–6.
20. Bonnin S, Sandali O, Bonnel S, Monin C, El Sanharawi M. Vitrectomy with internal limiting membrane peeling for tractional and nontractional diabetic macular edema: long-term results of a comparative study. Retina. 2015;35:921–8.
21. Chhablani JK, Kim JS, Cheng L, Kozak I, Freeman W. External limiting membrane as a predictor of visual improvement in diabetic macular edema after pars plana vitrectomy. Graefes Arch Clin Exp Ophthalmol. 2012;250:1415–20.
22. Murakami T, Nishijima K, Akagi T, Uji A, Horii T, Ueda-Arakawa N, Muraoka Y, Yoshimura N. Segmentational analysis of retinal thickness after vitrectomy in diabetic macular edema. Invest Ophthalmol Vis Sci. 2012;53:6668–74.
23. Wong TY, Sabanayagam C. Strategies to tackle the global burden of diabetic retinopathy: from epidemiology to artificial intelligence. Ophthalmologica. 2020;243:9–20.
24. Bandello F, Parodi MB, Lanzetta P, et al. Diabetic macular edema. Dev Ophthalmol. 2017:58:102–38.
25. Patelli F, Radice P, Giacomotti E. Diabetic macular edema. Dev Ophthalmol. 2014;54:164–73.

Index

A

Autologous retinal transplant, 125, 151, 152

B

Blue dyes, 4, 16, 23, 26, 27, 29, 30, 33, 35–37, 111
Blunt ocular trauma, 157, 163
Brilliant blue G, 16, 26, 29, 34, 134, 135, 213, 220

C

Central fovea, 65, 68, 70, 72, 74, 97, 215
Chromovitrectomy, 16, 23, 24
Close study group classification, 101
Cone bouquet, 65, 71, 72, 75
Corneal staining, 9, 10

D

Diabetic macular edema, 4, 239–243, 247
Diabetic retinopathy, 2, 4, 19, 111, 121, 122, 208, 239, 240
Dye toxicity, 35

E

Electronic retinal prostheses, 1
Epiretinal membrane, 2, 4, 10–12, 19, 23, 24, 40, 54, 55, 57, 58, 65, 66, 68, 69, 79, 99, 102, 124, 142, 160, 177, 179, 206, 207, 209, 217, 240–242, 244, 247

F

Flap technique, 2, 5, 111, 124, 130, 220, 223, 226, 227

G

Gass classification, 96, 97, 103

H

High myopia, 80, 121, 135, 142, 148, 150, 170, 174, 176, 180, 182, 197, 208, 209, 217–219, 222, 224, 230
Human amniotic membrane, 102, 106, 129, 130, 162
Hyalocytes, 81, 239, 241, 243, 244

I

Indocyanine green dye, 12
Internal Limiting Membrane (ILM), 9–12, 17, 23, 24, 40, 66, 73, 74, 79, 81, 82, 86, 93, 99, 111, 142, 143, 158, 178, 179, 182, 185, 205, 206, 208
Internal Limiting Membrane (ILM) peeling, 4, 157, 213, 247
Intraoperative OCT, 51, 53, 54, 60, 62
Intravitreal dye, 9
Inverted ILM Flap, 5, 39, 106, 111, 112, 114–126, 143, 144, 161, 226
IVTS classification, 100, 103

L

Lamellar macular hole, 5, 55, 58, 65, 69, 75, 183, 205, 206, 209, 215, 216

F. Patelli et al. (eds.), *Macular Surgery*, https://doi.org/10.1007/978-3-031-63508-3

Large macular hole, 57, 61, 93, 99, 123, 129, 130, 144, 150, 161
Lutein-based dyes, 23, 29, 30, 34

M
Macular buckle, 199, 200, 212, 222, 225, 226, 228–231
Macular edema, 4, 11, 40, 65, 69, 70, 73, 79, 80, 82, 83, 151, 244, 245, 247
Macular hole, 2, 5, 6, 10, 11, 15, 17, 28, 40, 54–57, 61, 70, 93–108, 111–115, 117, 118, 120–126, 129, 130, 133–135, 137, 141–152, 158, 159, 161, 164, 165, 174–176, 179, 182, 183, 189, 198–200, 205–213, 215, 217–219, 222, 229
Macular hole classification, 93, 94, 96, 108
Macular hole failure surgery, 130, 136, 138
Macular hole recurrence, 130, 138
Macular hole retinal detachment, 150, 179, 215
Macular hole surgery, 2, 4, 9, 10, 12–14, 17, 55, 73, 105, 130, 142, 147, 162
Macular proliferative vitreoretinopathy, 79
Macular pucker, 2, 4, 12, 65–69, 72–75, 79, 80, 88, 208
Macular retinoschisis, 176, 183, 209
Macular surgery, 1–7, 10–13, 15, 16, 74, 205, 206, 239, 242–245, 247–249
Macular traction maculopathy, 205
Maculopathy, 18, 28, 54, 66, 73, 123, 143, 150, 169, 171–177, 183, 185, 192, 200, 205–207, 209
Medical devices, 23–25, 30, 42
Membrane peeling, 2, 4, 5, 54, 55, 83, 85, 143
Müller cell, 11, 12, 31, 32, 67, 70–74, 81, 144, 160, 162, 216, 217, 240
Multi-layer ILM plug technique, 161, 165
Myopia, 6, 55, 111, 121, 169–171, 174, 176, 177, 181, 206, 207, 219
Myopic foveoschisis, 5, 69

N
Neuroregeneration, 7

O
Ophthalmic imaging, 51
Optical coherence tomography, 3, 41, 51, 52, 54, 66, 82, 93, 96, 112, 134, 151, 159, 171, 205, 207, 242, 244–246

P
Pars plana vitrectomy, 1, 23, 24, 40, 55, 58–61, 80, 82, 83, 86, 93, 95, 105, 106, 147, 157, 160, 205, 206, 209, 211, 212, 242, 247
Persistent macular hole, 130
Posterior staphyloma, 170–173, 176, 177, 179, 180, 182, 197, 205, 206
Posterior vitreous detachment, 24, 80, 96, 97, 177, 181, 182, 207, 208, 241, 247

R
Recurrent macular holes, 101, 162
Refractory macular holes, 129, 130, 138, 143, 144, 148–150
Retina, 1, 2, 4, 5, 10, 12, 15–17, 19, 25–27, 31–36, 41, 51–53, 57, 61, 66, 67, 70, 74, 79, 80, 82, 84–86, 95–97, 99, 105, 106, 108, 119, 121, 123, 126, 130, 134–139, 142–145, 147, 149, 151, 152, 158, 169, 170, 175–180, 182, 184, 185, 196–198, 208, 209, 211–213, 216, 222, 223, 226, 227, 229, 231, 240, 241, 245, 246, 248, 249
Retina schisis, 56, 69, 175, 176, 178, 182, 183, 184, 205, 209, 231
Retinal detachment, 6, 12, 17, 51, 54–56, 80–84, 86, 89, 121, 122, 124, 125, 134–137, 142, 147–150, 159, 165, 172, 174–176, 178, 182, 189, 197, 199, 200, 205–207, 210–212, 217, 223, 226, 243, 247
Retinal gene therapy, 2
Retinal transplantation, 7, 102, 144, 148, 150

S
Secondary macular holes, 157

T
Temporal flap, 5, 200
Traumatic macular hole, 157, 158
Triamcinolone, 3, 16, 23–25, 28, 31, 35, 40, 198, 212
Trypan blue, 16, 18, 25, 26, 29, 33, 74, 85, 89, 105, 115, 134, 135

V
Vital dyes, 9, 12, 13, 15–17, 19, 23–27, 30, 32, 34, 36, 41, 42, 130, 134, 135, 245, 247
Vitrectomy, 2–5, 9, 10, 12, 15, 17, 19, 54, 66, 72, 75, 80, 102–104, 111, 112, 115, 118, 121, 123–125, 129, 130, 132, 135, 138, 139, 141, 142, 148, 149, 179, 180, 182, 196–200, 211, 215, 239, 243
Vitreoretinal surgery, 2–6, 23, 24, 33, 80, 89, 130, 131
Vitreous cortex, 11, 24, 81, 96, 176, 182, 198, 208, 213, 217, 241, 243
Vitreous staining, 24, 28

GPSR Compliance

The European Union's (EU) General Product Safety Regulation (GPSR) is a set of rules that requires consumer products to be safe and our obligations to ensure this.

If you have any concerns about our products, you can contact us on ProductSafety@springernature.com

In case Publisher is established outside the EU, the EU authorized representative is:

Springer Nature Customer Service Center GmbH
Europaplatz 3
69115 Heidelberg, Germany

Batch number: 10756376

Printed by Printforce, the Netherlands